While Science Sleeps

A Sweetener Kills

Woodrow C. Monte, PhD

Illustrated by Becky Miller

Published in the United States of America

While Science Sleeps

It has been thirty years since the U-shaped curve of alcohol consumption was trepidatiously berthed and set afloat in the backwaters of the river of collective scientific knowledge. Until this day, the healing power of ethanol has yet to find either explanation or, more importantly, exploitation. The most significant curative force to come from over a hundred years of scientific investigation of the horror of chronic disease has taken a back seat to a taboo born of temperance, prohibition and the need to protect the unprotectable from their own destinies. This is an impossible scenario and will stand in the eyes of history as an inexcusable blunder done in the name of God by those who practice medicine... while science sleeps.

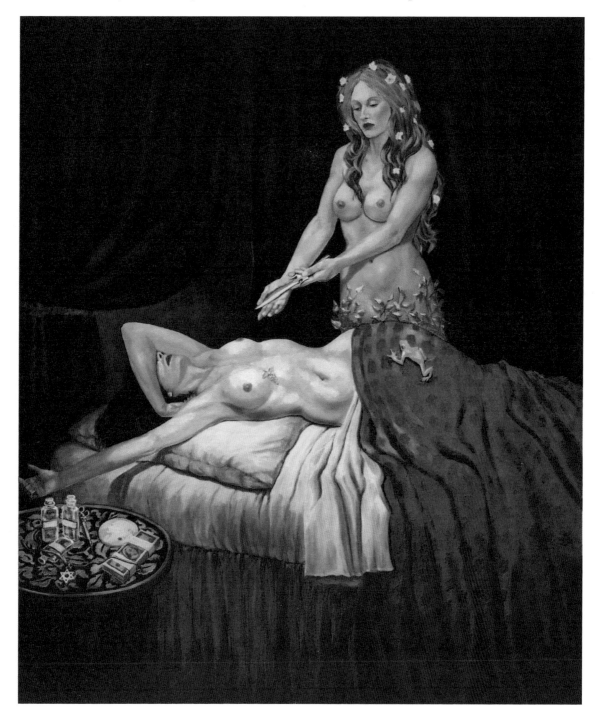

About the Author

Dr. Woodrow C. Monte has decades of experience in food science and nutrition as a researcher, teacher, inventor, industry consultant and consumer advocate who is committed to food additive safety and the prevention of food-borne diseases. For over thirty years he has studied the link between artificial sweeteners and the diseases of civilization, including Alzheimer's, heart disease, multiple sclerosis, numerous forms of cancer, autism and other birth defects.

Dr. Monte's testimony before Congress was instrumental in preventing sulfites from receiving the status of US FDA GRAS (Generally Regarded As Safe) and in the implementation of mandatory labeling for most foods that contain this dangerous additive.

Through his research, Dr. Monte has been awarded 22 US patents. He has shared his technical expertise during hundreds of television and radio appearances, including a special feature on the CBS Evening News with Dan Rather and on 60 Minutes. He is the author of numerous scientific publications and the book <u>While Science Sleeps: A Sweetener Kills</u>.

Dr. Monte is a dedicated scientist with both a Ph.D. and M.S. in Food Science and Nutrition and a B.S. in Biology. He has been a Registered Dietician, Certified Nutrition Specialist AIN, professional member of the American Chemical Society, and emeritus member of the American Association for the Advancement of Science. In 1985, he was chosen by the Council for International Exchange of Scholars as a Senior Fulbright Scholar.

As Professor Emeritus of Nutrition who taught at Arizona State University for over 25 years, Dr. Monte continues his study of the damaging effects of methanol in our food supply.

More information about Dr. Monte and his work can be found on his website: www.WhileScienceSleeps.com.

Table of Contents

Acknowledgements

Nature lives in all of us… I thank her gentle hand for the inspiration, intuition and revelation that guided this humble intellect through the massive clutter of literature, logic and lies that would bring me finally to the truth.

This book comes too late for many. Your sorrow is my sorrow; your dead are the numbers that made this writing possible. I did what I could. I never gave up, but the tide took so very long to turn.

There are those who need thanking but that will have to wait 'til we are done – 'til there is no danger that might go part and parcel with the platitudes of a grateful scholar. Your time will come, you know who you are… I love you all.

'Til all the demons are dead,

Woodrow

Introduction

Rather than dive immediately into the science of methanol poisoning, I am going to introduce you to the subject in the manner that I became involved with it, by way of a series of coincidences and encounters from which emerged a riddle that inspired deductive detective work in the tradition of Sherlock Holmes and Dr. Watson.

The following intriguing question was at the heart of this investigation: *Why did diagnoses of multiple sclerosis increase markedly with the increased consumption of aspartame?*

The Laboratory at Arizona State University

I was not, in the beginning, keen to study methanol toxicity. In fact, by the time aspartame became a major player in the food sweetener industry, I had already, early in my career, antagonized a number of my fellow food scientists by going public with one of the food industry's dirty little secrets. For many years, food manufacturers attempted to mask the age of plant produce, such as salad greens and avocadoes, and some animal food products, such as ground beef, with the addition of harmful substances called sulfating agents. These powerful chemicals, which, for example, were used to keep lettuce looking green and healthy for months at a time, also decimated its vitamin content. Arcane food laws, many of which still exist, helped hide this deception from the consumer.

I had joined several public interest groups in an effort to stop the Food and Drug Administration from listing sulfating agents as GRAS (an acronym for generally recognized as safe), a designation that would have increased their use and facilitated their concealment. Our campaign to prevent the reclassification of these dangerous chemicals, featured on the influential television program *60 Minutes*, eventually prevailed, yet I was not entirely satisfied with the results. I advocate the banning of sulfites altogether. About 10 percent of asthmatics are susceptible to a severe allergic reaction to food tainted with sulfites. If anaphylactic shock, a potentially lethal response, occurs at, say, a restaurant, the patron's sudden inability to inhale air can easily be confused with choking. When the Heimlich maneuver fails to bring relief and death ensues minutes later, an autopsy may not detect any of the long-gone sulfating agents and may instead determine the fatality resulted from cardiac failure. Although I was committed to pursuing this public health issue and had donated many hours as a pro bono expert witness for plaintiffs who had lost loved ones to death by sulfites, another dietary danger of burgeoning scope would soon capture and subsequently consume my attention.

A Brief History of the Aspartame War

The complete history of aspartame and how it came to be accepted as a food additive is well documented on the Internet.[39] I will fill in here only a little missing piece in this puzzle – some additional intrigue in which I played a role. This chapter in my career began on July 22, 1983, when, as a young assistant professor of food science at Arizona State University, I showed up during my summer break from ASU at the Food and Drug Administration's office in Washington, DC to review the documents submitted by G. D. Searle & Company demonstrating how safe aspartame was and why it should be allowed in diet soda. The previous ten years had been controversial for the sweetener. Because aspartame had the disturbing tendency to produce malignant brain tumors in rats, the FDA initially rejected it, and several noted scientists from prestigious universities thwarted lobbying efforts to have the product approved for the human food supply. The ensuing debate culminated in an ostensibly final refusal from an expert panel of scientists impaneled by the FDA in 1980,[57] the first time such a prestigious board of inquiry did not approve a food additive.

The next year, however, on January 21, 1981 – not insignificantly, the day after Ronald Reagan's inauguration – the CEO of G. D. Searle & Company, Donald Rumsfeld, took time away from his additional duties on the transition team for his good friend, now President Reagan, to see to it that the new application for aspartame's approval was, yet again, resubmitted to the FDA. Rumsfeld, who was not lacking in markers to summon or political connections to exploit, had been made President of Searle for just such an exigent and lucrative enterprise. It is not my intent to tell the whole sordid story here but merely to highlight the controversial history of the sweetener and to suggest an excellent review of the politics of its approval by G. Gordon of the *United Press International.*[39] At any rate, I was unaware when entering the FDA office that I was, as a late arrival and foot soldier, entering the aspartame war, which had already been raging for fifteen years and still persists today, although the battle lines have been redrawn.

As part of the process for this new and much expanded use for the sweetener, all the research had to be made available to the public for a short period of time before a final decision was made. This collection of papers, which includes the application, is called the docket file. The national soft drink industry had asked me, through one of its lawyers in California, to examine this file and evaluate the safety of aspartame. I was not aware at the time of the internal competition to become the first company to market carbonated beverages with aspartame, a privilege that looked as if it would be awarded to Coca-Cola. Although I cannot prove it, I am convinced that factions in the beverage industry were seeking leverage in these negotiations.

As I mentioned earlier, I had previously been involved in a successful and high-profile campaign of the Center for Science in the Public Interest to limit the use of sulfites as food preservatives. Food scientists willing to challenge the food industry are few and far between. This reluctance is not surprising given that government provides very little money for food research; food and, to a greater extent, drug companies keep many of the larger university laboratories in operation. I believed, however, that I could get my research accomplished with my limited university budget as director of the Food Science and Nutrition Laboratory for ASU. Since I had no great fear of the food industry and no desire to grow my laboratory with blood money, I was an ideal recruit to dig up dirt. Little did I know at the time how dangerous aspartame would prove to be to me, professionally.

It was a miserable, humid day at the Capitol when I arrived at one of the many offices of the U.S. Food and Drug Administration's Bureau of Foods and was met by someone who identified himself as chief toxicologist for the aspartame project.[14] Dispensing with the preliminary niceties or small talk, he immediately asked me what reservations I had about the artificial sweetener. I explained that I was troubled by the fact that aspartame quickly released the poison methanol after consumption. I will never forget his terse and stern reply intended to summarily dismiss my concerns: "Why, methanol is a food." Needless to say this was a distressing exchange with a man who claimed to be an epidemiologist (poison expert), who worked for a governmental agency mandated to protect public health and welfare, and who either knew nothing of the dangers methanol posed to humans or who, for political reasons, refused to acknowledge them. The encounter left me speechless.

Even though I had made this appointment several weeks in advance, the toxicologist left me in a dingy waiting room to cool my heels for five hours, until another FDA bureaucrat finally appeared to escort me all of twenty-five or thirty yards to the files in question. In this large windowless room with insufficient light, I was confronted with approximately twenty large tables piled sky-high with paper, the entire body of research that purportedly deemed aspartame safe. Each stack of documents was at least 3 feet high. Folders and papers were strewn about the floor, blocking the already limited pathways between the tables. They were not going to make this easy for me.

While poring over the largely unorganized mounds, out of the corner of my eye I noticed others passing in and out of the docket room. At first I paid little attention. The job ahead of me was daunting and beginning to seem quite impossible, but when a folder suddenly appeared on the table where I was working, I noted that the corner of a page had been folded back to single out its contents. I asked an older gentleman who had been in and out of the room if it was his. He smiled, took a quick look around, then responded, "No, sir. That's for you." The volume to which I had been directed was a complete copy of the heretofore unknown "52-Week Oral Toxicity Study in the Infant Monkey,"[229] an aspartame safety study funded by Searle in 1972 and conducted by Doctor Waisman from the Department of Pediatrics at the University of Wisconsin Medical Center in Madison. The results of this neglected study were deeply disturbing: all the infant monkeys fed aspartame developed seizures, and some even died. Little research gifts like this one kept coming that day, transforming an initially solitary exercise in frustration and futility into a fruitful, even collaborative, enterprise – a most memorable docket-file experience. I was to learn 25 years later that the most damning information – tests that showed aspartame had caused birth defects of the brains of test animals – had been removed from the docket file long before either my mysterious friends or I could have discovered them. More details on these studies will follow where their teachings can best be applied.

A Battlefield Casualty

I was not to last very long in the official ranks waging war against aspartame. My stripes were summarily, if only figuratively, stripped from my lab coat for what was deemed a transgression.

It began when I was interviewed in 1983 for a *CBS Evening News* feature on aspartame. I had already learned from previous experiences with other national television shows like *60 Minutes* that you never know when, or even if, your interview will be aired, and you never know how it will be edited. They were also interviewing other scientists from the G.D. Searle & Company, who would obviously be taking the other side of the issue. At this point, it occurred to me that it might be interesting to make an educated guess about, and a small accompanying wager on, the public's response to what had become a hot news item. Those of you unfamiliar with the machinations of the stock market may find it interesting to know that you can invest against any company listed on the major exchanges by purchasing options that gain value as their stock goes down, which is exactly what I did with G.D. Searle. After months of researching their sweetener and finding it unacceptable, I bought a few hundred options against the stock, for some two thousand dollars. I called it "putting your money where your mouth is," or as the *Wall Street Journal* was to correctly, but embarrassingly, quote me as saying, "It's the American way." I considered my wager so trifling that a few days after purchasing the options, I casually mentioned it to an attorney who represented Searle in Arizona, when by chance I found myself sitting beside her on a flight to Washington, DC.

Well, I hope that this confession does not discourage you from following the scientific counsel of this book, having decided that you now question the judgment of its author. Admittedly, my decision to bet against this company turned out to be a rather stupid thing to do, not only because of the bad publicity it generated, making me a persona non grata with the food establishment, but also because of the very deep ties folks on the other side enjoyed with the U.S. Treasury. Broadly interpreting the rules governing insider trading, this department decided to investigate my momentous $1900.00 investment. I treated the two Treasury Department investigators from the Securities and Exchange Commission to a two-hour slide presentation explaining the dangers of aspartame. They were actually two very pleasant women, one of whom was pregnant and had entered the warm federal conference room set aside for the interrogation with a diet soda in her hand. At some point during my presentation, she tellingly tossed her unfinished can into the trash bin. The investigation went nowhere, despite claims on the Internet about my spending time in jail or losing my university position over this minor indiscretion. These stories, like most Web legends, were simply not true. I was wholly exonerated of any wrongdoing and maintained my position at ASU for many more years until my retirement with the status of Professor Emeritus. Indeed, this brouhaha may have even been for the best, as it reduced my speaking engagements and gave me more research time in the library and laboratory, where I learned all that I could about the complex and fascinating poison, methanol.

The Diagnosis Is Multiple Sclerosis

The publicity from this series of events raised my profile considerably, in ways both positive and negative. Since my first public declaration questioning the safety of aspartame, many hundreds of individuals with stories to tell about their experiences with this dangerous sweetener have contacted me. A high percentage of these complaints are from women who had been, or who were soon to be diagnosed with the neurological disease multiple sclerosis. There is no denying the veritable epidemic of autoimmune diseases throughout the world over the last three decades. Multiple sclerosis, once almost unknown in Japan, now menaces a large segment of the population. The lower latitudes and warmer climates, once "mysteriously" protected from the full brunt of this tragically debilitating disease, have seen the incidence and prevalence of MS climb to as high as four times the rate that prevailed before cooling summer drinks were sweetened with aspartame. The United States, which has long had a relatively high MS incidence, has seen at least a 50 percent increase. Medical journals in Australia[263] and New Zealand[90] both report seemingly inexplicable increases in what now constitutes inordinately high[168] incidence rates. During the thirty years of exposure to methanol from aspartame, the incidence of this terrible disease has reached epidemic proportions, and its distribution has been shifting from a disease of primarily colder climates to one found anywhere where diet soda is consumed.

Let's now consider why this may be.

Chapter 1

A Time When All the Easy Questions Have Been Answered

Something very wrong is going on, something that is killing good people and causing untold suffering to families and communities around the world. Never has such a high percentage of us been afflicted with so many tragic and wasting illnesses. In the past thirty years, a group of diseases has reached epidemic proportions in the United States and many other countries. These afflictions, often collectively referred to as diseases of civilization (DOC), include multiple sclerosis, Alzheimer's disease, breast cancer, lupus erythematosus, rheumatoid arthritis, melanoma, and autism – a once rare birth defect. Because the incidence of these diseases has increased gradually over three decades, we are inclined to accept this as a natural, if unfortunate, part of modern life. But such a lethal trend is not natural; the changes that we have witnessed over the last generation are unprecedented in the history of medical science.

French physician Stanislaw Tanchou, the first to observe that cancer was rarely found in hunter-gatherer populations, is credited with coining the term "diseases of civilization" in a paper presented to the Paris Medical Society in 1843. His descriptive term survives to this day because certain diseases have still not been proven to have existed before the "civilized" era, and these conditions continue to be largely absent in modern hunter-gatherer societies.

These are the worst of times, as mankind endures a plague whose point of origin distinctly coincides with the Food and Drug Administration's 1981 approval of aspartame – an artificial sweetener containing methanol, which is metabolized into deadly formaldehyde within the brain and sinew of all who consume it. I am a food scientist who warned thirty years ago in the scientific literature of the hazards we court by adding large amounts of methanol to our food supply.[1] I am a professor who taught my students of these dangers. I am an activist who took the FDA to the Supreme Court in an effort to compel it to carry out its mandate and obligation to protect the public. I am still waging this battle and will continue to fight until the salient and suppressed facts have been revealed. To date, I have had little success in engaging the medical community, despite having presented at numerous professional meetings and published on this subject. I have even invented and received patents on novel means of addressing the problem – all to little avail, and with vexingly little explanation or substantive refutation of my central claim that dietary methanol may be the root cause of these and possibly other diseases.

Why, you may ask, hasn't the scientific community responded to what constitutes a clear and present danger? You may think it strange that the innovative ideas of a PhD from a good school, who was a professor in a major research university for twenty-five years and who has numerous scientific articles and over twenty-two patents to his name, would be excluded from consideration. The gatekeepers of the medical sciences are notorious, however, for impeding the academic access of those who are not members of their particular discipline, and the establishment has a number of reasons for not welcoming those who purport to reveal causes or propose cures for a malady. Exclusionary and dismissive behavior is, sadly, not the exception, but the rule in an age when legitimate cures are few and when marginal – even dangerous – treatments abound. Pharmaceutical corporations promise much but guarantee little, trafficking in false hope while extracting considerable sums for their coffers from desperate families.

Consider, for instance, the striking example of the Australian winners of the 2005 Nobel Prize in Medicine, gastroenterologist Barry J. Marshall and pathologist Robin Warren, who discovered that a bacteria, not psychological stress, causes stomach and duodenal ulcers. Until their groundbreaking findings were accepted, the lifetime administration of costly drugs blocking the production of gastric acid was the prescribed treatment for chronic and debilitating ulcers, which often relapsed because, as we know now, remaining bacteria perpetuated the inflammation. In the early 1980s, Dr. Warren first observed that biopsies of human stomach ulcers often coincided with findings of a spiral-shaped H. pylori bacteria, confirming the results of a neglected scientific paper published in 1940 by Dr. A. Stone Freedberg at Harvard, who had independently identified similar bacteria in 40 percent of patients with ulcers and stomach cancer.

When Dr. Warren first reported his findings in 1980, many doctors and drug companies were unconvinced, a point acknowledged by the Nobel Committee in its praise of Drs. Marshall and Warren for "tenacity and a prepared mind that challenged prevailing dogmas." [111] The Nobel Committee noted, "it is now firmly established that H. pylori causes more than 90 percent of duodenal ulcers and up to 80 percent of gastric ulcers," yet the young Dr. Marshall had been compelled to put his own health at risk in an effort to persuade earlier detractors. He infected himself with the disease-causing bacterium and underwent four biopsies that proved conclusively he had developed a type of severe stomach inflammation known to be a precursor of ulcers. It ultimately took over twenty years for a segment of the established medical community to recognize that antibiotics could quickly cure gastritis and most stomach and duodenal ulcers.

Some of you may think this was the happy ending to the story, that the Nobel Committee had said it all, and now a CURE for ulcers had been confirmed! But the tragedy of this story is that the cure is not being widely implemented. Big Pharma, the medical industry, and practicing physicians have little use for cures. They make a very good income treating ulcer patients with high-profit acid blockers and office calls. It has been five years since these scientists won their argument in arguably the highest court of the scientific community, but the cure is not being widely prescribed by practicing physicians, who often insist the patient continue self-administration of profitable palliatives – even after the patient has asked for the administration of the cure.

The above example demonstrates how big medicine treats its own when they dare to threaten income streams. The real tragedy here is that the patient with an ulcer can only be cured by his physician, since two of the antibiotics needed for the cure are prescription drugs which may only be administered by a trained medical professional. In contrast, the cure for methanol poisoning, as you will learn in the next chapter, is a straightforward dietary recommendation that is easy to learn and follow and will cost you nothing. Remember, the poorest people in the world are free of the DOC primarily because they cannot afford the foods that cause it.

It is essential to understand from the outset that we are proposing that we have discovered the direct cause for a series of diseases that the medical community has been investigating for the last 150 years – with a breathtaking lack of success. In five generations of what would appear to be relatively intense scrutiny, no one has found a cause for any of these diseases, much less a cure. The death certificates of 75 percent of people in today's world will list one of the DOC, the symptoms and consequent treatment of which often continue for decades before death.[587] That is big business. Prevention could considerably reduce the billions raked in by the drug and biotech companies of Big Pharma – or even put them out of business altogether. As the road to perpetual profit is most certainly not paved with cures, corporate medicine does not necessarily embrace recovery.

At this time, most of the easier questions concerning the origin and cause of disease have arguably been answered. To tackle the more difficult and persistent questions, scholars must be allowed to transcend the artificial barriers that separate the traditionally isolationist disciplines of scientific practice and thought. Generalist inquiry holds great hope for revealing vital secrets of the natural world, yet we provide no forum for the exchange of universal concepts, no means for their evaluation, no reward for the Herculean effort required to filter common truths from the vast heap of data and lonely facts doggedly milled by experts – those specialists whose single-minded laboratory environment often blinds them to the real world. The taboo of forbidden trespass – originating in a primitive communal mindset evolved for survival through competitive hunting – hobbles free interpretation, interdisciplinary thinking, and the pursuit of Nature's truth for the common good.

It is time to breathe new life into the practice of medicine and develop a sustainable basis for the foundation of the next generation of discovery. Sit back, relax, and consider an alternative perspective. Let a food scientist show you where his intuition and research have taken him. Your efforts may be rewarded with the insight necessary to understand a diverse, yet strangely similar, group of maladies.

Diseases Linked to Diet

You may be surprised to learn that most diseases are caused by what we put into our mouths. Diseases, after all, are not the result of life's normal wear and tear. Each disease requires an agent that causes a living system or systems to malfunction, producing the symptoms and the eventual outcome of the disease. We are all aware of certain bacteria and viruses that trigger illnesses. We are perhaps less knowledgeable of other deleterious living organisms – the worms, amoeba, protozoa, and prions found in our food, for example. Non-living things can also, of course, promote disease through either their unwanted presence, as with carcinogenic asbestos and formaldehyde, or their harmful absence, as with vitamin C, whose deficiency causes a long, slow death by scurvy. We call these causes of disease etiologic agents.

A very high percentage of etiologic agents are present in what we eat, and some of the most serious, complex human diseases can be attributed to the advent and evolution of food processing. Minor changes in how food is processed can be catastrophic and have been responsible for untold human suffering and death. For example, the simple process of milling off the outer layer of rice to give the final product a more pleasing white color also removes much of the vitamin thiamine, a seemingly small loss that can result in beriberi. Entire villages have died from this disease, which starts as a nervous system disorder and ends in heart failure and death. Conversely, pellagra, another deficiency disease, is caused by neglecting to process food, more specifically corn, through the simple application of a little rock lime the night before consumption. Killing thousands of Americans as recently as 1929, pellagra has symptoms that mimic many other diseases, including diarrhea, dermatitis, anxiety, depression, hallucinations, and headaches. Scurvy, pellagra, beriberi, rickets, and all the vitamin deficiency diseases would have been classified as diseases of civilization, had the term existed then. Today, the possibility that a simple nutrient deficiency or metabolic poison might result in conditions as diverse as Alzheimer's, multiple sclerosis, and atherosclerosis may seem improbable to you, but to a scientist trained in the history of nutritional sciences and familiar with the evolution of vitamin deficiencies, these modern diseases show all the outward signs of a common dietary cause.

My Research Orientation

I submit that the diseases of civilization we will be considering have been linked for years to diet and that we are dealing primarily with an issue of food safety and nutrition – my area of general training and subsequent specialization. I believe that the application of reason, logic, and old-fashioned common sense can resolve the most difficult of problems. I love reading scientific articles, picking out the good from the bad, and then reassessing the experimental results when disentangled from what may be a certain bias on the part of the researcher. Although this proclivity has not always made me friends in the scientific community, it has always proved useful in my pursuit of the mysterious origin of DOC.

Nature withholds nothing from us. She knows nothing of stealth. She keeps no secrets. The miracle of the newborn baby we hold in our arms, with its beating heart and compelling murmur, are the workings of a vision 4 billion years in the making. The parts are all there, no strings attached, no batteries required. Life's mechanisms and depths are free for us to fathom, if that is our wish. Humans are born tinkerers capable of understanding all that Nature has accomplished in the evolution of existence. The basic scientific rules that govern the natural, living world are, for the most part, clearly understood and taught as a matter of course in our institutions of higher learning. Still, Nature can be elusive, working at a scale so small as to mask life's finer elements. Even here, much may be learned from inference and generalization, which have contributed to our mastery of the subatomic world and the advancement of electronics.

Science has struggled for generations to identify the elusive and insidious etiologic agents responsible for diseases of civilization. Some historians date the beginning of civilization to the discovery and use of fire; in civilizations where fire has been a luxury, DOC have been remarkably rare. These are places where the population barely subsists, with incomes well below the poverty level by any standard. I have lived among the "dirt poor," where I witnessed such scarcity that even a discarded, empty oil can became a coveted item over which grown men came to blows. Much can be said about the tragedy of this subsistence lifestyle and the deprivations suffered by the inhabitants of these communities. In great contrast, we in the First World are the fortunate of the earth; we consume the lion's share of its available resources and spare ourselves few luxuries. But even with all this abundance, there are many among us who suffer from disease and who, in moments of deep despair, would gladly trade our luxuries for something common to the poor of the Third World – virtual freedom from diseases of civilization. The illnesses I will be discussing do not thrive in the environments of the truly destitute. How can this be?

I have spent the better part of my career studying this very issue, exploring dietary and food science to make sense of the disparity in afflictions that affect the "haves" and "have-nots." It is my ardent belief that diseases of civilization are the consequence of long-term consumption of methanol, a poison whose most damaging effects are specific to humans. It is exceedingly difficult to find methanol in any of the food consumed by primitive cultures, whether Paleolithic man or present-day foragers, all of which are known to be free from DOC. Methyl alcohol is also conspicuously absent in the diets of the poor, a menu that does not feature diet soda, canned fruits or vegetables, bottled or boxed fruit juices, or smoked meats and fish. Often a single cigarette, another major source of methanol, costs as much as they spend each week to survive. Eating from hand to mouth pretty much precludes methanol consumption. Although methanol, also called wood alcohol, has been with us since we first took a fancy to food flavored by the smoke of a wood fire, only in the early industrial age did it become dangerously prolific in our diets, making it a poison to be reckoned with.

Why Methanol

Methanol is a true nemesis of the human constitution. It is a chemical to which only humans are sensitive and from which we suffer greatly. Because of this it should have always been a prime suspect as the cause of the long list of diseases to which humans alone are susceptible – diseases which we do not share with other animals on the planet. The chapters that follow will take you one by one through these diseases in detail along with the possible reasons why methanol has been ignored from consideration as their cause.

You need to know what it is about methanol that makes it dangerous. The simple answer is that methanol is a bomb, very much like a hand grenade, that can do no damage unless and until it explodes. Luckily, it is very difficult to get methanol to explode; in fact, only two important enzymes in living things are capable of pulling the pin of methanol's hand grenade to start the explosion. We will explain what these enzymes are in more detail later, but for now one is called catalase enzyme and the other is called alcohol dehydrogenase enzyme, which we will shorten to ADH from now on. Pulling the pin of the little methanol molecule causes it to open up into a diabolical killing machine, much as visualized so well in one of those Transformer movies your kids watch.

The name of that killing machine is one you will recognize: formaldehyde. Yes, the very same formaldehyde that is now known to be a powerful cancer-causing agent – the one that we are warned to avoid at all costs. I describe methanol as a bomb, not because it explodes, but because the damage that it inflicts when it does convert into formaldehyde is very local and confined to a small area... just like a hand grenade. The reason for this is that formaldehyde itself is very quick to react to tissue in the immediate area where it is produced. You will see the importance of this in later chapters.

Why Are Only Humans Harmed by Methanol?

The two enzymes that can pull methanol's pin and make it explode are found in very different locations within the living cell. The catalase that animals use to explode methanol is located in a very special spherical shaped organelle within the living cell called a peroxisome. This peroxisome is shaped very much like the device that bomb disposal units use to safely explode terrorist bombs. Within this very special cellular contraption are other enzymes that are capable of breaking down the formaldehyde produced from methanol into safe components, thereby protecting the rest of the cell from contact with the very active formaldehyde itself. This arrangement makes the breakdown of methanol so safe for animals that the peroxisome in conjunction with the powerhouse of the animal cell, the organelle called mitochondria, can work together to safely burn methanol all the way to carbon dioxide, thus successfully using methanol as a food.

Unfortunately, although humans have catalase and peroxisomes, our catalase has been mutated over time and cannot pull methanol's pin. So here is the rub: in humans, the only enzyme that can explode methanol is the ADH. Unfortunately, the ADH enzyme is dissolved in the liquid of the cell and can float around just about anywhere inside it. This creates a much greater danger to the human from methanol poisoning. ADH can produce formaldehyde just about anywhere in the cell, meaning the formaldehyde is then free to do damage to all sorts of cellular components. If the formaldehyde is produced close to the nucleus of the cell, it can easily slip into the nucleus where the chromosomes are and act as a methyl molecule, causing autism. If produced close to the outside of the cell it can escape from the cell and do damage to nearby tissue, as happens in the case of MS and Alzheimer's. Luckily for humans, not all cells contain ADH, but the ones that do are all in places where the Diseases of Civilization originate.

Ethanol and Methanol Fight for the Attention of the ADH Enzyme

The one fact that can be used to save us from developing the DOC is this: ADH enzyme prefers to interact with ethanol (drinking alcohol), not methanol. ADH can, therefore, be prevented from converting methanol into formaldehyde. You see, ADH was originally designed by Nature to metabolize drinking alcohol, so if it has a choice, it will always choose ethanol.

Enzymes follow strict rules and they all have to do with relative concentrations. The rule of thumb with ADH is if the concentration of methanol is 16 times higher than the concentration of ethanol, then the ADH will finally be compelled to start turning methanol into formaldehyde. It all comes down to preference and compatibility. In this way our enzyme ADH is much like a fickle suitor. As Stephen Stills might have sung, "If you can't be with the alcohol you love, honey, love the one your with."

If you had to choose between someone who meets all your requirements and someone who is nowhere near as attractive, what would it take for you to have a relationship with someone you really didn't like that much? What if the unattractive one was twice as wealthy as the one you preferred? Not good enough? What about sixteen times as wealthy? Hmmmmm... now maybe those eyes look pretty nice! This is how it works with the ADH enzyme. If ethanol is available, it will ignore methanol completely and spend all its time helping turn ethanol into vinegar. This is a very good thing for us. All we need do is to see to it that there is always a little ethanol in our blood, and no formaldehyde will ever be made. Perhaps easier said than done.

What Damage Can a Sip of Diet Soda Do?

When you take a sip of aspartame-sweetened diet soda, you are consuming as much methanol as you would if you took an average puff of cigarette smoke. **A liter of diet soda contains as much methanol as you would inhale from a pack of cigarettes.** We have irrefutable proof that cigarette smoking is a cause for most of the diseases we will be discussing in this book. No one has ever discovered what chemical in that smoke actually causes these diseases. Methanol has never been tested as a cause, even though it constitutes a considerable percentage of the poisonous compounds in that smoke. I consider methanol to be the most deadly component of cigarette smoke. Smoking cigarettes and drinking diet soda constitute the two primary methods of consuming methanol.

A sip of diet soda containing aspartame is broken into methanol within a few minutes of consumption. All of the blood that flows from the heart through the entire digestive system, from the mouth to the anal sphincter, serves two functions. One is to provide oxygen to the cells that line the digestive tract. The other is to supply a river of blood to carry away all of the nutrients, minerals and other substances, both good and bad, that our very efficient digestion manages to suck out of the numerous things we chose to put in our mouths. Methanol from diet soda eventually passes down the digestive tract and into the small intestines, where the little alcohol molecule is easily absorbed into the river of blood on its way to the liver.

The next and last segment of the digestive tract is the most poorly understood. The large intestine, or colon, is primarily responsible for removing the water from what remains of the material not absorbed by our small intestines. The colon is a five foot long tube that behaves very much like a wine fermentation vat. It supports the lives of a vast and diverse population of microorganisms living in an often complex relationship with us and each other that has defied any meaningful scientific elucidation. Half the weight of the average stool sample expelled from the colon at the bowel is made up of living microorganisms to which we are not related, but without which we seem incapable of living. These microscopic creatures that foster colonic fermentation are fed by the waste products of our digestive process. Many chemical byproducts are produced by these little creatures, the most important of which, for our discussion here, is ethanol. It appears that ethanol is a fairly consistent, but not guaranteed, component of colonic fermentation. Proof of this lies in the fact that although our bodies have no genetic mechanism to manufacture ethanol, most people – even rabid *teetotalers* under most, but not all circumstances – are often found to have ethanol in their bloodstreams.[64] This is not usually enough ethanol to cause even a hint of intoxication,[186] but it is enough to help protect us most of the time, but not always, from methanol.

The river of blood flowing from our gut digestion is burdened by all of the nutrients, minerals, poisons, methanol, ethanol, and other substances that are dissolved in it. This blood is far too contaminated to allow it to be sucked directly into the heart, where it would mix with the general circulation. First, it must be cleaned and the nutrients balanced so that sensitive organs are not damaged. A special network of veins drains the entire digestive system and converges into a large vein called the hepatic portal vein. This large vein takes the contaminated blood to the only place in the body that can clean it up – the liver. The blood from our small intestine, which contains the methanol from our diet soda, travels to the hepatic portal vein and mixes with the ethanol from fermentation in the colon. This blend of ethanol and methanol now flows into the liver to be processed. It is very important to note here that although the liver contains a great deal of ADH it can not pull the pin on any of the methanol molecules because of the presence of the ethanol from the gut. This is how small amounts of methanol from diet soda make it into the general circulation and become available to cause disease in other parts of the body. Most scientists do not realize this and are under the wrong impression that the liver removes all traces of methanol from the blood before it can do any harm in say the brain.

Once past the liver, the methanol flows directly into the largest vein in the body – the superior vena cava

– just before being sucked into the heart and pumped directly to the lungs, where it joins the methanol being absorbed from the puff of cigarette smoke you might have taken between your last sips of diet soda. Once methanol gets into the blood and starts circulating to the brain you are dealing with a biochemical game of musical chairs. The methanol goes around and around in your bloodstream waiting for the ethanol level in your blood to reach zero, at which time it can have its pick of any of the ADH sites in the body where it can be turned into formaldehyde. This would not be a good thing. This formaldehyde is what causes all the diseases of civilization. You will learn the details of this after you have a little chemistry lesson in Chapter 4. Only two things can happen to methanol to remove it from the general circulation: one, it can slowly leave the body by way of urine or sweat, or two, it can just keep on circulating around the bloodstream until it finds a place to turn into formaldehyde and cause disease. There are no other choices.

Only a handful of places in the human body contain ADH. Look ahead, if you like, to Table 2 in Chapter 5 (Target Organs of Methanol Toxicity). It points to all of the locations where ADH can be found, along with the diseases which might be associated with each location. At these sites, methanol is converted to formaldehyde. This conversion takes place under one of only two circumstances: either the concentration of methanol in the bloodstream must rise to a much higher level than the concentration of ethanol, or, during the night or at some time during the day, your body must suddenly find that all of its precious ethanol has been metabolized and has vanished. In either case, the ADH will begin to be attracted to the methanol and convert it to formaldehyde on the spot.

Why Would the Ethanol in Your Blood Vanish?

What about the ethanol being generated by the colon? Won't it keep on protecting us throughout the day? Well the truth is that ADH and other enzymes are constantly using up the ethanol in our blood. Scientists have never studied how much time the ethanol produced by the colon can last after a meal before it is all metabolized, so we have no idea how long the protection lasts. We have only recently learned about the apparent universality of these low levels of ethanol in the human bloodstream.[363] As with the case of many of the observations that I use to support my hypothesis, the data was an accidental discovery made during the search for something else. It is possible that some individuals – and perhaps all of us under certain circumstances during some time of the day or night – may have no detectable ethanol in our blood. When the level of ethanol in the blood reaches zero, we are guaranteed that any methanol that is present will be made into formaldehyde – a very bad thing indeed. Studies have substantiated this, finding methanol alone in the blood of certain individuals with no ethanol to keep it from becoming formaldehyde.[188]

As you can see, ethanol can be a double-edged sword when it comes to preventing methanol from causing disease. A very small amount of ethanol in the blood can prevent the liver from removing methanol from the food we consume, thereby putting us in harm's way by allowing this methanol to pass into the circulation to the brain and other organs. On the other hand, the same ethanol concentration in the blood can prevent methanol from turning into formaldehyde within the brain and elsewhere, thus preventing the same diseases. The caveat is that ethanol must be sustained in the bloodstream continuously with no interruption if it is to prevent disease. We know this is true because when a human accidently consumes a dose of methanol that would normally kill him, only one antidote can keep that person alive. The only known antidote for methanol poisoning in humans is ethanol – enough ethanol to keep every molecule of ADH in their body occupied for as long as it takes for the kidneys (or dialysis, in some instances) to eliminate a sufficient amount of poisonous methanol from the bloodstream. Ethanol works perfectly as long as it is administered in time, before too much of the methanol has been converted to formaldehyde at all the body's ADH sites. It is not unusual to have to keep a methanol poison victim inebriated with ethanol for four or five days to save their lives.

The relationship of these two alcohols is actually even more fascinating than this. One more level of interaction with ethanol goes a very long way to proving my hypothesis without my having to go very much deeper into my very deep stack of evidence. If it is true that ethanol in the bloodstream prevents damage from methanol, then it would be logical to surmise that the daily administration of ethanol should, by increasing the amount of time ethanol spends in the circulation, reduce the incidence of the Diseases of Civilization. Amazingly this has been proven to be the case. Much to the surprise of every major laboratory that has discovered it, the incidence of atherosclerosis,[485] Alzheimer's,[534] lupus,[73] rheumatoid arthritis,[295] and other DOCs is less than half that in individuals that consume one alcoholic drink a day as compared to those who abstain from alcoholic beverage consumption.

Though you might find this a little confusing right now you, will soon see that no better explanation exists that could account for some of the serendipity of the incidence and timing of attacks of the various DOC. The development of these diseases in any of us depends first and most importantly on our intake of methanol, a factor over which we have complete control. Next, sufficient sites of ADH must be located in susceptible organs, a variable that is bound to be both hereditarily and sexually determined, and which has been scarcely studied. Third, the local influence of other enzymes that may be able to convert formaldehyde quickly into the safe formic acid would surely be an important factor, but once again we have no history of scientific elucidation. Ethanol levels in the blood from any source would constitute another variable that further overlays the complex interactions in play on a 24-hour basis. Do you see now why the DOC take years to fully develop? This is just the beginning.

In the next chapter you will learn where methanol can be found and how to avoid it. Then we will go into the history of methanol and how this plays an important part in why most physicians have no idea of the danger posed by this etiologic agent of the DOC. If your stamina continues, we will then go on to learn some of the chemistry of methanol and formaldehyde. The remaining chapters will present the exact details of how I believe each of the DOC are caused by methanol and what considerable scientific evidence I have to prove my point. If you have no stomach for science, but think some truth might be found in what I am saying, then all you need to do is read the next chapter, tear out the page of dietary recommendations, and attach it to your refrigerator door.

Chapter 2

Methanol: Where Is It Found? How Can It Be Avoided?

In order to impress you with the ease of removing all methanol from your diet I place this chapter early in this book. Do not wait...remove methanol from your diet now!

Methanol causes disease through metabolic processes that transform it into formaldehyde in your brain and other organs. An accidental legacy of civilization, methanol can be replaced in most industrial uses by ethanol (drinking alcohol), a relatively harmless alcohol. Tellingly, only in the production of commercial formaldehyde is there no replacement or substitute for methanol. Preventing methanol from entering your body is the best method of poison prevention. This chapter provides incentive about why and information about how to avoid this chemical in your daily life, practical advice that also fosters a better theoretical understanding of methanol-placed formaldehyde and its critical role in the origin of disease.

Environmental Methanol

At room temperature, methanol is a liquid and often used as a solvent to clean various items in industry. Like ethanol, it has a low boiling point and can easily evaporate into a dangerous gas quickly absorbed by the lungs. Since exposure to methanol gas has been responsible for both blindness and death in the workplace, its use is now strictly regulated and must be closely monitored. Although a comprehensive guide to methanol at the worksite is not within the scope of this book, anyone who works with methanol should request pertinent information from management and, if necessary, wear protective clothing.

Fortunately, this kind of environmental contamination is not common, a fact that affected my research to a significant extent. I spent considerable time looking for groups of individuals who worked with methanol uncontaminated by ethanol. Ironically, it was the teaching profession that provided me with the best group of documented subjects. In the age before Xerox, primary and secondary school teachers, and even some college professors, made copies for their classes on a hand-cranked Ditto machine that, employing almost pure methanol to transfer images, became a serious health concern in its day.

The paper and wood product industry has also been guilty of methanol exposure in the workplace. Wood alcohol is, after all, the original name for methanol. At temperatures close to burning, wood releases methanol, a method first used to create commercial methanol 200 years ago, when wood was heated by fire in iron retorts, producing methanol gas condensed in a still, just as one would produce ethanol from corn mash. Processing wood products and manufacturing paper occasionally exposes employees to methanol.

In the course of my research on various industries, I discovered a particularly grave situation in a small Ohio town where a foundry used methanol as a solvent to clean oil from hot molded metal parts and released it into the environment as air pollution. This abuse occurred over a number of years, and the Environmental Protection Agency was eventually called upon to investigate because of the community's increased incidence of multiple sclerosis – tenfold over what was accepted as normal. In a later chapter, I will elaborate on my study of involuntary human exposure to methanol.

Cigarette and Cigar Smoke

Cigarette smoke has been conclusively identified as the direct cause of many diseases of civilization.[345] Cigarette smoke is also a major source of methanol. Despite these well-established facts, research attempting to identify the specific chemical compound responsible for DOC has overlooked or dismissed methanol. It has managed to avoid detection in many years of animal testing because it is the only component in cigarette smoke without a viable animal model for determining its toxic potential. As early as 1939, researchers in Germany reported that cigarette smoke contained potentially dangerous levels of methanol,[62] findings that contributed to Adolf Hitler's decision to institute a popular Nazi health initiative educating the German public on the dangers of cigarettes. There is no doubt that cigarette smoke is causally linked to atherosclerosis,[345] lupus,[73] Alzheimer's disease,[535] and rheumatoid arthritis.[332] After 150 years of research, it also constitutes the only generally accepted causative agent of multiple sclerosis.[68] Unfortunately, the single article that more specifically posits methanol as a potential cause of MS[8] is never cited in the MS or smoking toxicology literature.

The particular production of methanol in cigarette smoke is noteworthy in this context. Tobacco leaf used to make cigarettes comprises considerable pectin, known to contain tightly bound methanol. Harvested leaves are hung in barns to ferment naturally for months at a time. The bacteria responsible for this fermentation process have enzymes capable of freeing the chemically bound methanol from the pectin. When a cigarette is smoked, this methanol is vaporized and quickly absorbed into the bloodstream. It travels directly to the brain and the rest of the body, bypassing the liver on the first pass. Cigarettes have a higher methanol content than cigars[62] because the tobacco leaf wrapping the cigar is often aged for up to three years, which reduces its methanol concentration through evaporation and may account for what research has indicated to be the somewhat reduced risks associated with cigar smoking. [513,410]

Methanol in the Food Supply

Absent in all but a handful of foods, methanol does not appear in the primitive diet of the Pleistocene and is almost unheard of in the diet of present-day foragers. Its presence is insignificant in major human food staples such as milk, cheese, fish, meat, eggs, fresh vegetables, beans, and any of the many grains or grain products. In the natural world, measurable, but typically inconsequential, quantities of methanol can be found only in ripe fruit. In fresh squeezed fruit juice, this amount is insignificant, but higher methanol content in rotting fruit and other spoiled plant material can pose a problem. As with the fermentation of tobacco leaf mentioned in the previous section, bacteria that cause fermentation may strip the methanol directly off the pectin found in most plant cells. Almost all primitive cultures share the long-held taboo about eating rotting or overripe plant material, a prudent policy for any of us who want to eliminate dietary methanol.

Methanol, a naturally occurring chemical, can be found in all living things in quantities typically too minute to pose a problem. It is not these trace amounts of methanol I am addressing here, although opponents have exaggerated my position in an effort to discredit legitimate concerns, critiques that, if taken seriously, could jeopardize corporate profit margins.

During a heated television debate on a Los Angeles news program some twenty years ago, another professor of food science, who represented the companies making and using aspartame, rebuked me for "next wanting to remove cheese from the market . . . because it contains methanol." This was news to me, the first time I had heard of methanol in cheese. Given that the source of this surprising information was a faculty member from a well-regarded university and an expert in dairy, I carefully reviewed the cheese literature, only to conclude that my opponent's comment probably said more about the integrity of the aspartame industry than it did about the composition of cheese. I found just one obscure article that mentioned an exceedingly small concentration of methanol in the gas escaping from aging cheese.[426] When I calculated the maximum possible amount that could have been in the cheese itself, it turned out that over a metric ton of cheese was required to produce the amount of methanol in only one can of diet soda, some 2000 pounds of cheese that would take a lifetime of almost continuous constipation to consume. (If you visit my website, thetruthaboutstuff.com, you can find our debate archived in the video section.)

Bad News about Blackcurrants and Tomatoes

In only two fresh fruits is the methanol content high enough to merit a warning. The first is the blackcurrant berry – despite persistent arguments about the safety of dietary methanol that often point to blackcurrant juice as an exemplar. Support for this dubious assertion has typically taken the form of a French conference paper based on a presentation to vendors concerned about the methanol in certain wines. Authors Francot and Geoffroy[19] explain that the data presented "may not" represent their work but that of "other authors." They identify only the lowest and highest methanol sources, respectively grape juice at 12 milligrams/liter and blackcurrant juice at 680 milligrams/liter. The other fruit juices used to generate their purportedly low average of 140 milligrams of methanol per liter are left completely to the imagination. The authors conclude their paper by blithely insisting that "the content of methanol in fermented or non-fermented beverages should not be of concern to the fields of human physiology and public health," so "drink up." A hearty but questionably all-encompassing toast: the fact remains that blackcurrant juice is dangerously high in methanol, and abstaining would probably not present any great hardship for imbibers.

Abstinence may prove more difficult, however, with the second more popular fruit. Providing as much methanol per glass as diet soda, tomato juice is just not worth the risk. Of particular interest here is the history of the tomato, another of those plants the Spanish conquistadors brought to Europe from the New World. Unlike corn, though, the indigenous people considered the tomato poisonous, cultivating it in their gardens strictly for its beauty. The wisdom of hindsight suggests they were right to be wary. The observational abilities of a people who devised the lime treatment of corn in order to avoid pellagra would have been ample to discover the beautiful and sweet-tasting tomato's toxic little secret.

If you are a fan of the tomato, as many are (particularly those of Italian extraction like myself), no need to throw down this book in disgust. You do not have to give up pasta sauce. The next section explains some European culinary means of removing methanol, thus restoring tomato sauce as a safe choice on your menu. Furthermore, there is no reason not to indulge in the occasional slice of uncooked tomato in a salad or on a cheeseburger, since it takes three full-size tomatoes to produce the methanol in a can of diet soda. Let moderation be your guide, and as you will see later, a glass of wine a day may even cancel out these potentially minor negative effects.

Canned, Bottled, Jarred, and Aseptically Packaged Fruits and Vegetables and Their Juices

With the invention of the canning process in 1806, civilization first began to encounter methanol on a significant scale. It is significant to note that diseases of civilization were rare before Nicolas Appert of France commercialized canning, a process that incidentally traps methanol derived from the heating and storage of plant materials containing pectin.[1] Coincidentally – or, as I argue, not so coincidentally – some twenty years later in 1828, the anatomical descriptions of a new disease began to appear in the medical literature. Jean-Martin Charcot, also of France, would be the first to fully describe this new affliction and name it multiple sclerosis.

A considerable capacity for methanol exists in the pectin found naturally in fruits and vegetables. Although the bonds in this chemical structure are so tight that digestion does not free potential methanol, the process of canning ensures methanol's release into a container from where it has no place to go except your stomach upon consumption of the can's contents. Whether commercially produced or home processed, canned or preserved fruits and vegetables and their juices are the worst non-diet foods you can consume; their methanol content greatly exceeds that of their fresh counterparts. Methanol is not present in canned meat and fish, however, making these safe to eat. As a general rule of thumb, a canned product that lacks pectin can be enjoyed with impunity. Quick-frozen or individually frozen products, a popular alternative to canned fruits and vegetables, are a great choice, with methanol contents as low or in some cases lower than the fresh products.

Canning fruits and vegetables increases methanol by staggering amounts, a topic I treat in great detail in a 1984 article.[1] Consider, for example, two more commonly consumed fruit juices: orange juice and grapefruit juice, both of which were the subject of scientific study by the U.S. Department of Agriculture in the 1950s. It found fresh squeezed orange[28] and grapefruit juice[362] to contain respectively 0.8 and 0.2 milligrams of methanol per liter of juice; compare that to the previously reported 680 mg. per liter of black currant juice. The study also canned these same batches of juice, then stored them at room temperature, as is typically the case with the product purchased by actual consumers. Retesting the juice samples at the end of this experiment revealed that the orange juice had jumped to 62 mg. of methanol per liter, increasing by a factor of close to 80 times, while the grapefruit juice had risen to 23 mg. of methanol per liter, a factor of over 100 times.

While there is probably nothing better for you than a glass of fresh squeezed juice, you should think twice about this beverage in canned form, contrary to popular belief about the health and nutritional benefits of all forms of juice. Fresh juice, properly defined, is juice that you have squeezed yourself or have watched someone else squeeze for you. **This warning about canned fruits or vegetables holds true for home-canned as well as commercial products.** Fresh juice with its live native yeast and bacteria, and with little or no methanol, is the best option. Juice that is bottled or aseptically packaged in a box or pouch, typically with a straw, is a bad choice because pectin at room temperature releases methanol into the container just as it does during the canning process.

Even before bottling, most fruit juices are processed with an industrial enzyme that, while ensuring a less cloudy liquid more attractive to the consumer, liberates methanol. All processed fruit juices, except for frozen concentrates such as those that come in cardboard cylinders, contain methanol and lack the natural microorganisms that may help your body protect itself from methanol. Freezing remains the best way to preserve fresh fruits and vegetables. It can be done with any container, including jars, and still be safe. I reluctantly say this, but it must be said: if your only choice is between a glass of water or fruit juice in a bottle, box, pouch, or can, water is by far the more prudent selection.

The Italian and French Exception: Long, Slow Cooking with the Lid Ajar

"What about canned tomatoes? How can I live without pasta sauce?" you may ask with dismay. Being of Italian descent, I appreciate the distress such a restriction could cause. Before the introduction of diet soda twenty-five years ago, Italy had an extremely low incidence of MS and certain other DOC, even though Italians consume per capita more canned tomatoes than any other population in the world. The explanation for this is enlightening. Even though canned tomatoes are hazardously high in methanol, you can make them safe by doing exactly what the Italians have been doing ever since Columbus introduced them to tomatoes from the New World: simmer the hell – or, in this case, the hellish methanol – out of the sauce.

My mom would empty cans of crushed and diced tomatoes in the saucepan early in the morning, simmering the sauce for at least two hours as it developed flavor and thickness. Hours of simmering with the cover slightly ajar leaves methanol, an alcohol whose boiling point is much lower than water, undetectable in tomato sauce. Similarly, the French cooking technique of reduction evaporates at least half the moisture from a sauce while removing the methanol that may have been present. It is amazing to me how cultural variations in food processing can make so critical a difference, even between life and death in some instances. Recall, for example, pellagra from the last chapter?

Aspartame – a Very Big No!

Every molecule of the artificial sweetener aspartame (a.k.a. NutraSweet, Equal, Canderel, or E951) turns into a molecule of methanol.[660] Aspartame has been the civilized world's most significant source of dietary methanol since the late 1980s. Although the recent introduction of methanol-free artificial sweeteners has reduced its U.S. market share, its worldwide consumption has risen dramatically.

Unscrupulous vendors of carbonated beverages in Third World countries profit from the low cost of patent-free aspartame, a considerably cheaper sweetener than natural sugar, and in some cases they have used their political influence to lobby for legislation that would legalize handing a diet beverage to a customer who had not specifically requested the non-diet variety. In New Zealand, for instance, so great was the political clout of the major beverage manufacturer that it succeeded in mandating the replacement of all carbonated beverages with diet versions in food programs for school children, a move embraced by health and food safety authorities, as well as certain parliamentary committees.

Smoked Foods

Fish and meats such as bacon are traditionally smoked by slow exposure to the condensation products of heated wood or wood chips in the exact manner that methanol is manufactured. A fire purposely set to produce smoke simultaneously liberates large amounts of methanol. Still, I admit that I do from time to time consume commercially made North American bacon, whose methanol content is relatively minimal due to its much shorter exposure to wood smoke. Processing relies more on heat generated by electricity than by combustion of hardwood. As always, the devil is in the details, and a thorough knowledge of exactly how food is smoked is key to determining its safety. The way food is conventionally smoked in countries like Scotland and Ireland produces excellent flavor but extremely high methanol, particularly if peat is used to generate the cooking heat, since peat smoke[180] contains up to three times more methanol than wood smoke.

It is no coincidence that in countries where you find the highest incidence of DOC over many years, you also find these traditional methods of food processing that can result in extensive methanol dosing. This is particularly true of multiple sclerosis. Scotland, where traditionally smoked food is consumed at most meals, has the highest incidence of MS anywhere in the world. Moreover, in the Faroe Islands – settled by the same basic stock of people but where, given the absence of peat, air drying is used to preserve fish and meat – multiple sclerosis had not been recorded until the English navy introduced cigarettes and canned fruits and vegetables during the Second World War (much more on this later).

Liquor or Schnapps Made from Rotting Fruit

The U.S. Department of Alcohol, Tobacco, and Firearms, the governmental agency in charge of the importation of alcohol beverages, will occasionally reject shipments of traditional fruit liquor imported from Europe due to excessive methanol content. My earlier warning about the danger of consuming traditionally produced food products that could cause methanol dosing extends to a whole class of liquors, schnapps, and slivovitz products made throughout the world from culled fruit. Frugal farmers often retrieve the fruit that falls to the ground before it can be picked, storing it in vats until the end of the season when it is processed into a strong distilled alcoholic liquor that goes by many names. The problem here is that this fruit is often contaminated by spoiling bacteria that strip pectin of its methanol, as discussed above. Once methanol mixes with ethanol produced by yeast fermentation, the final results can yield 3 or 4 percent methanol, a hazardously high concentration that can remain in the body for some time after the ethanol is metabolized away.

There you have it. The above constitutes the entire inventory of methanol sources, but in short, you should avoid the following:

1.	Cigarettes
2.	Diet foods and drinks containing aspartame
3.	Fruit and vegetable products and their juices in bottles, cans, or pouches (including home-canned fruits and vegetables)
4.	Jellies, jams and marmalades not made fresh and kept refrigerated
5.	Black currant and tomato juice products, fresh or processed
6.	Tomato sauces, unless first simmered at least 2 hours with an open lid
7.	Smoked food of any kind, particularly fish and meat
8.	Sugar-free chewing gum (most sugared gum sold in the United States also contains aspartame for "longer-lasting flavor")
9.	Slivovitz: You can consume one alcoholic drink a day on this diet - no more!
10.	Overly ripe or near-rotting fruits or vegetables

Man and Methanol: A Tragic History of Mutation and Deceit

Methanol, also known as methyl alcohol or wood alcohol and a component of methylated spirits, is extremely toxic. In its pure form it must, by law, be handled as a dangerous substance. A special extravagant placard bearing the skull and crossbones must be posted in plain sight to warn users of its potential to cause permanent blindness. If you find yourself in a hardware store looking for a cleaning solvent, those containing even a small amount of methanol will clearly stand out among the benzene, toluene, methyl ethyl ketone, and other dangerous and deadly solvents because, aside from bearing a special warning label, they must also be colored very brightly in a manner prescribed by law. Testament to its toxicity is the legal maximum percentage of methanol allowed in such methylated spirit products when they are made available to the general public for cleaning and such. -

Methanol was not always classified as dangerous. In the early 1900s it was considered safer than ethanol because laboratory animals showed no health effects of exposure. We have learned the hard way that animals of all kinds are completely immune to the deadly effects that methanol has on humans. To this day, all safety testing done using methanol on laboratory animals has consistently shown that methanol is treated as a food by their bodies. Humans, on the other hand, have gone permanently blind from consumption of less than a teaspoon of methanol, and have died from little more. The symptoms of methanol exposure in humans are so very different from those in animals that they are given the name "toxic syndrome."[107]

Strict laws specifically governing the use of methanol, but few other dangerous solvents, may be found in all countries of the industrial world. These laws originated in the first half of the Twentieth Century when thousands died from methanol being substituted for the more expensive ethanol in patent medicines and food flavor extracts. The tragedy proved for the first time, through human suffering and death, that the only test animals that can ever be used to determine the safety of methanol to humans are humans.

Surprisingly, while industrial methanol is treated as a deadly poison, methanol in food is presently being ignored. The artificial sweetener aspartame is 11% methanol by weight and constitutes a major source of methanol for those who consume it,[626] yet the lion's share of the laboratory testing done to prove the safety of aspartame was performed on laboratory animals rather than on humans.[1] Could it be that ignorance of the past has caused one of the greatest missteps in the history of human health? Humans have once again become unwitting test animals to prove just exactly how a little formaldehyde, produced from methanol, can cause disease.

A Curious Matter of Some Considerable Consequence

You might think that the discovery of the *only* known natural molecule that is simultaneously deleterious to human health and harmless to all other laboratory animals would surely have captured the attention of researchers with an interest in human health. After all, a number of well-known diseases and maladies mysteriously afflict humans but are impossible to replicate in an animal model. We might expect someone along the way would have put two and two together and asked whether methanol could have played a role in the etiology of these diseases. The common knowledge that methanol must be metabolized into formaldehyde, that it is associated with the industrial revolution, and that it is found in considerable quantity in cigarette smoke should have only enlivened the debate on the role of this poison in the evolution of diseases in modern times. Yet methanol is never even mentioned when toxic agents from smoking are considered as causative agents for the many diseases associated with that vile addiction.

That methanol is an "industrial" chemical seems, unfortunately, to have afforded it protection from serious critical investigation by the scientific community. In fact, since the beginning of the Nineteenth Century when methanol was first discovered to be particularly poisonous to humans, a much greater financial investment has been dedicated attempting to prove it safe than to determine the specifics of its toxicity. Indeed, industry-financed institutes and foundations have been established to ensure a favorable view of methanol and its sister compound, formaldehyde, a fact that goes a long way toward explaining how little scrutiny these substance have faced. These organizations are the dogmatic equivalent of the now-infamous Tobacco Institute, spending large sums of money to fund questionable research intentionally designed to muddle the truth, not foster it.

The Ancient History of Methanol

For millions of years, humans had scant contact with methanol, a natural, but rare substance. This was fortuitous, since very early in evolution the human race underwent a mutation that prevented us from safely consuming this little alcohol molecule, making us unlike all other animals.

The mutation produced a minor change in the way our cells build a very important enzyme called catalase. Found throughout the body, catalase is most abundant in the liver. It is used by all animals to protect against many poisons such as methanol. The bodies of all laboratory animals, including monkeys, treat methanol as a food because the catalase in their livers is capable of removing dietary methanol before it can reach their brains. Human catalase, on the other hand, has a slightly different shape, which prevents it from binding with methanol. Small amounts of methanol consumed in the human diet, therefore, have a very good chance of getting past the liver and reaching the brain and other organs.

Had this mutation never happened, humans would not suffer the diseases of civilization. Unfortunately, it did happen, and we can surmise, due to the universality of methanol sensitivity, that the mutation occurred in the chromosome of an individual who was a relative to every human who now lives.

The Mutation of Eve

Please bear with me as I weave a little yarn of how the mutation might have happened. I chose to call this unknown woman, whose child would become the mother of all modern humans, Eve.

A cool evening breeze filtered across the sultry fall savanna. An exquisite young female lay naked in the slow-beginning night, resting after an unusually long afternoon of love making. The sky was bright with no moon, but the glorious Milky Way provided light enough for the trees to shadow. The stars twinkled even through the clean, pollution-free air of the middle Pleistocene. As Eve lay dreaming about her strange new lover, events were unfolding that would change the fate of the new species that lay maturing in her womb.

Many millions of years before her fateful cross-species tryst, one of those stars had sent off in the direction of Earth a small gift of itself. Traveling at the speed of light through the vast vacuum of space it would make no great commotion as it entered her perfect little body. She felt nothing… not the slightest touch of the star's presence. Eve was never to know the terrible harm that was, that night, to be passed to her child, the alpha prime female of an evolving species. The strike was perfect, as bad luck so often is. Eve's child and the new species she would begin would forever bear the curse of that peaceful night.

The worst outcomes would be hidden until the great brain that was to mark Man's branch of the Tree of Life would devise to begin to challenge an unforgiving Nature. Progress would guarantee that never again would Eve's people be free from a complex strangeness of behavior and disease that would rise and fall with diet and season until few would survive long enough to ply their rightful purpose. So much to come would set man apart from other creatures, but none of it would be as elusive as this one tragic flaw. To this day, we have no name for it or for the misery that it has wrought. The mutation caused a small change in the shape of the enzyme catalase, just enough to prevent methanol from sticking to its surface. Because of this, the ultimate end result of methanol consumption in man is its conversion to formaldehyde in the most inopportune of places.

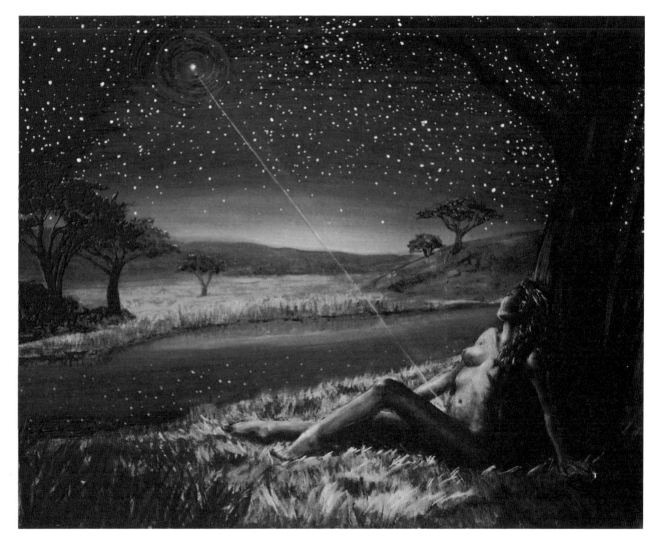

What Is the Meaning of This Human Mutation?

The first step in the digestion of methanol is always the production of formaldehyde, a very dangerous compound which, if not carefully controlled, can wreak great harm within a living cell. The two most important enzymes in the animal kingdom that are responsible for metabolizing methanol are catalase and ADH. But man's catalase enzyme cannot metabolize methanol,* leaving only ADH to do the job. The most important difference between these two enzymes is their precise locations within the cell. It is this, and this alone, that accounts for the great disadvantage that man has compared to all other animals. It also accounts for why animals can use methanol as a food and energy source, while for humans it is a deadly poison and etiologic agent of disease. Let me explain.

The ADH enzyme is found dissolved in the cell's fluid, or cytosol.[531] This makes ADH a free agent that can float around the cell unencumbered, releasing formaldehyde from methanol wherever it happens to be within the cell at the time. Nothing can then restrain the reactive formaldehyde; it is free to leave the cell or travel to the nucleus or other sensitive areas within the cell, where serious damage (such as methylation) can be done. Whether within the cell or outside it, the necessary enzyme that would convert formaldehyde to the next metabolite, formic acid, is, at the very least, a considerable distance away. The odds are quite slim that the very reactive formaldehyde will somehow avoid doing damage before reaching that enzyme.

Unlike humans, animals utilize catalase to metabolize methanol. Catalase is an enzyme associated with the detoxification of many poisons, which is likely why nature locates it in a special structure inside the cell, called a peroxisome. It is within the structure of the peroxisome that catalase transforms methanol into formaldehyde, thereby limiting its travel and keeping it retained long enough to allow for further metabolism. These peroxisomes are linked closely with another very important cell body that we will discuss later, the mitochondria,[664] a cigar-shaped cell body found in extremely high concentration in liver cells (they are what give the healthy liver its dark color). Mitochondria are the powerhouse of the living cell, containing in separate compartments the enzymes necessary to convert formaldehyde to formic acid and then to produce energy (in the form of ATP) and carbon dioxide, among other things.

The loss of the ability of human catalase to metabolize methanol put humans at very great risk by passing off the job to ADH, an enzyme not meant to do that work which is located in some very compromising parts of our anatomy. We understand very little about all the uses of ADH in the human body or why the distribution of this enzyme varies greatly by race and sex and heredity. But we do know that the locations within the human body where ADH is found have a great deal to do with the origin and epidemiology of disease.[216,501] Unfortunately, epidemiologists studying this well-known phenomenon give no credence to the fact that every site of ADH in the body is capable of producing formaldehyde. They apparently suffer from the delusion, likely fostered by the formaldehyde and methanol lobbying groups, that it is actually the vinegar* produced from ethanol at these sites that might be dangerous,[187] as silly as that sounds.

Vision is the one major responsibility of ADH that is well understood, and the retina is one of the sites where ADH is located. In fact, ADH is the enzyme that makes vision possible[663] by metabolizing the alcohol form of Vitamin A, which begins the process that initiates the eye's signal to the brain. This connection of ADH to vision can account for the phenomenon of blindness, both temporary and permanent, and other strange visual signs and symptoms associated with both methanol toxicity and multiple sclerosis. Yet, due to the fact that formaldehyde has never been actually found, per se, in the human eye, researchers have generally failed to explore any possible link of these symptoms to formaldehyde. By ignoring the chemistry of formaldehyde creation, they have become unwitting contributors to the continuation of the "Big Lie" about formaldehyde: that what we can't see won't hurt us.

To encourage common understanding throughout this book I will use the term vinegar to represent acetic acid and or acetaldehyde which I consider food substances of low toxicity.

Chapter 3

The Sordid History of Methanol in the Industrial Age

A century ago the scientific community believed methanol was benign and swore to its safety with disastrous consequences.[21] In the early 1900s, industry wanted to use a newly developed inexpensive and odorless form of wood alcohol to extract vanilla and other flavorings, and then add it to medications as a replacement for the expensive, heavily taxed ethanol.[17,21] Over the previous fifty years, numerous studies performed by reputable laboratories had shown that more methanol than ethanol was required to kill laboratory animals.[15,30] Testing of methanol toxicity was repeated with monkeys, dogs, rabbits, mice and laboratory rats.[17,30] Each time the results were the same: methanol consumption was found to be safer than ethanol consumption. These data were interpreted by industry scientists to support the safety of human methanol consumption. Accordingly, the much less expensive methanol soon replaced ethanol in many patent medicines and food flavors and extracts.

Not long after the first bottles of methanol-laden consumables appeared on the market,[25] many consumers became blind and others even died. Stories linking methanol with this suffering, blindness and death[165] were for years discounted by the pharmaceutical industry as "anecdotal" and unrelated to methanol, which "had gone through such intensive testing."[17] When incidences of death[16] and permanent blindness[37] continued to mount, the chemical industry and their paid experts surmised, with scant evidence, that some "impurity" had found its way into the methanol used to produce individual products linked to tragedy. A similar assertion is often made today when, for example, severe reactions to diet soda are blamed on phantom allergies. Then, as now, the scientific community, encouraged by industrial money, maintained that nothing was wrong with methanol, per se.[17,30]

A few noteworthy physicians had the courage to speak out against industry. They published articles and gave lectures that presented irrefutable evidence against the use of methanol in drugs and food. In 1904, Casey Wood and Frank Buller[189] reported on 235 cases of blindness and death due to methanol exposure. Their damning article, published in the *Journal of the American Medical Association*, exposed both the economics behind the use of methanol by the food and drug industry, and the exact details of the strangely delayed process by which methanol kills and blinds humans.

The pleading of Wood and Buller went unheeded for many years; researchers could not, in good conscience, test a suspected poison on humans. The true death toll will never be known, but thousands must have perished by horrible deaths from methanol[120] before Dr. Olaf Roe, in a comprehensive study of a mass accidental human poisoning from methanol, finally showed in 1946 that animals and humans do not metabolize methanol in the same way or with the same enzymes.[3] It took many human deaths and forty years of debate to prove the obvious, that humans are exquisitely sensitive to methanol, and to end its use as a food and drug additive. The food and drug industry finally did the right thing when it came to methanol in that case, but sadly, it was not to be the last time that their decisions regarding methanol consumption by humans would cause suffering and death on a large scale.

The details of the issue have never been fully resolved, due to the ongoing attempt by Industry to hide the fact that formaldehyde production within the brain and elsewhere in the body is what is ultimately responsible for the human symptoms and fatalities from methanol. It was in the summer of 1952 that the celebrated biochemist and physician Albert M. Potts put everything eloquently into perspective in a published statement that stands as true now as it did then: "Whenever methanol poisoning appears one finds avarice and greed and the placing of financial gain above human life itself."[171]

The "Real" Killer Is Formic Acid: A Fairy Tale if Ever I Heard One

If you research the methanol literature today using the usual scientific resources or the Internet, you will find an overwhelming consensus that formaldehyde is not responsible for causing blindness and death from methanol poisoning. Recent review articles and all of the medical literature published over the last thirty years consistently point, not to formaldehyde, but to formic acid as the real toxic agent of methanol. Yet formic acid is a food,[365] not much more poisonous than vinegar, and considered to be only slightly toxic by ingestion.[661] How could it be that formic acid – an acid that is so mild[365] that I have used it to make salad dressing when I ran out of vinegar in my laboratory – is a killer? Such a claim is nonsensical, ignores basic chemistry and is at odds with my own experience as a practicing food scientist who is familiar with the many uses of formic acid and its sister acid, acidic acid (vinegar), in the food industry. Who would even propose such a ridiculous scenario, and more importantly, why?

From the first time I researched the issue years ago, this interpretation of the body of methanol-related scientific literature made no sense to me. I could not understand how anyone in the scientific community could take something like this seriously. Surely, I thought, this must be some kind of misunderstanding. But what I discovered was that the exact metabolic anomaly that makes the human relationship to methanol distinct from all laboratory animal models, including primates,[26] has always been muddied by industrial agendas[27] with a vested interest in proving that the formaldehyde produced from methanol in the human body does no harm.[28,29]

Most of the literature cited to prove this impossible scenario comes from one group of researchers at the University of Iowa's medical school and was generated over a relatively short period of time. How could this have happened and how did this nonsense embed itself into the scientific literature so indelibly in the midst of a longstanding legitimate and thoughtful debate?

First, scientists are not immune from the social naiveté that plagues the general population. Their strict adherence to a pecking order based on seniority and publication status may make them even more susceptible to the slight-of-hand that pharmaceutical companies long ago learned to perpetrate on medical practitioners when the first detail-person plied her magic over a five-star meal in some quiet little place far from a doctor's practice. To borrow from the first page of the *Pathogenesis of Multiple Sclerosis Revisited,*[615] "The fact that an opinion is widely held is no evidence whatsoever that it is not utterly absurd; indeed in view of the silliness of the majority of mankind, a widespread belief is more likely to be foolish than sensible." – Bertrand Russell

Thirty years after Dr. Roe's seminal work establishing a biochemical basis for human sensitivity to methanol, the discovery of a potentially highly lucrative artificial sweetener initiated an urgent effort to redeem methanol's reputation, and within the pharmaceutical community, this effort exploded into a cause célèbre. The no-holds-barred competition was spearheaded by a major drug company previously well-known for the development of the first, and arguably most dangerous, of the birth control pills (the implementation and approval of which proved good practice for the daunting job ahead when it came to winning FDA approval of its new sweetener, aspartame).

It seems that one of the G.D. Searle's subsidiary company's chemists, in the process of synthesizing a new drug for the treatment of ulcers, accidentally discovered (while licking his fingers) that one of his new chemical creations had a powerfully sweet flavor. Aspartame, thus born out of ignorance and bad laboratory technique, began its path toward becoming a very popular new artificial sweetener. The downside was that this potentially profitable new product, aspartame, was made with methanol, which was released quickly into the stomach when it was consumed.

In the 1970s, Searle began pouring millions of dollars into trying, once again, to convince the scientific community that methanol was safe.[39] Conveniently, the laboratory that chose to do Searle's bidding was only

200 miles from the G.D. Searle headquarters in Skokie, Illinois, at the medical school of the University of Iowa in Iowa City. We will never know for certain exactly how much research funding Searle poured into the work done at the University of Iowa in the years since the late 1960s to prove methanol and, therefore, aspartame is safe.[39] We do know, however, that the team at this laboratory did everything it could to prove that it was formic acid, the chemical produced by the body from formaldehyde, and not formaldehyde itself that was the cause of the toxicity of methanol.[274]

To reach the goal of removing formaldehyde from consideration as the cause of death from methanol poisoning, the laboratory researchers had to successfully accomplish three tasks, utilizing scant evidence and questionable experimental methods:

1. Assert that a monkey is a valid animal model for human methanol poisoning, even though the rhesus monkey is 100 times less sensitive to methanol than humans and is far more similar to the rat in this regard.[17]
2. Identify a marker (formic acid) measurable in the human bloodstream that could be used to indicate "chronic" exposure to methanol, even though it is only measurable in the most extreme poisonings (formaldehyde vanishes too quickly).
3. Falsely blame formic acid as the culprit responsible for doing all the damage from methanol poisoning. Even when it is clear that formic acid, when administered alone to monkeys, causes no such changes.[462]

The fact that they were successful in convincing the medical/epidemiological community to believe all of the above goes more to show the lack of adequate chemical training of our modern medical professionals than anything else.

A careful reading of their work and, more importantly, the criticism of their work by scientists from other laboratories working on formaldehyde produced from methanol,[7,240] reveals that they never convincingly proved anything. True, they never found formaldehyde in monkeys poisoned by methanol, but then again they never established their methods were capable of finding it in biological systems. In their enthusiasm to find that monkeys would develop the toxic syndrome of methanol found in humans, they tortured their experimental monkeys by placing them in small glass bell jars, severely restraining them, and covering their heads in hoods for long periods of time until stress produced the symptoms and slow deaths they sought.[132] This technique was severely criticized by none other than Oluf Roe,[52] who originally discovered the difference between human and animal metabolism of methanol.

The University of Iowa's laboratory results, however, continued to find easy publication in "friendly" journals that were accustomed to working with the pharmaceutical industry and the elite group of toxicologists who were deified by virtue of the money and awards freely provided by a fawning pharmaceutical lobby. Big Pharma has a disturbing legacy of providing almost unlimited private funding to laboratories whose researchers will then have not a single meaningful bad word to say about methanol and who will flood the scientific literature with inaccuracies. The otherwise well-regarded lab at Iowa City did not disclose in these seminal articles its financially intimate ties to a large pharmaceutical company.[121]

I implore other scientists reading this to review all the work from this "prestigious" laboratory and see for themselves. Formic acid is a food and has nothing to do with human death from methyl alcohol. Formaldehyde is the culprit!

The Tortured Toxicology of Methanol

Toxicology is a study in contrasts; substances that may be beneficial or at least harmless in low concentrations can prove poisonous in larger doses. Similarly, medicine assumes that most of the curative agents it dispenses also have fatal potential. The origin of these two sciences predates humanity. Creatures in the wild, particularly mammals, will occasionally purposely consume plants they know to be toxic in order to receive some beneficial end, such as killing parasites in their gut. The Chinese emperor Shen Nung, who is considered the father of medicine, is credited with having written the very first toxicological treatise *On Herbal Medical Experiment Poisons* five thousand years ago. He studied 365 herbal medicines and tellingly died from an overdose of one of them. Evaluating the risk of administering a known poison in order to better prescribe its potential as a cure exemplifies the highest mission and best application of toxicology. Shen Nung gave his life so that others might be saved.

In the last fifty years I have witnessed the science of toxicology devolve from a noble endeavor dedicated to helping save lives to a tool of industry used to facilitate and justify the proliferation of poisons for profit. Nowhere in the literature is this better portrayed than in the vanity publication *Aspartame,*[121] a book funded and distributed by Searle. Lewis Stegink and L. J. Filer from the University of Iowa College of Medicine were remunerated by Searle to edit and contribute to the treatise, which featured chapters authored, for pay, by many of the professional members of the Iowa State toxicological team they headed. This was the very same group of scientists noted above who significantly changed the way the world thought about the formaldehyde produced from methanol poisoning. After being subpoenaed by a congressional committee chaired by Senator Howard Metzenbaum investigating approval of aspartame, Filer admitted during questioning that he had helped Searle win FDA approval for the methanol-containing sweetener. Most damning of all, University of Iowa records show that Lewis Stegink had received well over a million dollars in grants and gifts from Searle beginning in the early 1970s.[39]

Stegink, a pediatrician turned toxicologist, revealed a dark side of toxicology by twisting its meaning in the first sentence of his chapter in *Aspartame,* declaring, "Toxicology is based on the premise that all compounds are toxic at some dose, salt, water, sugar, and even a mother's love produce deleterious effects when given in inappropriate amounts." The statement defines a new toxicology, which calls everything a poison so that manufacturers of dangerous, but profitable, chemicals might point to any other substance as also toxic, linking the two in an effort to confuse the public. Why else would Stegink insist on calling salt, water and sugar "toxins" when it is obvious that they are not toxins? They are not poisons, they are nutrients – foods – and essential for life. His cynical aside about a mother's love is a telling statement that defines the man and his laboratory. This is not the toxicology that I learned years ago at lectures by good scientists dedicated to the prevention of harm to their fellow man from real poisons. This is the toxicology of scoundrels who would play with definitions to hide the real truth.

I cannot protect you from scholars who chose to use their considerable talents to espouse the merits of an unhealthy additive. So let me simply take you to where you will be able to understand the basics of the chemistry and toxicology of methanol sufficiently to make your own informed decisions.

Minimum Lethal Dose

The single lowest dose of a poison needed to cause death is called its minimum lethal dose (MLD). This number is always given as the weight of a substance per kilogram weight of the subject killed. The reason it is expressed in this way is that the concentration of the poison in the blood causes the death; therefore, a larger animal will require proportionately more poison than a smaller one to get the same concentration in its greater volume of blood. This method of expressing lethal dose allows for easy comparison between species as divergent as mice and elephants. Thus individual animals may have the same lethal dose for many poisons, but require different amounts of that poison based on the weight of the particular animal being killed. Usually one can expect that a poison will have a similar lethal dose across many species.

This implies, of course, that all species metabolize and otherwise process the poison in a similar manner. It is unusual when the MLD varies greatly between species, but when it does it indicates that the poison in question is being handled very differently within the bodies of those organisms. This becomes extremely important in the case of methanol, as revealed by the data in Table 3.1. For example, the MLD of methanol for a rhesus monkey is 6 grams per kilogram, while that for a human is less than 0.3 grams per kilogram. Such a large difference in MLD should raise red flags. The fact is that humans are far more sensitive to methanol than any other living thing, making methanol unique among all the world's poisons and eligible for extreme scrutiny – the type of scrutiny that industry has tried to prevent for over a hundred years.

Table 3.1
Minimal Lethal Dose of Methanol

Species	Dose: Grams/Kg	Grams to Kill 70kg Male
Rat[17]	9.0	630
Dog[17]	9.0	630
Rabbit[17]	7.0	490
Monkey[17]	6.0	420
Man[204]	0.089	6

As a food scientist, I begin any investigation into a substance to be used in food by finding out the minimum amount of that substance that is known to do harm or cause sickness to a laboratory animal. This number is vital since, as a general rule, we like to see that the daily consumption of any substance never goes above one hundredth of what that harmful dose might be. No general guidelines link consumption to MLD, since death is an outcome of ultimate harm.

If you search the internet for the MLD of methanol in humans, you will often find the following statement: "The lethal dose of methanol for humans is not known for certain. The minimum lethal dose of methanol in the absence of medical treatment is put at between 0.3 and 1 g/kg." I hope this statement strikes you as odd. Actually, it is patently misleading to the point of deception. Indeed, if any evidence exists that 0.3 grams/kg has killed a human, then by definition the MLD is 0.3 grams/kg, not the deceptive range given. We are, after all, dealing with human life. If, therefore, the first statement is true and "the lethal dose for humans is not known for certain," then we, as scientists, are required by the definition of minimum lethal dose and our responsibility to humanity to give the true minimum lethal dose known to kill. That dose would clearly be the lower figure of 0.3 grams per kilograms. Actually, the MLD of methanol *is* known, has been recorded in the scientific literature, and, in fact, is lower than 0.1 grams per kilogram, which makes rats a hundred times less sensitive to methanol than humans.[16]

To illustrate the teaching of the above chart relative to the toxic dose of humans and laboratory rats, visualize a rat grown to the size and weight of a human. The human would find that a shot glass full of methanol would be lethal, while the oversize rat would require 100 such doses to end to its life. For those who prefer visuals, our illustrator has portrayed a suicide standoff between a young lab technician and a 60 kilogram monster rat.

Two Ways for Humans to Die from Methanol

An early indication of the human MLD for methanol was provided through the tragic death in 1951 suffered

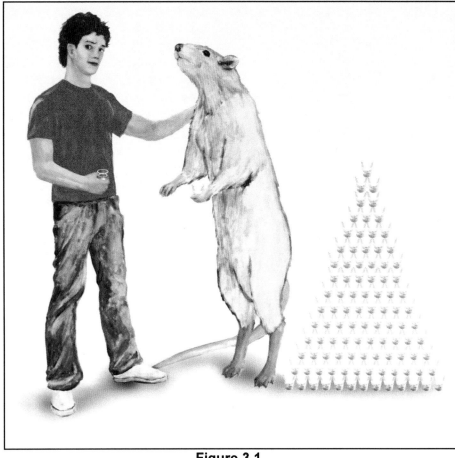

Figure 3.1

by a young black woman, who was unaware of the significance of her sacrifice. We know her only as Patient 17, twenty years of age, who tasted only a tablespoon of methanol-contaminated whisky, then refused to drink any more. Her cruel death three days later in hospital in Atlanta, Georgia, was brought on by an ignorance of the extreme danger of methanol that still exists throughout the world today, just as it did then.[204] Along with her died forty others who were sold whiskey diluted with methanol.

The episode was carefully chronicled by physicians from the Emory University School of Medicine in a comprehensive publication in the prestigious journal *Medicine.*[16] The lethal dose of methanol that killed Patient 17 was calculated by determining the weight of methanol in a tablespoon of 40% methanol solution at 4.75 grams and then dividing by her weight of 53 kilograms (117 pounds). This produced the published MLD of methanol in humans at 0.089 grams per kilogram, or more significantly, one hundred times less than that required to kill a laboratory rat. It is awkward to have to compare this young girl to a laboratory animal but it is important to understand that a lethal dose of methanol kills laboratory animals in minutes. It required three days to kill Patient 17. The others who died with her took between two and four days to finally and tragically succumb to the toxic syndrome of methanol, the exact symptoms of which will be presented in a later chapter.

The human's response to an MLD of methanol is very slow with a reprieve of at least 12 hours, but more often 36 hours that pass with no symptoms, save the rather dizzying and often pleasant giddiness that methanol shares with its sister alcohol, ethanol, and described as the solvent effect. Animals, including humans, can die from the consumption of both methanol and ethanol solely from the solvent effect. When they consume methanol at 9g/kg of their body weight or ethanol at 7g/kg, they lapse quickly into a sleep that lasts until the solvent anesthetizes their brain to the extent that vital functions stop and they never wake. If Patient 17 had consumed 1.3 quarts of the contaminated liquor rather than one tablespoon, her death would have been mercifully peaceful and she would have probably passed before arriving at hospital.

All laboratory animals and humans have the identical MLD for ethanol. It has been shown time and time again that no lower dose of ethanol can be administered and kill either man or beast over a longer period of time. Ethanol can be administered to humans and animals at daily doses very close to the lethal dose for months at a time and not cause death. The minimum lethal doses of both ethanol and methanol in a laboratory rat are very similar, 7 grams of ethanol per kilogram and 9 grams of methanol per kilogram, with methanol, therefore, being the less harmful of the two.

Why is man almost a hundred times more sensitive to methanol than all the other life forms with which we share the earth? The answer is simple. Men can die in one of two ways from methanol. Methanol can kill like ethanol does by acting as a solvent, but this requires very large amounts of the alcohol. The other way that men can die from methanol is actually not from methanol at all, but from a chemical into which methanol can be transformed within the body: formaldehyde. This transformation requires time as does the process formaldehyde uses to kill.

There is little doubt that ethanol is a food to both men and animals and, like any other food, it can be abused and cause death. Methanol is also a food – one that is even safer than ethanol to laboratory animals – but not to man. Man is disabled in his ability to use methanol for food by a catalase mutation. He must treat methanol as a true poison. Science should have tried in every way possible to elucidate the details of this problem even without an experimental animal model and come up with a prudent course of action. Methanol has not been, and may never be a priority for the scientific community due to the intense pressure from industry and lobbying organizations such as the Methanol Institute and the Methanol Foundation. One thing is certain: presently, we have no reasonable way to extrapolate anything about the lethality of methanol to humans from research on laboratory animals.

The Hard Way to Die from Methanol

You would never forget watching someone die from methanol poisoning. I have never seen it myself but have read enough descriptions in the scientific literature to have had the scenario indelibly etched into my memory.[16] One time, I lay down on a table in a large lecture room to demonstrate the terminal details of the endless inhalation that marks the unique death from methanol to my assembled students. By the finale, tellingly, they had all left the room and I found myself quite alone.

I hold absolutely no morbid curiosity about the tragic end of a human life. I would much rather forget forever the details of what I am about to describe, but it is here in the final act of living that a poor soul, her life cut short by a poison whose treachery is so often protected by the consummate greed of American industry that the ultimate truth, the confirming ferocity of methanol's power to do metabolic harm, is revealed by a Nature that hides nothing from us. No other poisons or torture can produce an ending that duplicates human death by acute methanol poisoning. I am of the opinion that we would have never have known about the fascinating anomaly that constitutes the toxic syndrome of methanol in man[401] if it were not for the accidental deaths of innocent individuals such as Patient 17. The details of the suffering of these individuals must be scrutinized to the point that we can explain every detail.

The last moments of living for Patient 17 began with a violent series of inhalations, each filling her lungs with more and more air. In the end, the muscles of her chest that worked the inhalation mechanism could not relax even in response to the most potent muscle relaxants. [16] Death finally came with a massive terminal inhalation and sudden "freezing" of the chest in a position of her deepest inhalation followed several minutes later with cessation of the heartbeat. Her death was frozen thus with rapid rigor mortis.

As we look for a reason for this unusual response the first thing that comes to mind is that her brain was calling for more oxygen. Why this ravenous insatiable appetite for air? Laboratory testing of her blood clearly showed saturation of her blood hemoglobin with oxygen. To understand the plight of this young girl we need to know why her body thought it needed oxygen and how it was used. The brain and all of Patient 17's other organs required vast quantities of energy to perform all its functions, including sight and memory. In all humans, this energy comes mostly from the burning of the simple sugar glucose in the cell, a process which requires oxygen.

Individual protein molecules in the brain that require energy to do their jobs are not equipped with their own furnaces in which to burn glucose. The furnace that all living things use to produce the energy of life is the mitochondria that we discussed earlier. The origin of the mitochondria is unknown, although it is thought to have once lived on its own, much like bacteria. It is a complex structure with its own genetics which require that it must be transmitted as a complete unit to us from our mothers only, fully formed in the egg cell from which we develop.

I haven't the time to do justice to this fascinating structure, which calls every cell in our bodies its home and distinguishes animal cells from those of plants, but I will tell you what it does, which is intriguing enough. The mitochondria acts just like a powerhouse attached to a big factory! It absorbs oxygen and uses it to burn fuel (glucose) to produce useful energy. Some of this energy is heat, which we can use to keep up our body temperature, but the lion's share is used to charge a very small biological battery, enabling easy distribution and utilization of the energy by any molecule in our body that needs it to perform a function. The most important of these fully charged batteries is called adenosine triphosphate (ATP). To avoid chemistry that you won't need I will put it simply and say that the TP stands for three phosphates.

When one of the phosphates is removed by a cell process that requires its energy, the result is the uncharged version of the battery, adenosine diphosphate (ADP). After the battery has been discharged, the undamaged phosphate and ADP are attracted back to the compartment of the closest mitochondria where they can be reassembled and recharged with the energy produced from combining the oxygen and glucose. This conversion from ATP to ADP is extremely crucial and is the basis of life itself. Formaldehyde has the ability, in extremely small concentrations, to prevent the mitochondria from reattaching the phosphate back to the ADP,[113] a process called phosphorylation, which we will talk about again. Basically formaldehyde damages one of the enzymes that make our battery charger, the mitochondria, function.

With no charged batteries available for high energy functioning, such as vision and thinking, Patient 17 went blind and sank into a terminal coma. Her confused brain made one final attempt to call for more ATP by doing all it knew how to do, all it ever had to do in the past; it called for more air to stoke the flame of life, but to no avail. It is this last fruitless inhaled scream that tells us all we ever needed to know about why and how humans die their strange and frightening death from methanol poisoning. All those who are asked to accept as safe the use of methanol in foods to be consumed by pregnant woman and children should first be made to watch someone die from methanol. Might I suggest some subjects?

How Dangerous is Methanol?

Just how dangerous is methanol? I was asked to present two lectures in March of 2010 to the Multiple Sclerosis Society of Southland New Zealand. I was invited because some of the members who were MS sufferers had read my Medical Hypothesis article[586] and convinced the leadership that I should be asked to speak. I am of the opinion, as you will see as this book proceeds, that the formaldehyde produced from methanol in the brain is the sole cause of MS and other autoimmune-appearing diseases. Although I had been working with two friends who had MS and were following my dietary suggestions for over a year with what appeared to be extremely encouraging results, it was a very difficult decision for me to go public. Once convinced that I could do no harm with my plea to stop smoking and avoid the consumption of diet products and canned foods, I began preparing the hundred slides that I would require to give my lay audience the science they would need to understand the logic behind my dietary regime.

I contacted the kindly woman who was the director of the society and told her of my acceptance and gave her the general plan of my presentation. When I mentioned that I would need at least two hours in front of the group she let out an audible sigh. I told her that I had considerable university lecturing experience and would do all I could to make the presentation "spellbinding." What that meant to me was that I had to have a table full of interesting stuff next to the lectern that would keep their attention at least until I explained to them what it all meant. I learned in the early days of my teaching career that when I brought a bag full of show and tell items into a lecture hall my audience was more likely to pay attention. The little trick worked perfectly and the two lectures I gave in Invercargill and Gore both went on for over three hours, if you add the question and answer periods.

The search for items worthy of the presentation was another matter. No problem finding a liter or two of vodka to represent the human lethal dose of ethanol. Canned vegetables, both commercial and homemade, were easy to find in New Zealand, which shares with Australia the dubious statistic of consuming more canned fruits and vegetables per capita than any other country in the southern hemisphere (interestingly, they also share the highest incidences of MS for that region). But to my great surprise, the one thing I couldn't find was a sample of the subject of my lecture – methyl alcohol.

If you go to just about any hardware store in any country in the world you can find something called methylated spirits or red alcohol, which is a mixture of ethanol and methanol. The reason it is called red alcohol is that it is usually brightly colored to warn consumers of its deadly nature. I found many bottles of what was labeled methylated spirits on the shelves of hardware stores in New Zealand, but on closer inspection each bottle and brand, although containing brightly colored liquid, declared proudly on the label that it contained no methanol.

In 1855, Great Britain became the first country to "denature" ethyl alcohol with methanol to make it unfit for consumption (getting drunk) so that it could be sold without a tax and, therefore, be more affordable for use in cleaning and burning in cook stoves. In the 1800s, methanol was considered safe. The reason wood alcohol was chosen as a denaturant was that it had a repulsive odor and taste, as a method had not yet been discovered to deodorize it. Denaturing was accomplished by mixing ten percent of wood alcohol with ordinary drinking alcohol, the resulting mixture being called methylated spirit.

Various countries have methylated spirit with varying amounts of methanol. In Egypt the methanol content of their red alcohol can go up to ninety percent methanol. It was quite a surprise to me to learn that the New Zealand methylated spirits did not contain any methanol. I decided to use for my presentation what the hardware stores had to offer, even though it was not methanol. The explanation to my audience of the story of how and why the decision was made by their government to completely remove methanol from easy reach of the consumer was revealing. The maximum allowable methanol content of New Zealand denatured alcohol was for decades set at only 5 percent of the final product. Even at this low concentration, a number of doctors throughout the lovely land of the long white cloud (a country that practices its own very successful form of universal health care) reported permanent blindness and death from consumption of this considerably watered down version of methylated spirits. The result of this was that in 1995 the New Zealand Environmental Risk Management Authority (ERMA) ordered that no methylated spirits produced from then on could contain any more than 2% methanol. This is lower than any other country in the world.

What happened during the years that followed this major decision says more about the sensitivity of humans to methanol than anything in the present day scientific literature. In 2007, New Zealand barred any use at all of methanol in methylated spirits. The Chief Executive in charge of such things, Rob Forlong, noted that methylated spirits containing up to 2 per cent methanol had been available to the public for over a decade as a cleaner, solvent and fuel. Mr. Forlong said Chemical Injury Surveillance Reports had attributed the deaths of three people in 2002-03 to drinking methylated spirits, while a total of 24 poisonings were recorded in various New Zealand city hospitals during 2005. However, concerns raised for years by coroners, medical practitioners, social workers and the public about damage to the health, and in extreme cases death, of people drinking methylated spirits had prompted New Zealand to reassess the substance. "The result has been the decision that only formulations of methylated spirits without methanol should be available for sale to the public," Mr. Forlong said. "Methylated spirits bought over the counter from 21 June, 2007 will no longer contain the poisonous substance methanol."

Standing in stark contrast is another government agency in New Zealand, the Food Safety Authority, which is for the most part staffed by those who apotheosize for the food industry, as are all such agencies throughout the free world. This agency has consistently given a clean bill of health to aspartame, which contains in pure form no less than 11 percent methanol. In many parts of the world, including New Zealand, a sugar replacement tablet called Equal, which contains over twenty one percent aspartame (951), or 2.3% pure methanol, sits on grocers' shelves, readily available to the public. One has to ask the question how qualified scientists in the same country can, on the one hand, for dire safety considerations, remove from the market something that is used to clean floors solely because it contains less than 2% methanol, while on the other hand, allow and encourage the use of a food product often used to sweeten children's cereal, containing over 2.3% of the very same substance?

Infant Deaths from a Touch of Methanol

Few realize just how sensitive humans are to methyl alcohol. The real MLD is really still unknown. The fact that Patient 17 died from a minimum lethal dose of methanol a hundred times less than that of laboratory animals means little to the average person. To truly appreciate an issue such as this we need to express it with an up close and personal example. Most stories of death from methanol revolve around alcoholics, who make an unfortunate choice of something to drink and pay with their lives. Sympathy for these poor souls is often not forthcoming. But no one (except a modern toxicologist) would ever take the death of a child lightly. When an infant exuding an insatiable love for life succumbs to a bad end we pay attention and seek answers.

So it was in a small Egyptian farming village miles from the crowded capital Cairo. Three two-month-old infants slept in the arms of their doting mothers, who waited in nervous anticipation of what was to be their babies' last encounter with non-ayurvedic medicine. The nurses and doctor who were preparing to administer vaccinations as part of a national health schema were not knowledgeable about and had no training in methanol poisoning. Of course, why would they have been? Modern medicine considers methanol poisoning a thing of the past. It would mean nothing to them that red alcohol was subsequently used by the babies' families when they returned to their homes as a compress to swab the little arms after their therapeutic jabs of vaccine. The vaccinations all went flawlessly with the usual youthful protests and crocodile tears. Nothing gave even the slightest hint of the horror that was to follow.

Methanol is the smallest alcohol molecule – half the size of ethanol, which gives it a superior ability to travel through the skin. Only a small portion of the methanol on a cotton swab applied to a vaccination site would actually pass into the infants' bodies, and who would ever think it could be enough to kill? But within the first hour of its application, methanol had entered the infants' circulatory systems and traveled everywhere throughout their bodies. Hours passed with no symptoms, no pain, and no indication of the troubles ahead that would be caused by the methanol slowly turning into undetectable formaldehyde. Sadly, the outcome for three of the children from this village and three from another not far off would ultimately be fatal.

Because methanol leaves no evidence, autopsy samples show nothing of the cause of death from methanol poisoning. Years passed before the true story was finally pieced together. It was not until dedicated investigators had analyzed the contents of red bottles discovered in the homes of each affected child that they found the only evidence that linked all the deaths: methanol.

The scientists who wrote the article that appeared in the Journal *Vaccine*[204] were much more interested in proving the safety of the vaccination program than informing the world of the dangers of methanol. They spent little time on the plight of the children or their families, treating the details of their suffering with the aloofness we have grown to expect from such professionals. Because of this we can only surmise what happened after the latent period passed and the beginning of twenty or so hours of intermittent coma and suffering that led to the final excruciating terminal inhalation that often marks the last moments of human methanol poisoning. A child's scream locked forever in time is the legacy of man's encouraged ignorance about his only true chemical nemesis – methanol.

The Big Lie

A tacit takeover has occurred in the toxicological community, its societies and professional journals, including a conquest of its political advisory role as to public safety. The conquerors have been industrial interests, pharmaceutical lobby groups and those in general who would benefit financially by understating the negative health implications of anything chemical, including drugs, genetic modification, and methanol. It has been a brilliant strategic success that represents an ingenious implementation and spin of *Große Lüge*.[621]

We are today witnessing an apparent universal acceptance of the previously untenable null hypothesis* and the implementation of the risk benefit statistic to excuse and legalize corporate murder of the gentile flock with which we share the planet. The result is that it is nearly impossible to categorically prove to politicians and their bureaucratic henchmen that any profitable chemical can do sufficient harm to justify banning it completely from use.

Political transitions are often far more complex than they may, at first, appear, but simply stated, the most visible sign of this sea change in the role of democratic government from caring for its people to catering to its industry is the diminution of the publicly-funded search for – and implementation of – cures. From the perspective of Big Pharma, treatment pays over and over again during the course of a tortured lifetime, while cures are an endgame to be avoided.

From a distance, the added cost of the considerable health care burden of such folly appears to run counter to the best interests of the governments involved. The ingenious method used to implement this machination by corruption at the intellectual core of a once trustworthy, but thinly populated scientific discipline such as toxicology leaves no easy route to its reversal. The methanol/formaldehyde lobby should serve as an elegant example of how the distribution of surprisingly small perks and the diligent application of creative advertizing can pervert the brain trust of a society and cloak all manner of high crimes

The Null Hypothesis

The "null hypothesis" is a statistical method demanding that there is no relationship between exposure to a poison (for instance) and a disease. Rather than trying to prove methanol is the cause of the diseases of civilization, you must show that the null hypothesis is wrong – you have to refute the null hypothesis. Unfortunately you have to assume that methanol is safe until you find statistically significant evidence to the contrary. So the poison is always innocent until proven guilty. This approach makes it virtually impossible to show that any toxic substance is causing disease. You wind up with the best outcome being a possibility, but never a certainty, even when there is no reasonable doubt. For instance, if you hold your breath for over an hour, there is only a *possibility* that it would cause your death, so why not give it a try? This way of thinking about poisons was ready-made for Big Pharma and is totally unacceptable.

and misdemeanors.

Barring insurrection, your health and the health of your family will be, at least for the foreseeable future, in your own hands; therefore, it is essential that you take the time to evaluate the evidence presented in the remainder of this book. If funding of the scientific community were not now under the thumb of Big Pharma, and if brilliant minds were trained in the language of chemistry and the ways of nature and were capable of devoting their lives completely to the freedom of mankind from suffering and disease, with no quarter given to prejudice or profit, their publicly-supported laboratories would be abuzz with the promise of success on multiple fronts. Their mantra would be, "methanol/formaldehyde kills."

Chapter 4
Formaldehyde is the Real Problem

The Look of DOC

When one looks through a microscope at slides of diseased organs made from the remains of individuals who have suffered and died from the various diseases of civilization (DOC), one is struck repeatedly by the remarkable similarities between what should be very different tissue samples. Ever present is the sense that one is flying over a series of battlefields and viewing the aftermath of many different skirmishes between identical combatants. Every slide, be it of atherosclerosis, lupus, rheumatoid arthritis, multiple sclerosis, or Alzheimer's, always reveals the preserved remains of a fearless, ferocious defender of our well-being, the cell without which we cannot live, the amoeba-like white blood cell, our friend the macrophage, looking suspiciously like it just might be responsible for most of the damage. But is it?

A closer look confirms that the now-transparent white blood cell was caught in the act by the pathologist who prepared the slide, busily digesting bits and pieces of our myelin, our connective tissue, an LDL, or some other tasty component of the very cells it has been programmed to protect, with its own life if necessary, from the day of our conception. Appearing more often than not is the dreaded foam cell, a normally rare transformation of the macrophage into an unstoppable warrior with no control over its appetite, whose fate is to gorge itself until it explodes, spilling its enzyme contents to do even more damage to the enemy.

When looking at these slides full of the dead warriors of an immune system seemingly bent on attacking its master's healthy tissues, the question is and has always been, "Where the hell is the enemy these cells were sent to fight?" A million scientists over two hundred years have stared endlessly at tissue samples like these, taken from those who suffered from DOC. They have used every tool known to science to visualize all manner of bacterial, viral or prionic interlopers in a fruitless attempt to find the enemy. Yet the enemy was there and has always been there, in every tissue sample, on every slide – it was just too small to be seen.

The formaldehyde made from methanol is not much bigger than a water molecule, and no matter how hard you stare or what type of microscope you use you will never come close to seeing the real enemy or the changes it makes that cause disease.

Methanol's Formaldehyde

When the body begins to turn methanol into energy, the first substance produced is always formaldehyde. But this process cannot happen just anywhere in the body; it can only happen in the locations where the ADH enzyme is found. Only a very small percentage of cells in the human body contain the ADH enzyme necessary to turn methanol into this dangerous reactive substance.

The ADH in these cells is always dissolved in the free flowing fluid that makes up the blood of the cell (cytosol). It is essentially freely floating around within the cell's fluid, which means that ADH can come into contact with methanol almost anywhere within the cells where ADH is located. This, in turn, means that formaldehyde can be produced almost anywhere within those same cells. Only a moderate statistical possibility exists that when the formaldehyde is produced in this manner it will be able to fly past the many other tasty proteins available to attack and instead find itself close to an aldehyde dehydrogenase enzyme (ALDH), which has the ability to convert it safety to formic acid, a harmless food additive.[365] This very low possibility of production of formic acid from formaldehyde is what accounts for the fact that an increase of formic acid is only found in the bloodstreams of those who have been poisoned with very large, lethal doses of methanol.

For the most part, formaldehyde is far more likely to find itself in a position to attach itself to cellular proteins or DNA, doing damage to them in the process. Looking for appropriate prey, the small formaldehyde molecule could very likely leak out of the cell in which it was produced, easily slipping through pores or other gaps that allow for passage of moisture and nutrients between the cell and the plasma of the bloodstream, or worse, would leak into the unprotected nucleus of the generator cells.

Once liberated from its ADH-containing generator cell, formaldehyde, which strongly wants to bond with other molecules, would not be expected to travel very far at all in the body before finding and chemically reacting with some protein or DNA. The thought that formaldehyde that has been generated by the large store of liver cells containing ADH could ever travel the great distance to the brain, eye, breast or fetus, which are known targets of methanol poisoning, is ludicrous, to say the least. The notion that the non-toxic formic acid (which actually *can* travel those distances) is the toxic cause of methanol poisoning is also ludicrous, and has its origin in the desperate attempts of scientists who have been paid to show methanol as less dangerous than it really is.

This chapter will teach the chemistry of formaldehyde, which will be indispensable in helping you understand why its generation from methanol within a living body makes such a fascinating etiologic agent in causing the DOC.

An Untraceable and Invisible Killer

Smallness and stealth are important advantages of successful etiologic agents. They are indispensable traits when infiltrating the most intimate parts of the body to initiate disease. Formaldehyde wins the stealth competition by disappearing completely after it strikes its target, but it is far too reactive to reach anywhere deep inside the human body. Methanol, on the other hand, is water soluble and nonreactive, and it can travel long distances before finding itself being metabolized inside a cell containing ADH. In fact, it travels so well that it can be found inside the developing brain of a living fetus within an hour of her mother's having taken a sip of diet soda.[103]

The transformation of methanol into formaldehyde within the living cell would be the etiologic equivalent of a long haul B-2 stealth bomber letting loose a laser-guided payload. Nothing could be more perfectly destructive or more difficult to trace, particularly for a scientific community trained to soak its tissue samples in formaldehyde solution before examination!

The smallest living thing that we know to be a disease causing agent is the prion that is responsible for mad cow disease (BSE). It is 100 times smaller than the most petite of bacteria and makes a virus seem enormous, yet the prion dwarfs formaldehyde, weighing over 1000 times more than a molecule of formaldehyde. Even as molecules go, formaldehyde is among the smallest of molecules, containing only one carbon atom. It disappears (not in the good way) within a few minutes of being introduced into any compartment of the human body and is completely undetectable by any known medical diagnostic technique after it attaches to a protein or DNA target molecule.

Formaldehyde is not often found in the food supply, and even if it were, it is far too reactive to get past the stomach lining and travel into organs such as the breast, bones or brain. The only way that reasonable amounts of formaldehyde can reach organs deep within our protein rich bodies is in disguise. The very best disguise is the one carbon alcohol, methanol. Methanol is the Trojan Horse for formaldehyde.

Methanol is the Mother of the DOC, Not Their Cause

If Methanol did not exist, then neither would DOC; yet methanol does not cause disease by itself. In actuality, it is a pathetically inert little alcohol that is harmless under all but one circumstance. It is only when formaldehyde is produced from methanol that the disease processes can begin. This metamorphosis requires some very special circumstances and will only occur in parts of our body that contain the enzyme ADH. And to underscore that point, the locations in the human anatomy where this enzyme is found coincide exactly with the sites where the DOC are known to originate! *No other mechanism* can bring formaldehyde to the exact critical sites within the body where the DOC begin.

Methanol's undeniable impression of chemical innocence and convoluted route to disease causation, along with its danger only to the human species, with no laboratory animal that can be used for testing, have gone a long way toward keeping methanol below the radar of its potentially greatest enemy, the young untainted scholar eager to cure disease and save lives.

Why is Formaldehyde a Danger?

It would be very handy at this point if you knew some chemistry. I am going to be using every trick that I know to teach you the intriguing and surprisingly complex chemistry of formaldehyde, but first let's just get directly to the heart of the matter: What is the big deal if methanol is converted to formaldehyde within the body?

I will explain the problem first in biological terms without the chemistry. Formaldehyde's effect actually amounts to four very big deals, one representing each of the types of damage that it can do to living human tissue when it can get close enough to attack it:

1. Formaldehyde Causes Human Cancer

Formaldehyde is known to be a human carcinogen in every country of the developed world, with the notable exception of the USA until just recently – June 15, 2011, to be exact. Of course, Americans are just as susceptible to getting cancer from exposure to formaldehyde as other people are, but in the USA, formaldehyde is protected by the lobbying of the Formaldehyde Institute and the Formaldehyde Council.[605] It has the ability to damage DNA in ways that can directly cause cancer. It is officially a Group I carcinogen, a member of the same group as plutonium and asbestos.[11]

Formaldehyde is most commonly known to cause cancer of the lining of the nasal passages, but the notion that this limited type of cancer is all that it is capable of causing is a misconception. The reason many people believe it is that all formaldehyde cancer studies that are done on individuals and animals expose them directly to formaldehyde in its gaseous form. The formaldehyde gas then makes contact with living human cells when it is inhaled into the nose. Formaldehyde is so highly reactive that it disappears into the nasal passages and is known to produce cancers affecting the upper part of the throat behind the nose, where it immediately binds to the tissue there and virtually disappears. Essentially none of it survives to reach further into the body to make contact with other organs. The blood-brain barrier, for instance, prevents any formaldehyde that does manage to leak into the blood from entering the brain, even though the nasal passages are so very close. This explains the strong association of formaldehyde to this particular malignancy.

To this day, due in part to powerful industry lobbying groups such as the Formaldehyde Council and Methanol Institutes, which use their money and political clout to protect the reputations of their namesakes, no laboratory has ever seriously considered the carcinogenic effect of the formaldehyde produced from methanol deep within the body in the tissues of the breast, brain, skin, lung, kidney, etc. This is very unfortunate, since this mechanism is the only logical way that formaldehyde can ever reach these organs in quantity sufficient to have a carcinogenic impact. Certain cancers of these organs, which are considered DOC, have increased dramatically in incidence since the introduction of aspartame into the diet in 1981. Once Science finally wakes from its slumber, it will realize that no intellectual or biochemical barrier exists to accepting the truth: that formaldehyde from methanol is the most important etiologic mechanism in the evolution of these human cancers.

2. **Formaldehyde Activates the Immune System**

In the case of formaldehyde, that which is unknown to man is well-known to Nature. Living organisms, including humans, use formaldehyde in a very limited way to do important work within their bodies. Its use is similar to many other potentially dangerous reactions, such as the burning of glucose in the mitochondria of animals to produce heat and charge ATP. Though formaldehyde can be produced and used by living organisms, mechanisms like peroxisomes are genetically engineered into the biological system to prevent its leakage into more vulnerable tissues where it could cause harm.

Three hundred million years ago, about two billion years into the evolution of life on Earth, Nature evolved the so-called innate immune system and, in particular, the white blood cell, or macrophage. This amoeba-like gentle giant of a cell is designed to destroy and consume any threat to the life of the organism of which it is a part. Among other features, it has built into its outer membrane an intricate biochemical structure that has a way of detecting proteins that have been attacked and changed by formaldehyde. Such proteins are sought out and devoured,[23] linking unwanted formaldehyde directly to the immune system. Thus, the macrophage is always found in tissue affected by DOC.

The innate immune system is composed of a group of white blood cells that prowl the body using the circulatory system as a freeway to take them to sites where they detect trouble may be lurking. The nature of the trouble could be anything from an invading bacteria to a splinter or some other foreign substance piercing the flesh, or even to one of our own cells that has been damaged and must be removed or cleaned up to make room for repairs. It is the detection of the perceived danger by the macrophage that is all-important in the discussion of its involvement in the evolution of autoimmune disease.

The exact nature of what attracts this free living cell to trouble is not at all clear, but we do know that Nature has imbued the macrophage with sites on its outer cell membrane that can specifically detect certain substances and cause it to propel itself toward those targets much like the nose of a bloodhound leads it toward a crime scene. One of these sites on the macrophage is specifically programmed for proteins that have been attacked and modified by formaldehyde. The clear implication is that Nature finds formaldehyde dangerous enough to provide for a very specific mechanism to rid the body of proteins which it has managed to change. This, I believe, is the reason we find macrophages ravaging tissue in close proximity to the only sites in the body where methanol transforms into formaldehyde.

The amoeba-like macrophage engulfs and digests targeted protein in a process called phagocytosis. As the damaged protein is digested by the macrophage, it is broken down into short bits and pieces that, under the right circumstances, can then be "displayed" on the surface of the macrophage attached to special molecules that will attract the attention of other immune system cells and thereby stimulate them to turn on antibody production against the savaged protein. This process is a required step for all human antibody production.

The immune system's reaction to formaldehyde has been put to positive use in the development of vaccines. In fact, without formaldehyde treatment the production of many of the vaccines used to protect us from various diseases would be much less potent. Jonas Salk first used formaldehyde to produce the polio vaccine in 1954. Pharmaceutical companies have since learned that when they treated disease agents, such as diphtheria protein, with very small amounts of formaldehyde,[26] the agents would react more reliably with our macrophages after injection into our bodies to guarantee the production of sufficient and potent antibodies that could impart immunity to the disease.

It is reasonable, therefore, to conclude from this that when the formaldehyde made from methanol attaches to our own protein, the response of the immune system can make it appear that we are becoming immune to ourselves by attracting macrophages to the damaged protein. This is exactly what occurs to protein in the blood of workers that are exposed to formaldehyde gas in the environment and produce antibodies against their own serum.[445] Absolutely no visible change to this protein would make it stand out from other proteins, either before or, in particular, after it had been soaked in histological grade formaldehyde solution to make it into a microscope slide. We would also expect that the macrophage might occasionally initiate antibody production to its unfortunate cannibalistic feast (our macrophages have our identical chromosomes).

You have heard many of the DOC described at one time or another as autoimmune diseases. This designation goes in and out of favor, depending on what faction of the medical community holds sway at the time. Without a doubt the immune system is in play during these diseases. The look of damaged tissue from a patient with multiple sclerosis or lupus is loaded with evidence that the patient's own immune system is "going mad" and destroying what outwardly appears to be healthy tissue. Often, autoantibodies are being produced against self proteins in many of the DOC just as they would be produced against attacking bacteria such as diphtheria, smallpox or the virus that causes the flu after vaccine inoculation. For lupus alone, more than a hundred of these antibodies against self protein have been identified.[520]

The truth is that if these diseases were truly full-blown autoimmune diseases with the immune system of your body waging war against one or several of your own tissues, the battle and suffering would be over very quickly, with the tissue marked for destruction having no chance of survival. Juvenile onset diabetes is the closest disease I can think of to exhibit such a complete eradication of specific tissue, where the cells that manufacture insulin in the pancreas are targeted by just such an attack, and the results are swift. In the days before insulin from other animals was available to treat the juvenile diabetic, death ensued very quickly after diagnosis.

Imagine, for instance, what would be the outcome if the body's immune system decided that the major protein that makes up the myelin sheath of the brain, myelin basic protein (MBP), was marked for destruction. This appears to be exactly what happens during the DOC multiple sclerosis. The problem with the theory that multiple sclerosis is an autoimmune disease is that not all the MBP is attacked simultaneously. There is a selectivity to the attacks. The MBP closest to the lining of the veins and arteries is attacked first, with a slow progression further and further away from the veins taking, in some cases, years to travel a centimeter. If the immune system had sent out a message to attack MBP, it would disappear simultaneously and rapidly over the entire brain. Such a message would be an antibody against MBP but this is only occasionally found in MS and when it is it is not particularly effective.[475]

This phenomenon can have only one explanation. Formaldehyde is slowly being produced within the lining of the circulatory system of the brain and diffusing outward into the tissue, and attaching itself to the MBP. The macrophages are then called in to remove all the formaldehyde-damaged MBP that is in its wake. It is the intermittent production of formaldehyde in the lining of the circulatory system of the brain, beyond the blood brain barrier, that turns on when methanol from the diet is high and ethanol from the colon is low, and that is more likely to lead to the slow progression of the perivascular plaque, which is the discerning feature of multiple sclerosis.

3. Formaldehyde Turns Tissue to Plastic

Man first discovered formaldehyde in 1886 and since that time its most important industrial use has been binding together molecules to make plastics. It is so reactive and anxious to grab onto other molecules that it can transform a small molecule like urea, a component of urine, into a tough urea-formaldehyde plastic by binding to it over and over again, producing long chains of alternate urea formaldehyde beads. This plastic, used often in the construction industry, is infamous for causing the formaldehyde contamination of trailer homes used to house flood victims in New Orleans after Katrina.

The ability of formaldehyde to plasticize extends to human tissue, both living and dead. The slides made by pathologists to study tissue from patients who have died from various diseases of civilization have all been treated with formaldehyde in the process of their production, turning them into a plastic that will not rot over extended periods of time; therefore, any changes made by formaldehyde in living tissue will not be visible through any microscope, no matter how closely observed.

A student of anatomy might first encounter the ability of formaldehyde to make plastic when first carefully removing the custard-like fresh brain of a laboratory animal. After the brain has soaked in the formaldehyde solution for a week or two, the student's next encounter with the brain will require a very sharp knife to cut the tough rubbery brain into slices for the microscope. Amazingly, although the nature of the tissue has changed dramatically, microscopically it is difficult to tell it from tissue that formaldehyde has never touched.

I believe that the plastic feel that formaldehyde gives to tissue is what is responsible for the term "sclerotic" that is given to several of the more important of the DOC. Once seen, one will never forget a famous wood etching of the French scientist credited with discovering and describing multiple sclerosis. The etching is quite crude, but it shows Professor Charcot formally dressed wearing a very tall top hat and a tattered apron leaning over a large kitchen sink. He is running his fingers through the custard-like freshly extracted brain of one of his kitchen servants who died from multiple sclerosis while under his hire. Charcot goes into great detail about how leathery and "sclerotic" the tissue feels that surrounds the veins of her MS brain and that make up the MS plaque.

During an autopsy I have with my own hands felt sclerotic arteries from a fresh cadaver of a man suffering for years before death from atherosclerosis, another major DOC. The leathery texture of these arteries felt identical to the comparable tissue from a disease-free patient that had been preserved in formaldehyde for teaching purposes.

Formaldehyde is the best way to bind proteins together. It has been implicated as a cause of Alzheimer's disease and has been shown to attach to basic proteins called Tau, found deep within in the axons of nerve cells, in such a way as to bind them together into useless knots called tangles.[234,235] Tangled Tau proteins eventually block the communication between cells so they cannot participate in the memory process. The mind is slowly but surely thereby robbed of its ability to remember. The fact that Alzheimer's, much like multiple sclerosis, is a disease that starts forming around the veins and arteries in the brain, which is exactly where formaldehyde is produced from dietary methanol, may explain why the incidence of Alzheimer's has increased 10,000% since aspartame became a major addition to the methanol component of the civilized diet.

4. Methanol Causes Birth Defects

When I wrote a scientific article in 1984 warning of the methanol in aspartame[1] I stated correctly that methanol had not been tested as a possible cause for birth defects although, unknown to me or the rest of the scientific community, aspartame actually had been secretly tested and did indeed produce fetal birth defects of test animal brains.[677] Unwanted methylation caused by formaldehyde is a frequent finding in both the chromosomes[558] and in the brain tissue[559] of autistic children. Unfortunately, formaldehyde, for reasons unknown to me, is now referred to as the "methyl molecule" by epigeneticists (scientist who study the chromosomal linked disease-causing effects of methylation). This makes their literature quite confusing to those of us who have concern for the disease-causing potential of formaldehyde produced from methanol in the human body. We will discuss this in more detail in Chapter 12, the last chapter of this book.

Why Is Methanol/Formaldehyde Being Ignored by Science?

Formaldehyde disappears with great speed and without a trace in the human body, foiling efforts to study its role in multiple sclerosis and other major human diseases. In spite of the fact that formaldehyde is now recognized as a cause of cancer in humans,[11] research laboratories in the world today are not studying methanol-produced formaldehyde as a possible agent of any human diseases.[586] Could this lethal oversight be due in part to the scientific community's ignorance of its mysterious chemical behavior?

To help answer this question, we need to consider the implications of a tragic incident recorded in a 1990 research article that is, I believe, the most important work on formaldehyde ever published in the scientific literature.[236] The disturbing episode involved a physician whose husband discovered her unconscious on the bathroom floor, a partially empty bottle of pure laboratory-grade formaldehyde solution by her side. In a dark Shakespearean twist, her husband consumed the remainder of the flask, determined to join his wife on her suicidal journey – that is, until the excruciating pain and second thoughts that soon followed made him seek emergency aid instead.

The quick-thinking internist on duty called for an immediate blood analysis, whose results showed no trace of formaldehyde in the blood of either subject. Incredulous, he then did something that had never been done before with human subjects. He had additional samples of blood drawn from the patients and treated to remove any living cells that might have had enzymes capable of metabolizing formaldehyde to formic acid. He also added formaldehyde solution to the cell-free vials of plasma before analysis, in a procedure called spiking. Even this formaldehyde did not appear in the test results, meaning that the additional formaldehyde had also quickly disappeared before it could be detected. These two individuals had clearly consumed enough of this poison to kill themselves only minutes before, yet no formaldehyde could be detected in their blood— an absence that should come as no great surprise given that a lethal dose of formaldehyde injected directly into a live laboratory animal also vanishes within minutes.[122]

Acute kidney failure developed rapidly in both patients, a result of what attending physicians concluded were "the toxic effects of plasma constituents altered by reaction with the formaldehyde."[236] Lobbyists for the Formaldehyde Institute[605] would likely at this stage be quick to ascribe their condition to the effects of formic acid rather than formaldehyde. This assertion, however, would be undermined by the fact that dialysis was prescribed for these patients very soon after admission, a treatment that would have quickly removed all formic acid.

Both patients survived the severe damage incurred by the direct contact of the formaldehyde with their digestive system, although the woman's stomach had to be completely removed. Unfortunately, however, they both died from protracted pulmonary and heart complications three and eight weeks after the formaldehyde poisoning, even though their lungs did not initially appear damaged. The details of just exactly what the formaldehyde did to kill those people will never be known because science is at a loss as to where to look and what to look for. Samples were saved for posterity, all preserved in formaldehyde. Nevertheless, it was undoubtedly their single exposure to pure formaldehyde that proved lethal for these otherwise healthy patients, leaving not a clue as to causation.

The Production, Use and Nature of Formaldehyde

I remember two encounters with methanol and formaldehyde from my childhood. The first was a news report I heard on the radio while waiting for my ride to grade school when I was 7 years old. An eye doctor in Europe was going to be recognized for his work, which proved conclusively that the blindness and death caused by accidental methanol consumption could be prevented by getting the patient drunk and keeping them drunk for a week or more. This was probably a report based on the work of Olaf Roe, the discoverer of the unique human susceptibility to methanol, and who was to become so very important to me thirty years later.[52,494] I am sure that I found this worth remembering because my fantasies in those days were all centered around helping people and learning helpful facts that could save lives.

The second incident happened while I was attending high school in New Jersey. It was Christmas and one of my presents was a magic hand warmer, an interesting little contraption that consisted of a shiny chrome case the shape of a large cigarette holder that would fit into your hand quite nicely. Inside was a reservoir which you were required to fill with methanol. The instructions emphasized very clearly that no other alcohol would work. The idea was simple; all you had to do was put a match close to the wick and light a blue flame. It had a platinum wire strand above the wick that brought the methanol vapors to the chamber in the top of the contraption, and the wire would start glowing red, at which time you blew out the flame. The platinum wire continued to glow red hot even after the flame was extinguished. Replacing the metal cover and returning the warmer to a red velvet carrying case was all there was to it. It worked like a charm, giving off heat for ten hours with each charge of methanol. The only thing I found unattractive was the smell it put off – a smell I remembered from biology class when we were dissecting fetal pigs.

On Christmas day I went out for a long walk with my trusty hand warmer in my pants pocket, where it gave off a lovely steady heat. Periodically, I would take it out to warm up my hands in the frigid December evening. When I got home it was time for bed and I remember bringing my trusty warmer under the covers with me on that cold wintry night. The next day it was off to the doctor's office with one of the worst asthma attacks I can remember. Asthma was the scourge of my childhood and such an episode was not uncommon or unusual, except perhaps for its severity. While at the clinic the doctor noticed that I was constantly scratching at my left thigh. Upon examination he discovered a reddening and severe swelling of the skin that would have lain directly under the hand warmer from the walk the night before. He asked about anything unusual that I could remember and I told him about the hand warmer. He advised me that it appeared I might be allergic to my hand warmer. The rash developed about week later into a classic granulomatous inflammation.[555] It took weeks for the rash to finally subside, but the hand warmer was never to be used again.

It was a very long time before I was to have my next encounter with methanol and its alter-ego, formaldehyde. This hand warmer was actually a formaldehyde gas generator. It worked on the principle that methanol really wants to be formaldehyde and all that is needed is a platinum wire catalyst. The abundant energy released from the conversion of methanol to formaldehyde was more than enough to keep the platinum wire glowing red hot for as long as the methanol lasted, with the excess heat providing the warming effect of the product. It is on the very surface of the catalyst wire that the methanol turns into formaldehyde just as it does in that little window of the ADH enzyme. The smell that had reminded me of dissecting fetal pigs was due to the only end product of this reaction: pure formaldehyde gas.

The scientific community has never fully fathomed the complex chemical nature of formaldehyde. It was discovered and first produced from methanol by A.W. Hofmann in 1868 using a hot platinum wire – thirty years after Robert Carswell's first depiction of multiple sclerosis in a 1938 atlas of pathologic conditions.[306] Formaldehyde was not believed to occur naturally. For years, it was simply considered a notorious laboratory oddity because of its penchant for turning flesh into plastic and killing all manner of living things. It was soon commonly used as a preservative for tissue samples prepared for microscopic study.[593] All the samples of multiple sclerosis brain tissue studied by the great histologist Dawson and his contemporaries were first preserved in formaldehyde solution before staining to reveal their structures and defects.[620] Formaldehyde treatment of histological specimens persists to this day, with rare exception.

Putting Formaldehyde into Perspective: Meet Venus!

In many matters where science remains ignorant, Nature seems – in design and in practice – omniscient. As I explained earlier, the bodies of humans and other living organisms have evolved to employ formaldehyde in very limited ways to do valuable work. But at some point, macrophages were designed to seek out and devour proteins that had been inappropriately altered by formaldehyde.

Why does Nature find formaldehyde such a threat? After all, it contains just one carbon atom. As molecules go, it is extremely small, too small for a physician to distinguish a large protein molecule that has been attacked by formaldehyde from one that has not. Trying to visualize the behavior of a virtually invisible compound is difficult. To see why Nature responds so forcefully to such a miniscule entity, we need to find a way to make life's molecules – and the biological systems they comprise and affect – more substantial and tangible so that you can relate to them more easily. So at this point in your reading, pour yourself a cup of coffee or tea (no diet soda, please), sit down, relax, and let's daydream a little.

First, we need to assign roles or personas to our key molecular and cellular players to make them easier to understand. Let's start with methanol. While I have likened methanol before to a Trojan horse, for our present purposes, such a creature would be too large in physical stature and too grand in character. Imagine a methanol molecule in this scenario as something more ordinary and less imposing. Let's think of it, for conceptual reasons that will become apparent as we go on, as a common pigeon in the order of things, a methanol pigeon that will set the scale for everything else in our analogy. See Figure 4.1.

We have to see everything in a relative size relationship before we can truly visualize the details that make the story of how a small molecule like methanol can cause disease. Bear with me as I bring the molecular reality down to components that we can relate to. Now picture a petite young woman about eighteen years of age and four feet nine inches tall, a charming person with whom I am sure you would enjoy chatting. Although she has multiple sclerosis, she has not yet experienced any serious symptoms other than the occasional headache. She has no idea what lies in store for her. Her name is Venus, and about an hour ago, she drank a diet soda sweetened with aspartame.

Figure 4.1

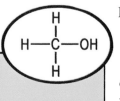

METHANOL

If a methanol molecule circulating in Venus's blood – a byproduct of her diet soda – is the size of a pigeon, then how big would Venus be? It might surprise you to find out that she would be exceedingly large, so tall that she would struggle to balance atop an Earth the size of her fist. And at approximately 250,000 miles tall, she would also need to duck a little to allow the moon, which would be the size of a golf ball, room to orbit. See Figure 4.2.

If you do some fairly exact calculations that keep everything in scale, you will be amazed to find that just one of her brain cells would become the size of Manhattan, the island that constitutes most of New York City. As anyone who has been to New York knows, pigeons love it there and can be seen flying in flocks all over the island. Interestingly, the nucleus of this enlarged brain cell would become the size and have the relative location of Central Park in the very heart of Manhattan Island. The mitochondria we talked about in the previous chapter that burn glucose and recharge ATP would correspond nicely in both size and shape to the many cargo ships or large ferry boats docked at the port of Manhattan or cruising down the Hudson River. See Figure 4.3.

Now it is time to introduce a protein molecule into our analogy. Proteins serve many functional and structural purposes in the body. The enzyme ADH is a protein. It is not necessary to understand the structure of protein in great detail. Just remember that proteins are much larger than methanol or formaldehyde and are made up

Figure 4.2

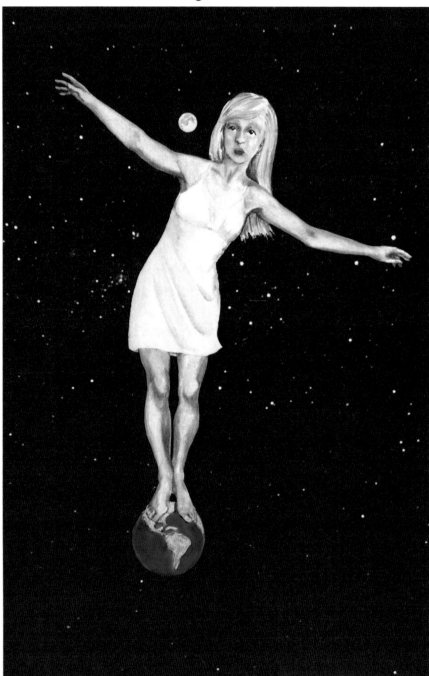

of many amino acid molecules bound together into very specific shapes. ADH would be about the size of a two story house. ADH is unusual and it is produced as a dimer, or two ADH molecules bound together, each with one active site the size of the average house window. So you can imagine it as two two-story houses attached to each other, each having one window. The active site is where our pigeons can turn into formaldehyde if no ethanol is available.

Let's envision the methanol molecules heading toward Venus's brain as pigeons flying down the vessels of her bloodstream looking for an enzyme where they can land for awhile. The pigeons travel quickly, being helped along by the bloodstream, where island-sized blood cells push the tiny pigeons along their way.

A quick peak forward to Chapter 7 will let you see illustrations of size perfect methanol pigeons floating along with red blood cells and macrophages in Venus's circulatory system. Once inside her brain, they get pushed quickly through the arteries and start back into the smaller arterioles, which are often where MS plaques begin to develop. The cells that line the vessels of Venus's brain are each as big as Manhattan with a thickness that would correspond to the height of the Empire State Building. These epithelial cells are thin and set quite close together in a layer one cell thick, looking from a distance altogether like the white tiles used to protect the major underground traffic tunnels around the world.

These cells in the brain, called the endothelium, constitute the blood-brain barrier. Their spacing is tighter than the lining of the vessels of most of the rest of the circulatory system of the body and this spacing acts to keep most dangerous substances from entering the brain. But they do not react with, stop or even slow down the inert little methanol pigeons. Pushed through the gaps between the cells and traveling with the plasma of the blood, the pigeons soon find themselves in the mass of cells that constitute the body of the blood vessel wall. It is here, within the cells that give structure to all the blood vessels throughout the body, where Nature, in her wisdom, has placed the largest cache of ADH enzyme in the body, outside of the liver. Remember, the ADH can turn methanol into formaldehyde.

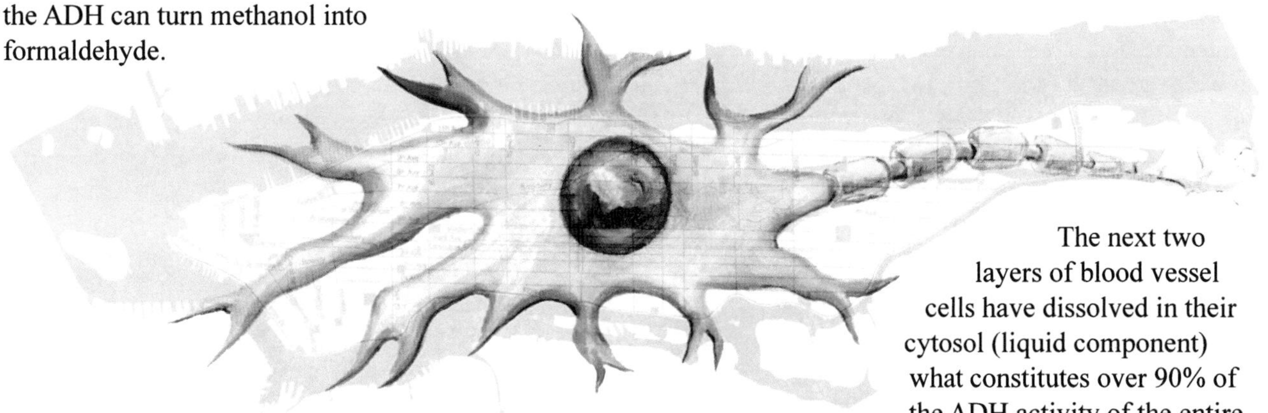

Figure 4.3

The next two layers of blood vessel cells have dissolved in their cytosol (liquid component) what constitutes over 90% of the ADH activity of the entire circulatory system.[220] The first of these layers is part of the endothelium and is called the intima (where 23.5% of ADH activity occurs), and right beneath is a thick layer called the media (where 74% of ADH activity occurs). The exact distribution of this cache of ADH has not been thoroughly explored by the scientific community, but we do know it varies a great deal, even within the same individual.[220] We will revisit this phenomenon again, so pardon the repetition but please put it to memory.

In the mean time, our pigeons have their destiny in sight. Entering cells in the media or intima of the arteriole is a breeze; the blood plasma liquids in which our little birds are dissolved bring nutrients easily into these cells – as easily as they will carry out the formaldehyde that remains after the pigeons find the ADH that will someday make our Venus a martyr to corporate greed. Once inside the cell, our pigeons are lucky because our young girl is on a diet and hasn't eaten much in the last few days, meaning no ethanol pigeons (which we will represent as giant New Zealand pigeons) are hovering around at the active sites to scare the methanol pigeons away. Since Venus's blood contains no ethanol to keep the ADH busy it is free to give all its attention to turning the methanol into formaldehyde. The pigeons find empty window sills in the two-story home-sized enzymes, aptly structured to stand in for the active sites of ADH. See Figures 4.4 and 4.5.

Since cells in the human body are made up of over 95 percent water, this change should be understood as a sea change, in both the metaphorical and literal sense of this term. This means that our imaginary Manhattan is at once a familiar, yet fantastic location, a submarine city entirely submersed in water. Remember water has a potent effect on formaldehyde. Exposure to H_2O induces a personality change similar to that of the little creatures in the 1984 movie "Gremlins." Once wet, they morphed from harmless little pets into destructive, deadly monsters.

An enzyme, despite its large size, commonly possesses only one or two active sites that can perform a desired function. The window represents the only place on the enzyme that can function to convert methanol into formaldehyde. Picture our pigeon – a.k.a. methanol – flying into the open window of the floating duplex. Once inside, it undergoes a physical transformation as it undergoes the metabolic process of conversion. A short time later, out it flies reborn as a sparrow hawk – a.k.a. formaldehyde.

The Two Faces of Formaldehyde: Base or Acid - Bad or Worse.

Few scientists, even chemists, know or seem to care much about the significant transformation of formaldehyde from one form to another, a lapse that may help account for why, over the last 100 years, researchers have overlooked this little molecule as the ultimate cause of many diseases. This dimorphism allows each formaldehyde molecule to resonate and become either of the two forms of formaldehyde that exist in our bodies simultaneously, in the form of either an acid or a base. A formaldehyde molecule can either contribute hydrogen to a reaction or remove it. We overlook the duality of formaldehyde and its potential to wreak great havoc at our own peril. The innocuous little stick figure molecule that chemists draw as formaldehyde can only exist alone when formaldehyde is a gas. The second that formaldehyde makes contact with water and dissolves, much of it instantly combines with a water molecule to become formaldehyde

Figure 4.4　　　　　　　　　　　**Figure 4.5**

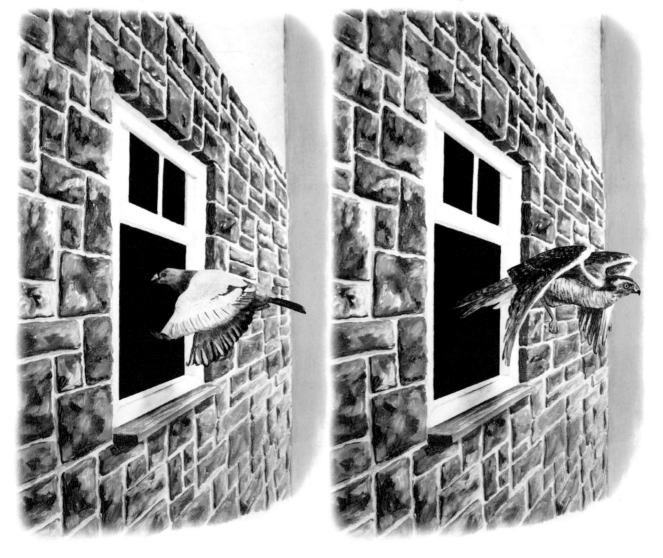

hydrate, a much more menacing persona.

For purposes of our analogy, we will show this morphing back and forth as being either a sparrow hawk (formaldehyde - see Figure 4.6) or being what we will call a Crazy Hawk (formaldehyde hydrate - see Figure 4.7). Formaldehyde hydrate, the acid form of formaldehyde, does not play well with others; it is a monstrous entity with the power to disrupt, disable, and or eventually kill every living thing with which it makes prolonged contact. It desperately wants to grab hold of anything within its reach and hold onto it. It will even attack its alternate form, formaldehyde, if it cannot find anything better, and it can change from one form to another at a moment's notice. This is a very important point for you to understand so please bear with me as I explain it further.

The pure formaldehyde gas that I produced with my hand warmer is highly reactive but will not react with itself to form the polymer paraldehyde. This is because the gas is all made up of the one molecular form of formaldehyde that we are calling the sparrow hawk. Usually, in chemistry, molecules that are identical will repel each other the way magnets do when they are identically charged. So in our illustration, our chemically identical formaldehyde sparrow hawks will not grab hold of each other and bond to produce a chain. They need to attach to something that is different from them in order to create a plasticized substance, such as what comes to mind when we think of tissues that have been preserved in formaldehyde.

Industry uses the gaseous form of formaldehyde to produce long chains called polymers by linking other small molecules together with the formaldehyde to make some tough leathery plastics, such as the urea-formaldehyde used in the building trades. Bonds made with formaldehyde, and in particular, the sparrow hawk, tend not to be as permanent as one would like and this may be why these plastics tend to give off formaldehyde gas for years after they are manufactured. The sparrow hawk will hold on tightly for awhile, and then release its grasp and return to its gaseous form. The temporary nature of these formaldehyde bonds is legend and gives some scientists the false impression that they are weak, but the truth is that not all types of formaldehyde bonds are weak. They are simply unstable, which is another matter altogether.

Figure 4.6

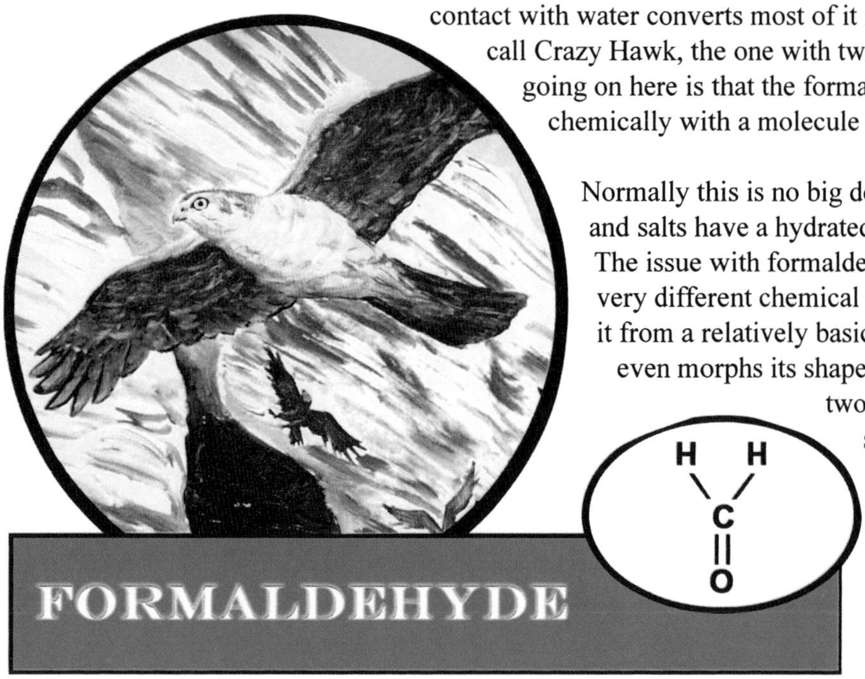

When methanol is turned into formaldehyde within our bodies everything takes place essentially under water. Our sparrow hawk emerges from the ADH and instant contact with water converts most of it into the hydrated monster we will call Crazy Hawk, the one with two huge claws. What is actually going on here is that the formaldehyde molecule is combining chemically with a molecule of water.

Normally this is no big deal; in chemistry many chemicals and salts have a hydrated form and a non-hydrated form. The issue with formaldehyde is that the hydrated form has very different chemical properties.[27] Hydration changes it from a relatively basic compound to an acidic one and even morphs its shape so that it is capable of forming two bonds, one on either side of the single carbon atom. See Figure 4.8.

FORMALDEHYDE

Now I said that most of the sparrow hawks are turned into Crazy Hawks. Well, it is actually much more interesting than that.

These hawks can and do switch from one persona to another in the blink of an eye. Imagine a sparrow hawk flying along and then all of a sudden it morphs into a Crazy Hawk and then back again. This is the reason the chemistry of formaldehyde in living systems is so fascinating and difficult to pin down. The fact is that under normal conditions in our bodies 99% of the formaldehyde present is in the acidic form represented by the Crazy Hawk, but at any moment its personality can switch back to the basic form, or sparrow hawk. See Figure 4.9.

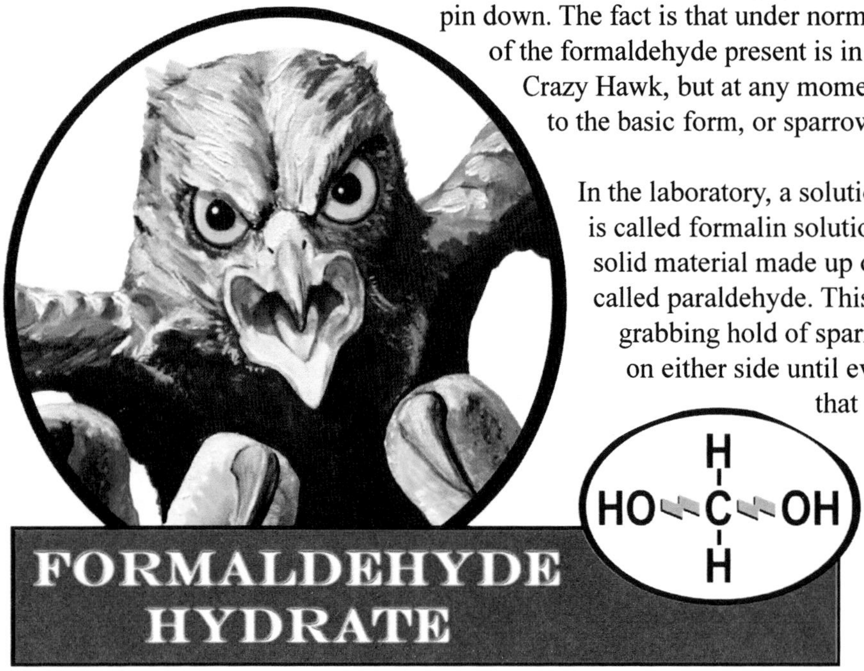

In the laboratory, a solution of formaldehyde gas in water is called formalin solution. When stored, it will produce a solid material made up of a plastic of pure formaldehyde called paraldehyde. This is produced by Crazy Hawks grabbing hold of sparrow hawks and bonding to them on either side until eventually a long chain is produced that is no longer soluble and falls out of solution to the bottom of the jar. This reveals and embodies the persistence of formaldehyde hydrate to bind to anything with which it makes contact, even its alter ego.

FORMALDEHYDE HYDRATE

$$HO - \underset{\underset{H}{|}}{\overset{\overset{H}{|}}{C}} - OH$$

Figure 4.7

This is the formaldehyde sparrow hawk that is produced from methanol pigeons in the lining of Venus's blood vessels by the ADH enzyme there – it flies out of the cells of the vessel lining, desperately wanting to combine with the closest basic protein in her brain, such as myelin basic protein (MBP), the very protein whose damage and loss is causing Venus's multiple sclerosis.

Figure 4.8

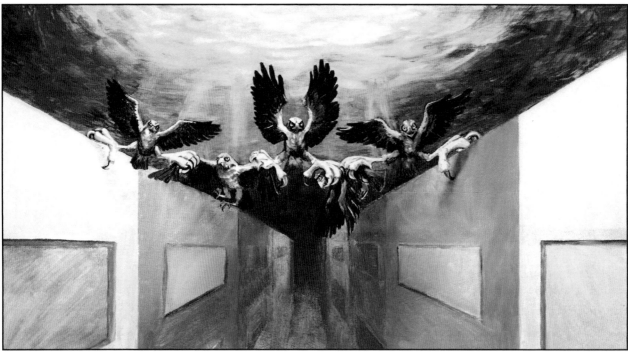

What Attaches to What and Why: the Many Bonds of Formaldehyde

I refuse to go into the extremely complex and confusing details of all of the ways that formaldehyde can change other molecules. This would discourage many readers. You are being fed here what you need to know, and no more.

The formaldehyde Crazy Hawk (Figure 4.9) cannot attach just anywhere on any protein molecule, nor can it bind to another Crazy Hawk. It must wait until a suitable basic form of formaldehyde or a basic protein comes within reach so it can attack it. Some parts of a large protein molecules repel our little monster hawk. When a landing place is found, however, contact is made and a chemical bond is formed between the protein and the formaldehyde. The hawk does what it must do based on chemical attractions between itself and the protein or DNA it is attacking. One important thing to remember is that after a protein is attacked by formaldehyde hydrate that protein always becomes more acidic.[594] (This explains why humans who are dying from a high dose of methanol poisoning will often experience an acidification of their blood.)

Figure 4.9

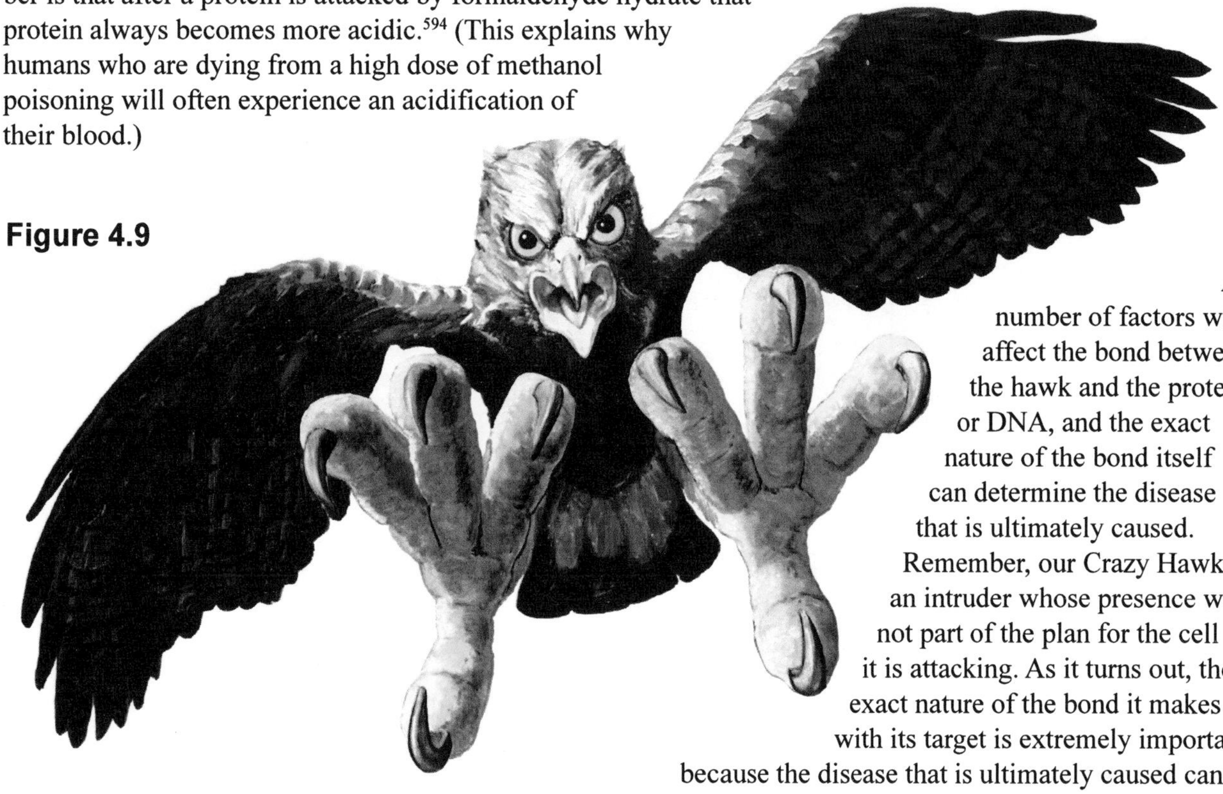

A number of factors will affect the bond between the hawk and the protein or DNA, and the exact nature of the bond itself can determine the disease that is ultimately caused. Remember, our Crazy Hawk is an intruder whose presence was not part of the plan for the cell it is attacking. As it turns out, the exact nature of the bond it makes with its target is extremely important because the disease that is ultimately caused can depend on the details of this interaction.

I will classify these bonds into three categories of my own making that have more significance relative to disease than to the exact details of chemistry. May all my chemistry professors, both living and dead, forgive me.

The "Tag...You're It!" Bond

This is the easiest bonding to understand on a very superficial level. A hawk can very quickly form a bond either with one of the amino acids or with one of the nitrogen bases that make up a protein or DNA molecule, and it can nest there for a period of time. In comparison to its host, it is so tiny that once it is nested, it becomes virtually invisible. It would be hard to guess at just how many of these bonds actually exist; perhaps it is hundreds. They have been studied for many years in test tubes, but never in a living organism. These bonds account for the disappearance of formaldehyde within a few minutes of its being injected or produced inside a living thing.

Why should this bond be studied? Because it is the bond that is the basis of all of the so-called autoimmune diseases caused by methanol's formaldehyde. It is this bond that changes a protein and tags it for elimination by the macrophage. It is also the bond used by vaccine companies to produce their best products.[26]

It was not until 1986 that researchers discovered that the macrophage, or white blood cell, had a specific, universal receptor site specially designed for protein that had been damaged by formaldehyde.[23] This receptor site was determined to be responsible for the special attention that the macrophage gives to formaldehyde modified protein.[24] The significance of this discovery will have tremendous bearing on all of the autoimmune diseases where macrophages, known to scavenge self protein, appear to be the only visible cause of both the symptoms and the disease itself.

The exact details of the specific targeted site on the protein, or even which proteins are susceptible to this targeting by formaldehyde, has yet to be clearly explained, due to the lack of attention given formaldehyde modified protein since its discovery in 1986.[23] Many different autoimmune diseases exist that may actually be the direct result of macrophages devouring formaldehyde damaged proteins. The specific disease induced by the formaldehyde would be determined by the location of the protein that is tagged. We can, however, give an educated guess and surmise that multiple sclerosis would primarily result from formaldehyde-damaged myelin basic protein; atherosclerosis would require the tagging of the protein shell of the LDL lipoprotein; rheumatoid arthritis would involve an unknown protein or proteins in the vicinity of the ADH-rich fibroblast of the bone and cartilage; lupus (SLE) would involve tagging of another collection of proteins surrounding the ADH layers of the general circulation and the numerous ADH-rich fibroblasts of the skin; and so on.

A fibroblast, by the way, is a type of cell that is responsible for making connective tissue. Since we mentioned the ADH in the fibroblasts of the skin, let me give you a close-to-home example of exactly what I am talking about. Fibroblasts are found almost everywhere in the body, and a handful (notably for our discussion here, those in human skin) have been found to contain ADH.[638] The implication here is that methanol in the bloodstream from diet soda could be responsible for producing formaldehyde in the tissue of the skin. This has serious implications relative to skin cancer and lupus (SLE) which we will discuss in the next two chapters.

For now, let's start off with my little run-in with the formaldehyde-producing hand warmer I received for Christmas 45 years ago. The type of skin rash that I developed was Granulomatous Panniculitis. Don't let the name frighten you; it refers to a rash that is defined by many puss-filled eruptions (pimples) that are filled with macrophages and foam cells. Curiously enough, this reaction was identical in every way to skin lesions that have been shown in certain individuals to be caused by consumption of food sweetened with aspartame.[228] I want to walk you through exactly what causes these two identical reactions, as they involve formaldehyde tag bonds and are good examples of the evolution of all of the so-called autoimmune diseases, from MS to rheumatoid arthritis.

My encounter with pure formaldehyde gas under high concentration was localized to the area of my left thigh. If I had been placed in a room with that concentration of formaldehyde I probably could not have lived for more than a few minutes. I mention the high concentration because normally, low concentrations of formaldehyde, our sparrow hawks, anxious to grab onto a protein as quickly as possible, would tag the protein in the top dead layers of skin called the epidermis. Plenty of protein would be available there to satisfy all of the sparrow hawks, so none would venture further into the skin where it could cause harm.

In this case, however, the concentration of formaldehyde gas was high enough for a long enough period of time to actually allow the formaldehyde to penetrate my epidermis and reach the living tissue of the dermis.

The sparrow hawks that made it past my epidermis reacted with the water in my dermis to evolve into Crazy Hawks that tagged protein there.

Interestingly enough, the dermis is where the ADH-containing skin fibroblasts reside. This means that the methanol from diet soda can also be converted to formaldehyde there as well.

How does formaldehyde, whether from a gas poisoning or the conversion of methanol from diet soda, still produce identical granulomatous inflammation? The definition of a granuloma is a compact collection of mature mononuclear phagocytes,[555] which is just a fancy name for our friends, the macrophages. It is clear that the macrophage is doing what it is programmed to do: devouring formaldehyde-modified protein. This is what always happens when formaldehyde tags and, therefore, modifies living protein. Since Dr. Novick published his article in the Annals of Internal Medicine, convincingly linking aspartame to the production of granuloma in his young female patient,[228] it has been proven conclusively that the methanol from aspartame does indeed transform into formaldehyde within the living organism.[7]

Methylation, the Most Important Bond: a Result of Formaldehyde Poisoning

The conversion of an attached Crazy Hawk into a permanent part of a protein or DNA molecule is called methylation and is a process of utmost importance. Methylation is used by nature to work magic with the timing and evolution of the entire genome of living things. It is what controls the timing of when the chromosomes perform what process. DNA methylation is one of the key factors involved in the regulation of genetic expression and stability, and is necessary for the maintenance of most cellular functions. If one of our hawks decides to nest on a DNA strand, it can alter its activity in ways that are harmful.

Methylation is the permanent attachment of formaldehyde to a protein or DNA. Our hawks can methylate a protein or a DNA molecule, but can only do this in living tissue – they can't methylate dead tissue or tissue in a test tube. It works like this: just as when methanol flew into the active window of ADH I enzyme and came out formaldehyde, so also can our Crazy Hawk, after it has attached to a protein or DNA with one claw, be changed back into a peaceful persona by other enzymes often found in the nucleus of living cells.

Suffice it to say that successful methylation takes a bit of teamwork on the part of several different enzymes. Just think of it like the mating of Grey Whales; the job cannot get done unless a third behemoth participates in the maneuvering. Luck – or the lack of it – plays a role in the process as well. From now on we will use a nesting dove to represent a methyl group which is made up of the single carbon atom from the transformed formaldehyde that has been bound to DNA or protein and is surrounded with the three hydrogen atoms, making it a very placid member of the chemical landscape. See Figure 4.10.

Figure 4.10

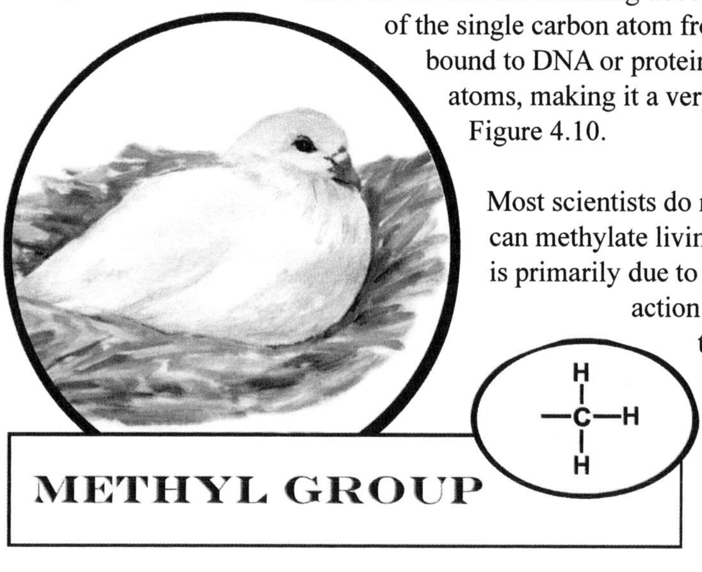

METHYL GROUP

Most scientists do not realize the ease with which formaldehyde can methylate living tissue. This ignorance is unfortunate and is primarily due to the fact that methylation requires the direct action of enzymes[225] located in parts of the living cell that are accessible only by formaldehyde that has been produced from methanol by ADH within that living tissue (in situ). Methylation cannot occur in a laboratory, when dead tissue is being treated with formaldehyde, or in a test tube where formaldehyde is being reacted experimentally with other molecules, such as protein and DNA. It can only happen inside a living body.

This methyl group, this dove, no longer has any of the chemical aggressiveness of our Crazy Hawk formaldehyde hydrate molecule, but it does stand as a permanent change to the molecule to which it is attached. It is one of the few permanent changes that formaldehyde can make until we talk about embalming. This process makes the hawk forever a permanent part of the protein or DNA molecule.

The Plastic Bond: Embalming Process and its Similarity to Alzheimer's

The Crazy Hawk can rest on a landing spot only to be knocked off it by other hawks, leaving insufficient time to form a permanent bond before it turns back into the sparrow hawk and flies away. This happens most often when formalin solution is used by embalmers to preserve dead tissue for medical and aesthetic purposes. During an autopsy the pathologist carefully removes the subject's delicate brain and gently places it into a jar containing formalin. After a week in the formalin solution, most of the proteins of the brain will be bound together by chains of sparrow hawks and Crazy Hawks, hardening it into a solid block of plastic that would bounce if dropped to the floor. This is mostly what goes on during embalming when there is an overabundance of formaldehyde and nothing but time.[593]

How does this process occur exactly? To give you a better example of what is going on let me give you a little visualization. I once visited a very beautiful place near my home in Arizona. Paria Canyon is a magical location where the Paria River from Utah winds its way and eventually meets up with the mighty Colorado River inside the Grand Canyon. The sandstone walls of the Paria canyon are steep and close together in places, rising more than 600 feet above the little river. There are places in the canyon that are so narrow you can stand in the water and easily touch both walls at the same time. The sandstone is flawless and monolithic except for occasional little niches here and there where a stone shelf provides a perfect spot for a bird of prey to nest.

Let's imagine each side of the canyon representing adjacent protein molecules. Picture now the release of a thousand formaldehyde hawks into the narrowest part of the canyon. Competition for the few nesting sites would be tremendous. Birds would be bumped off their perches by the competition and the end result would surely make it appear that the hawk does not bind quickly to protein.

The truth, of course, is just the opposite. The illusion was caused by introducing many more hawks than could ever reside in the small canyon. So it is when high concentrations of formaldehyde are used for preservation. The formaldehyde appears to take days to do its work but eventually the dominant hawks persevere and claim their rightful perches and bridge the gap between proteins. See Figure 4.11.

What does the Crazy Hawk do after landing? It can reach across the narrow canyon and grab the other side with its other claw. The little bird grasping both cliff faces, or holding together two protein molecules, is remarkable but this is exactly what happens when formalin is used as a preservative or when formaldehyde hydrate inside a cell grasps two proteins and won't let go. This link is called a methylene bridge. If the distance is too far for one Crazy Hawk to reach by itself it grabs the closest sparrow hawk, which is then grabbed by another Crazy Hawk and so on until the last hawk in the chain is close enough to grab the other canyon wall. This visualization might seem a little silly and not very birdlike, but this is exactly how formaldehyde hydrate, given enough time, can turn a dead body into a plastic statue, binding to every available site on all the available proteins.

This type of binding, interesting enough, is also what appears to be happening to the Tau proteins in the brains of those developing Alzheimer's Disease.[234] More on this subject later.

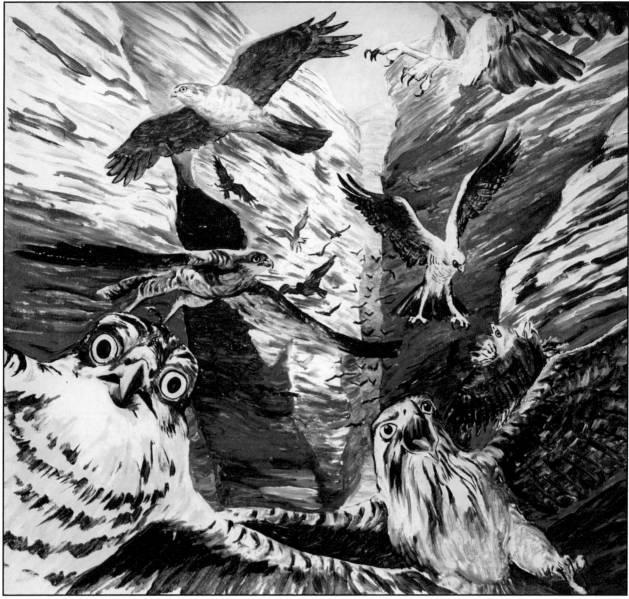

Figure 4.11

What You See Is What You Study!

Why has all this been so difficult to study? Why are these reactions so elusive? What is it that has kept science from seeing these important changes that go on when methanol turns into formaldehyde within the living cell? Perhaps the answers lies in the tremendous size differences between formaldehyde and the very large proteins and DNA to which it likes to attach itself. We saw the pigeon that represented methanol landing on the duplex-sized ADH I enzyme, but let's look at one more example.

Let's visualize the myelin basic protein (MBP) molecule that makes up an important part of the myelin in Venus's brain as a two-story, 3,000 square foot average American home. A sparrow hawk alighting on the roof barely makes any difference at all. Can you see now why scientists who are used to separating proteins primarily by their weights are not able to get their heads around the addition of a formaldehyde molecule? The larger the difference in weight between two molecules the easier it is to separate them.

For instance methanol and ethanol are two very similar molecules chemically, but ethanol weighs twice as much as methanol and, therefore, can be easily separated from it. A protein molecule that has a formaldehyde hawk nesting on it just does not weight much more than one that is formaldehyde-free, making the process of identifying the formaldehyde-modified protein very difficult for scientists, if not impossible, at least until very recently. See Figure 4.12. (Can you find the pigeon nesting on the roof?)

To bring this closer to home, I can look out the window of my office and see a house on pilings that just a week ago was moved from across the street, where its owner no longer wanted it, to a new lot owned by a guy who is a friend of mine and who likes to recycle. I was fascinated by the interesting array of hydraulic and earth-moving equipment that was needed to make the move. The house weighed 59 tons, according to the man who ran the hydraulic pump that lifted it off the foundation.

While I was watching the move I noticed a sea gull landing on the roof of the precariously balanced house in motion. I asked the big burley guy who ran the hydraulics if he noticed the landing. He smiled and said something about the bird leaving a little gift behind that was going to make the moving job a lot more difficult. We all laughed because it was a silly question.

What about That Other Aldehyde: the Ethanol Aldehyde?

It has always been very odd to me that my epidemiological colleagues have absolutely no time for formaldehyde but constantly worry about the dangers of its weakling cousin, acetaldehyde. Acetaldehyde is the aldehyde of ethanol and is a very chemically placid compound on its way to becoming vinegar.

Figure 4.12

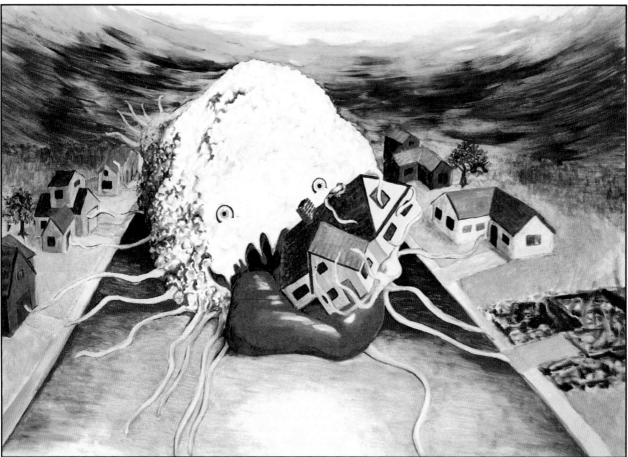

ADH was originally designed to metabolize ethanol, which is identical to methanol except for the fact that ethanol is made up of two carbons instead of one. We will be portraying ethanol also as a pigeon, but because it is larger, we will portray it as a New Zealand giant pigeon, which is twice the size of any pigeons you would see in the USA (see Figure 4.13). ADH removes a hydrogen atom from ethanol, turning it from an alcohol into an aldehyde, just as it turns methanol into formaldehyde. The giant pigeon molecule fits perfectly into the active window of the ADH enzyme, and because the ADH prefers ethanol, the process excludes methanol whenever ethanol is available.

But what about ethanol's aldehyde? It will be twice as big as formaldehyde. Does that mean it could cause even more trouble? The answer is an emphatic no. The aldehyde made out of ethanol is called acetaldehyde and it is a very peaceful molecule compared to its one carbon sister, formaldehyde. Acetaldehyde is quickly and easily turned into energy by all cells in the human. In fact, the danger presented by formaldehyde does not even compare to the peaceful aldehyde from ethanol. The extra carbon of acetaldehyde seems to allow for an additional outlet for the resonance of the electrons of this aldehyde and takes the edge off its bonding power.

We will not give acetaldehyde a persona because it has no bearing on anything we are studying. But what you may find surprising is that the entire epidemiologic and medical community appears to be much more concerned about acetaldehyde than formaldehyde. None of the articles debating the link of increased disease such as breast cancer to increased ADH activity in humans even mentions formaldehyde; acetaldehyde is the aldehyde that concerns them.[216] They are apparently unaware that formaldehyde, a known human carcinogen, can also be manufactured at ADH sites.

Figure 4.13

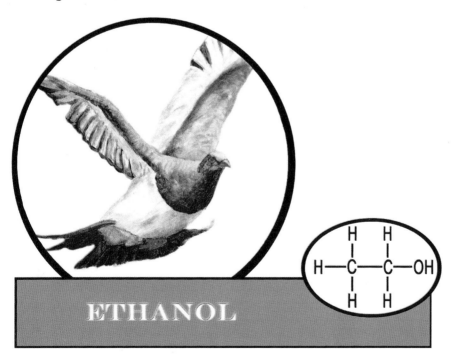

ETHANOL

Chemists will recognize that the behavior of formaldehyde hydrate is due to the resonance between the basic CH_2O and the acidic $CH_2(OH)_2$ structural configuration. Don't let the term "formaldehyde Schiff base" confuse you. In dilute aqueous solution at human body temperature the acidic hydrated form $CH_2(OH)_2$ predominates 99.99 percent of the time. Chemistry considers formaldehyde to be a strong reducing agent, yet it fixes proteins in aqueous solution by an oxidative reaction.[688] This resonance between an acid and base, oxidizer and reducing agent is part of what causes the complex biochemical outcomes of the dilute formaldehyde solutions that occur after methanol is oxidized to formaldehyde hydrate in-situ within the human circulatory system, outside the reach of aldehyde dehydrogenase, which is normally more easily available in the human liver.

Formaldehyde titration lowers the pH of a solution of protein.[594] This along with the lactic acid buildup caused by formaldehyde's ability to stop cellular aerobic oxidation by inhibiting cytochrome oxidase (formaldehyde is 100 times more powerful at this than formate)[676] is most likely responsible for the lowering of the pH of the blood often seen in cases of accidental human methanol poisoning. Formic acid levels have never been able to explain this phenomenon. The entire issue of ascribing formic acid or formate as "the toxic component of methanol poisoning" is ludicrous and amounts to disinformation of the worst kind.

Both these substances are classified by the US Food and Drug Administration as food additives on GRAS (generally regarded as safe) and have lethal doses on the same magnitude as table salt. Although commonly used in the food industry there is no published incidence of death caused by their consumption in the last 100 years. In a safety evaluation of both formic acid and sodium formate done in 1976 by an expert panel of the Federation of American Societies for Experiential Biology for the Food and Drug Administration it was determined that formic acid is a natural constituent of many foods and the tolerance of the human body to large amounts is relatively high with accidental overdoses of 50 grams or more not causing any of the symptoms in humans ascribed to it by the University of Iowa team in their many studies on their supposed monkey model of methanol toxicity[365]

The joint FOA/WHO Expert committee on Food Additives points out in their study that "2-4 grams of sodium formate daily did not produce toxic manifestations in human subjects, even if they were suffering from kidney disease, It has been stated that a daily intake of 2-4 g for therapeutic purposes could be tolerated for months without untoward effects".[678]

Chapter 5

The Silent Battle that Turns Methanol into Disease

A battle is raging in your body now as you read this book. Twenty four hours a day, seven days a week, every second of every minute that you live, your nemesis, methanol, is competing for dominance over your molecular friend, ethanol. The prize is the conjugal attention of the enzyme ADH. At wager is your health and wellbeing. If ethanol prevails, your will be free to fulfill your potential, free from the chronic effects of the diseases of civilization (DOC) and many cancers. If methanol is the victor you will join the 75% of the population of the civilized world to have listed on your death certificate one of the persistent diseases that plagues only the most advanced societies of our planet. The rules of engagement of the tryst between the enzyme and these two alcohols are now known to you.

The first and most important rule of this war, as it is in all wars, is that if the enemy doesn't show up, then no battle will take place. One sip of diet cola poisons you with hundreds of trillions of enemy pigeons, all of which must be kept from turning into Crazy Hawks or damage will be done. Constant vigil is required, for it only takes one of these methanol molecules turning into formaldehyde and finding the right spot at the wrong time to turn a healthy cell into a cancer that may eventually mean your untimely demise.

More usually, the damage is chronic, with the predominant involvement of one or more of the organs listed in Table 5.2. Your own genetics and the distribution of ADH throughout your body will make you more or less susceptible to each of these diseases, but given time and opportunity, the formaldehyde will eventually find your weakness and slowly work to cause disease.

The quality of your life depends on the outcome of this molecular free-for-all and your only defense, once methanol is consumed, is a chemical weapon that is as useful as it is dangerous. Ethanol – that is, the alcohol found in beer, wine, and liquor – is the only weapon you have. If used properly, it will protect you. But this protection is a double-edged sword. If it is overused or misused, it will make things worse…much worse.

As promised, I have explained my position much as it developed through my research over the years. My position has slowly evolved from being a hunch that aspartame contained something that was causing multiple sclerosis, to the present hypothesis that points to methanol as the etiologic agent for all of the DOC. Before we get to the nuts and bolts of specifically what happens in which location of the body that causes each of these DOC, let's review the basics.

Review

Methanol is a natural chemical that is rarely found in fresh foods. The few places where methanol is found in abundance are cigarette smoke, canned fruits and vegetables and their juices, and aspartame-sweetened food products, whose introduction into the food supply in 1981 has been associated with an epidemic of DOC.

The reason Science appears oblivious to the dangers of methanol is due, in part, to the fact that methanol itself isn't dangerous to laboratory animals, who can use it as a food. This is an anomaly due to a human mutation that leaves humans with only one enzyme to metabolize methanol – ADH, which turns it into formaldehyde, a very dangerous molecule known to cause cancer, but undetectable after its release into the human body.

Formaldehyde has all the attributes necessary to cause cancer, activate the immune system, cause tangles in tau protein identical to those in Alzheimer's disease, induce methylation, and otherwise cause birth defects in the areas of the brain known to be damaged in Autism. The only difficulty is that formaldehyde by itself is too reactive to ever reach the areas of the body where these defects need to occur to cause DOC. When ingested, injected or inhaled, it quickly bonds to the nearest proteins and disappears. However, methanol can reach these critical areas and then, under the right conditions, turn into formaldehyde on the spot.

Only one chemical is known to be capable of stopping this scenario from happening; the only cure for methanol poisoning that will prevent it from turning to formaldehyde is ethanol – thus the miracle of the recently discovered U-shaped curve of alcohol consumption. Those who refrain from consuming any alcoholic beverages at all are statistically twice as likely to get Alzheimer's disease, atherosclerosis or lupus erythematosus (SLE) as those who consume one drink a day. What would explain the protective effect of ethanol consumption if these diseases where not being caused by methanol turning into formaldehyde?[586]

The power of the methanol theory of disease causation lies in its simplicity and the undeniable and intuitively compelling links to the health realities of cigarette smoking, the elucidation of the U-shaped curve, and, perhaps most important of all, the link to the increase in DOC incidence in populations poisoned over the last 30 years by the methanol from aspartame.

The cause of DOC by environmental methanol's conversion to formaldehyde within the living body in the absence of ethanol is the only explanation that both survives every logical challenge and makes a perfect fit to the reality of the epidemiology of each of the DOC.

Bad ADH and Good ADH III

When at war, the most vital intelligence relates to the location of enemy weapons. Alcohol dehydrogenase class one (ADH I) is indeed the only weapon of the DOC. The ammunition is those little pigeons (methanol). As you can see, I am using the formal name of ADH. The reason is that this chapter will concern itself with the exact whereabouts of this enzyme in the human body.

The fraternity of scientists who study enzymes have a real problem with naming these vital biochemical factories. Like most other of the medical/scientific groups that spring up around narrow scientific topics, they tend to behave like siblings, twins usually, who have insufficient supervision and eventually develop their own language that no one else can understand. A good example of this the more recent epigenetics investigators, who took it on themselves to rename formaldehyde the "methyl molecule" (more on this in Chapter 12). For now, our problem is that Alcohol Dehydrogenase Class I (ADH) is the official name of the enzyme with which we are most concerned – the one that converts methanol into formaldehyde.

Another important enzyme has the ability to safely destroy the formaldehyde before it can do any harm. This may be what protects many people from developing some forms of the DOC, depending on just how it is distributed in their bodies. This good enzyme is "officially" called Alcohol Dehydrogenase Class Three (ADH III). Why do they name an enzyme that operates on aldehydes an alcohol enzyme? Well, I know the answer to that, but in telling you I will only confuse some readers and it is just not worth it.

To simplify this issue we will do what the enzymologists do. All you need to remember is that from now on I will continue calling the bad enzyme that turns methanol into formaldehyde "ADH." The good enzyme that destroys formaldehyde and turns it into the safe food additive, formic acid, I will call by its official name, "ADH III." I know it sounds a bit confusing, but if you can get it straight the scientific literature will be understandable to you in the future when you have finished this book and are all on your own.

ADH is bad. ADH III is good. Got it!

Chapter 5

Alcohol Consumption

Most ancient cultures know of ethanol and consider it a medicine. The reverence given this natural product by ancient peoples contrasts with its modern classification as a mind altering substance, carcinogen and agent of abuse. Interestingly, we as a culture continue to put a great deal of effort into ethanol's production, distribution and marketing and it is not unusual for governments who have strongly enforced its prohibition to be ridiculed, ignored or on occasion brought down.

Science has recently performed large and well-done epidemiologic studies of the diets of individuals with certain DOC. While analyzing the data they have purely by accident stumbled upon strong, undeniable evidence that abstinence from ethanol consumption is a very bad health choice and can double one's risk of contracting the DOC under investigation. Reading this literature as they very reluctantly release this powerful data makes one feel that it goes against everything that they believe, against perhaps even their religious beliefs.

Not every DOC has been studied for this association, but I believe that it would be a good test for evaluating the candidate diseases for potential methanol origin. The truth now appears to be on the side of those ancient peoples whose power of observation was not overwhelmed by bad science, Big Pharma and religious sentiment. The truth, based on my observations over twenty five years of study, is that ethanol is probably an essential component of the civilized diet. Like all other essential nutrients, it is required only in quantities sufficient to perform its biochemical roll. That role is to protect us from methanol's efforts to turn into formaldehyde.

Ethanol, like biotin and vitamin K, vcan be produced for us naturally by microorganisms in the large intestine; therefore, supplementation may not always be necessary. Like vitamin A, there is a rather narrow consumption that is safe and anything over that can produce poisoning and do damage and, in some cases, cause death. Unlike any other nutrient, ethanol absolutely cannot be stored in the body for later use, meaning daily supplementation or the complete removal of methanol from the diet is required.

The Brain and Alcohol

It is to our good fortune that scientists studying alcoholism have for years put considerable effort into revealing sites of ADH in the brain. Their reason for this has nothing to do with methanol; they are interested only in locating the places where ethanol is metabolized into acetaldehyde. The brain is one of the organs that are seriously damaged in some, but not all alcoholics and no clear explanation for this has been found. Laboratory animals can be fed ethanol or, more likely, be made to breathe high concentrations of ethanol to the point of inebriation for months on end without suffering the kind of brain damage (or liver damage, for that matter) that some human alcoholics suffer as contributing causes of their untimely deaths. This has always been a mystery, but one that medicine has consistently tried to blame on acetaldehyde.

Acetaldehyde, as you know well by now, is a relatively harmless aldehyde that ADH produces from ethanol. Acetaldehyde is produced at the same ADH sites as formaldehyde, but is a much less reactive aldehyde. It is more likely to find ADH III and be converted into vinegar, a substance which every cell in the human body has the ability to put through the citric acid cycle and burn for energy. The medical profession tells the acetaldehyde story as I paraphrase from several sources here:

Acetaldehyde is a highly unstable compound and quickly forms free radical structures which are highly toxic. These free radicals can result in damage to embryonic neural crest cells and can lead to severe birth defects. Prolonged exposure of the kidney and liver to these compounds in chronic alcoholics can lead to severe damage. The literature also suggests that these toxins may have a hand in causing hangovers and alcohol withdrawal.

This is a story that bodes better as a cautionary tale warning against the wages of sinful alcohol consumption than it does as hard science. It is an interesting story that has never been proven using laboratory animals. To the contrary rats have been given 40 proof alcohol solution as their sole source of fluid for up to 11 months with no observable signs of either physical withdrawal or dependence on cessation.[295] It could be made much more accurate merely by substituting the word formaldehyde for acetaldehyde. It would be interesting to see what old time chemists have to say about the instability of acetaldehyde and these "highly toxic" free radicals. Remember the minimum lethal dose of ethanol is identical in both humans and all laboratory animals, so it should be causing similar damage in each species. Why, then, doesn't it?

Of course, our interest in the location of the brain's ADH sites is due to their ability to produce formaldehyde, which, is far more dangerous and more likely to be the cause of much of the damage incessantly blamed by the medical community (who, by the way, have notoriously insufficient training in classical chemistry) on acetaldehyde. This issue might have been put to rest once and for all if it hadn't been for direct intervention of a group of scientists who were hired by Big Pharma to prove that formaldehyde has nothing to do with the consequences of methanol poisoning. We will refer to them as the "Iowa Team" from this point on. Here is an account of just one instance of their meddling with the normal course of scientific discovery.

The Diversion of Dr. Majchrowicz

Many wonder how Big Pharma can literally take over fields of endeavor such as toxicology. The answer is one scientist at a time. This is not accomplished through intimidation, torture or bribery, but rather by the logical extrapolation of the "detail person" concept invented by the pharmaceutical industry and used for years to advertize their wares directly to medical practitioners. The detail girl makes the doctor feel like he is very special. She gives him gifts, buys him a meal and more… sometimes, financially, much more. Soon he feels like he has friends at Big Pharma. Here is one variation that worked to win over a brilliant research scientist who was working on the link between methanol and alcohol withdrawal.[384]

One type of alcoholic, called a "binge drinker," appears to suffer much more serious consequences from alcohol abuse to their liver, kidney, brain and other ADH organs than alcoholics who maintain a consistent consumption of ethanol throughout the day and maintain some ethanol in their blood at all times. The latter form of alcoholics fare much better, health-wise – and in many cases appear to be protected from, say, atherosclerosis – than those who go on binges and abstain from alcohol for stretches of time between bouts of heavy drinking. The real cause of this, as you can probably surmise from what you have learned thus far, is formaldehyde, not acetaldehyde. But how can this be proved?

An acquaintance of mine, now deceased, was very close to proving just that before he was stopped in his tracks by some considerable attention paid to him by Big Pharma. Edward Majchrowicz is a hero of mine – a Polish Jew who, as a boy, escaped the Nazi's overthrow of his country to join the Polish Independent Carpathian Brigade after the start of World War II. He was wounded three times during the Italian campaign and nearly lost his life in street fighting against the Germans to control the Abbey of Monte Casino. He was a free-thinking brilliant researcher who, while working for the National Institute on Alcohol Abuse at the National Institute of Mental Health, detected accumulations of methanol in the blood and urine of alcoholics who were on controlled binges.[134]

Methanol accumulation in the blood does not usually occur under normal conditions because it is removed at a constant rate through urine, sweat and in the breath. However, during prolonged periods of high ethanol consumption, the high concentration of ethanol in the blood competes with the methanol for removal from the body via the lungs and filtration by the kidney and sweat glands. Consequently, both the metabolism and removal of methanol is delayed, and methanol accumulates in the blood of binge alcoholics each day their binge proceeds.

Dr. Majchrowicz had observed over the years that alcoholics who went on binges with high ethanol intake suffered and occasionally died from the more serious effects of alcohol withdrawal. The symptoms of alcohol withdrawal are much more severe than a hangover. They include all the symptoms of methanol poisoning – paresthesia (numbness, tingling, pricking of the skin), extreme headaches, insomnia, depression, anxiety, visual disturbances, seizures, and delirium tremors that can result in death.[387,669] The longer the binge, the more likely the alcoholic might die from the results of cessation of ethanol consumption. The public learned about this recently during the controversy over the untimely death of the jazz singer Amy Winehouse, who at some point was thought to have actually died from alcohol withdrawal.

The very important issue with alcohol withdrawal is that the symptoms do not start immediately when the drinking is stopped, or even after ten to eighteen hours afterwards, when much of the ethanol is gone from the blood. The symptoms start only some time after the blood alcohol level is low enough to allow for the metabolism of methanol to formaldehyde.[133]

Scientists who study alcoholics considered all symptoms to be caused by the withdrawal of alcohol from cells that had become used to its presence, much like what happens during withdrawal from opiates or amphetamines. This theory was severely rebuffed in 1969 when it was reported in the journal *Surgery* that a number of alcoholics who were prone to serious alcohol withdrawal symptoms were treated while severely inebriated with hemodialysis shortly before what should have been the onset of symptoms.[136] Dialysis removes ethanol from the blood very quickly and should have made things much worse if the "withdrawal" theory were correct. The results were stunning. None of the alcoholics experienced any symptoms at all. It is noteworthy that dialysis is also used to remove methanol from the blood as a treatment for severe methanol poisoning.

In order to put this issue to rest, in the early 1970s Edward Majchrowicz designed and conducted an audacious experiment that could never be repeated today. He enlisted nineteen alcoholic inmates from an alcohol rehabilitation facility. Each volunteer had been there long enough to be alcohol-free for some time. Each was admitted into a controlled hospital environment and allowed to get inebriated and stay that way for up to 14 days. Their blood was sampled often and tested for the major players – ethanol, methanol and acetaldehyde.

The levels of acetaldehyde barely changed during the entire experiment. Blood methanol levels rose continuously from a level of less than 1 milligram per kilogram of blood on the first day until it reached an average of between 20-40 milligrams per kilogram ten days into the binge. After the drinking stopped, it took between 10 to 18 hours for the remaining ethanol in their blood to be cleared. The highest levels of methanol were measured at the moment the drinking stopped and they did not change statistically until the ethanol in the blood began to approach zero. At that point, the methanol began to be metabolized by the ADH into formaldehyde. As the methanol level diminished in the bloodstream the withdrawal signs and symptoms began appearing. It took between 6 to 8 hours for the methanol to finally return to background levels.

The most severe signs and symptoms of the alcohol withdrawal syndrome were observed in those subjects whose blood methanol concentrations were highest and blood ethanol concentrations were approaching zero level. The temporal correlation between the withdrawal signs and symptoms corresponded more closely to methanol rather than to ethanol clearance from the blood.[133]

Majchrowicz had finally settled two important issues. Methanol, not acetaldehyde, caused alcohol withdrawal symptoms and, more importantly, he gave us a reconfirmation of the small amount of methanol that can cause serious symptoms and occasionally even death in the human. While the young black girl who gave her life set the minimum lethal dose of methanol at 0.089 grams per kilogram, Majchrowicz reinforced that 0.040 grams per kilogram can cause harm to humans, with occasionally a deadly outcome.[384]

Table 5.1
Minimal Lethal Dose of Methanol
Alcohol Withdrawal - Majchrowwicz

Species	Dose: Grams/Kg	Grams to Kill 70kg Male
Rat[17]	9.0	630
Dog[17]	9.0	630
Rabbit[17]	7.0	490
Monkey[17]	6.0	420
Man[204]	0.089	6
Man[134]	0.040	3

Lethal dose of methanol in the above animals and man is 7.0 grams/kg
The lethal dose of salt is 6.0 grams/kg

This reconfirmation of the small amount of methanol that could cause serious injury, prolonged symptomology and, occasionally, death was vital to reinforce the exquisite sensitivity of humans to this dangerous natural substance.

Why does no one use Edward's work to warn of the danger of small doses of methanol?

Twenty years or so after this work was published, as I sat in my office at Arizona State University, I received my first phone call from Dr. Edward Majchrowicz. As he introduced himself, I took an immediate liking to him. He sounded almost exactly like a man who was my mentor in high school and who had saved my life during a serious laboratory accident years before, my high school chemistry instructor, Dr. Oscar Weisberg. Edward's daughter had seen a segment of a special done by the CBS Evening News that featured me holding up a small flask of methanol and declaring it was the lethal dose and asking why anyone in their right mind would add it to soft drinks. Edward was calling to talk to me about methanol.

We talked for hours, after which we promised to send each other reprints of our work and talk again. I don't know how many times we spoke, but soon I felt comfortable enough to ask him some personal questions. I found that he was retired but still kept his interest in the literature. When I felt the time was appropriate, I asked him the question that I had wanted to ask since I first read his seminal article on methanol, which I describe above.

"Edward," I asked, "why didn't you continue with your methanol work?" After a long silence on the other end of the phone, he finally started telling his story, which I will relate as I recall it. His work had been well-received, at some point he was contacted by a scientist who, he said, introduced himself as the world expert in methanol metabolism. It wasn't long before he was invited to attend a very special "invitation only" seminar given by the Iowa Team. He was treated like a king, he said. He didn't have to pay for anything and they all treated him with deference. The way he described the encounter was reminiscent of what I had heard about time share sales encounters.

He continued that they had put up a very convincing series of presentations to show him the error of his ways: that methanol could in no way do this kind of damage, and no one had proven it turned into formaldehyde. He said they showed him their laboratories, which were fitted with the best equipment that money could buy. In short, they made him feel like a bit of a fool who was working in an area somewhat outside his field. To show that they "respected his approach and valued his thinking," they offered to assist him with some of his pet projects that needed funding… and they did what they could to keep him busy working on other projects, including the publication of an edited work that was to be his pride and joy.

I listened in silence during his telling of the story, only asking a question for clarity every now and then. When he had concluded, I hesitated for a bit longer than was comfortable while I gathered the courage to ask whether they had ever mentioned that they happened to be in bed with the company that was trying every trick in the book to get a methanol-containing sweetener approved by the FDA.

He replied sadly, "No. They said nothing about that connection." He went on to say that had he known, he would never have gone to their seminar in the first place. We said goodbye, and as I look back on that exchange, I think I might well have overstepped my bounds, for I never heard from him again.

The REAL Lethal Dose of Methanol

Let us determine your personal lethal dose of methanol. This will be easier than you think. Just go back to the methanol toxicity chart and take the higher of the two numbers – 0.089 grams per kilogram. Your weight in kilograms is whatever your weight is in pounds divided by 2.2 pounds. For a five foot seven inch tall male with a weight of 112 pounds, or 51 kilograms, multiply 51 times 0.089 and you will get 4.54 grams of methanol. That is the minimum lethal dose for you For the sake of simplicity, we will assume you are our sample adult male and round that figure up to 5 grams, which equals one teaspoon of methanol.

Now let's take a look at what Dr. Majchrowicz discovered in his comprehensive study to learn the concentrations of methanol that cause the sometimes deadly symptoms of alcohol withdrawal. From the same methanol toxicity chart, take the number that represents the highest concentration of methanol in his patient that had the very worst withdrawal symptoms[133] in his study. That would be 0.04 grams of methanol per kg of body weight. Multiply that by your weight, or in our case, a 51 kg adult male. That is just under 2 grams, or less than a half of a teaspoon of methanol, to guarantee that an adult will feel the very serious withdrawal symptoms (and possibly death) of methanol poisoning.

This is the amount of methanol in 20 liters of carbonated orange soda sweetened with aspartame.[1] This demonstrates very clearly how close the actual consumption of methanol from ordinary and casual consumption of diet products approaches toxic consumption levels. If Dr. Majchrowicz numbers had been used to determine the safe consumption levels of diet products (they should have been, since they are the only numbers that were derived from human studies) then at the very most no one could be allowed to consume more than one hundredth the minimum dose know to cause harm, any harm. The Majchrowicz numbers are high since they represent very serious harm. If we use them anyway as the criteria, then *the maximum allowed consumption of aspartame for an average adult male would be that contained in one half a can of diet orange soda or one can of diet cola per day*. A child would be restricted to a few tablespoons of such beverages. This criterion would have prevented aspartame from use in foods no matter who was made director of the Food and Drug Administration. Is it any wonder, then, that the population has reacted in such a disastrous way to the forced introduction of additional methanol into the world's food supply?

The symptoms experienced by members of the population who consume diet drinks were investigated by the Centers For Disease Control. The following symptoms were some of those listed in that study: paresthesia

Table 5.2: Target Organs of Methanol Toxicity

Methanol Target Organ	ADH 1 Site (reference)	Formaldehyde's Potential Target
Brain	Vascular tissue (218, 220)	Tau Protein
	Vascular tissue (218, 220)	Myelin Basic Protein
	Vascular tissue (218, 220)	Vascular Lining
Eye	Found with retinol dehydrogenase	Retina
Blood Vessels	Intima, media (220) Aorta	LDL
Skin	Fibroblast (221, 638)	Fibroblast
	Fibroblast (221, 638)	Fibroblast
	Skin and Perivascular	All ADH Organs
Breast	Epithelial (357)	Epithelial
Kidney	Epithelial Tubule (637, 640, 503)	Epithelial
		Epithelial
Bone	Synovial Fibroblast (563, 514)	Synovial Fibroblast
Pancreas	Langerhans Islets (637, 503)	Insulin Production
Lung	Fibroblast (221, 503)	Fibroblast
	Fibroblast (221, 503)	Fibroblast
Fetus	None in placenta (503)	DNA Methylation
	(503, 640)	Liver, Lung, Kidney
Liver	Highest in Body (503)	Various

(numbness, tingling, pricking of the skin), extreme headaches, hallucinations, insomnia, depression, anxiety, visual disturbances, and seizures.[58] The final report confessed that the investigators could not find a "constellation of symptoms" that would point to any of the components of the sweetener even though the Majchrowicz articles had been published 11 years earlier. One can only wonder how such a lie could stand for so long a time.

Where Methanol Turns into Disease: the Front Lines of the Battle for Your Life

Table 5.2 contains a great deal of information and leads you toward a good deal more. Figures 5.1 and 5.2 on the following pages show where these diseases manifest in the human body. The references that are presented tie together not only the location of ADH throughout the human body, they also reveal compelling evidence, such as the links to smoking, the U-shaped curve of alcohol consumption, and aspartame consumption that implicate methanol as the cause of various diseases that originate at these locations. This important chart brings together the evidence that will help us make a case for methanol as the etiologic cause for many DOC. We will discuss the information presented in these articles as we discuss the diseases specifically in the coming chapters. The numbers in parenthesis represent reference numbers for the scientific articles that reveal this information. These references can be found on my website (www.whilesciencesleeps.com). If you like reading science, I suggest you read them all.

(Bad ADH Sites)

Disease Manifestation	Incidence ↑ Last 35 Years	Reference Incidence	U-Shaped Curve	Smoking Methanol	Aspartame Causation
Alzheimer's	↑10,000% (100X)	540, 533	531, 534	643	
Multiple Sclerosis	↑100% Women higher	77, 214		332	586
Headache, Seizures	↑	471, 181		376	471, 328
Cancer Glioblastoma	↑200%	329			
Macular Degeneration	↑30-40%	668		667,3,37	
Atherosclerosis	↑	532	485	345	
Skin Cancer	↑400% Young women	95		645	229
Dermatitis	↑			227, 437	328,545, 630
Lupus (SLE)	↑300% Women higher	536	73	73	228
Adenocarcinoma	↑50% Adenocarcinoma	250, 193		242, 574	50,48,197
Kidney Cancer	↑200%	577, 646		652	50
Kidney Function ↑	↑100% (Aspartame link)	577, 646		651	588, 659
Rheumatoid Artritis	↑After decades of decline	635	295, 642	332	
Type II Diabetes	↑1000% Adolescent Females	629	650	648, 647	647
COPD	↑100%	523, 641		345	
Adenocarcinoma	↑With decreased smoking	655		655, 656	657
Autism other Terata	↑2500% (25X)	525		644	159, 659
Preterm Delivery	↑	653	654	654	617
Hepatic Cancer	↑300%	577		332, 345	657

Figure 5.1

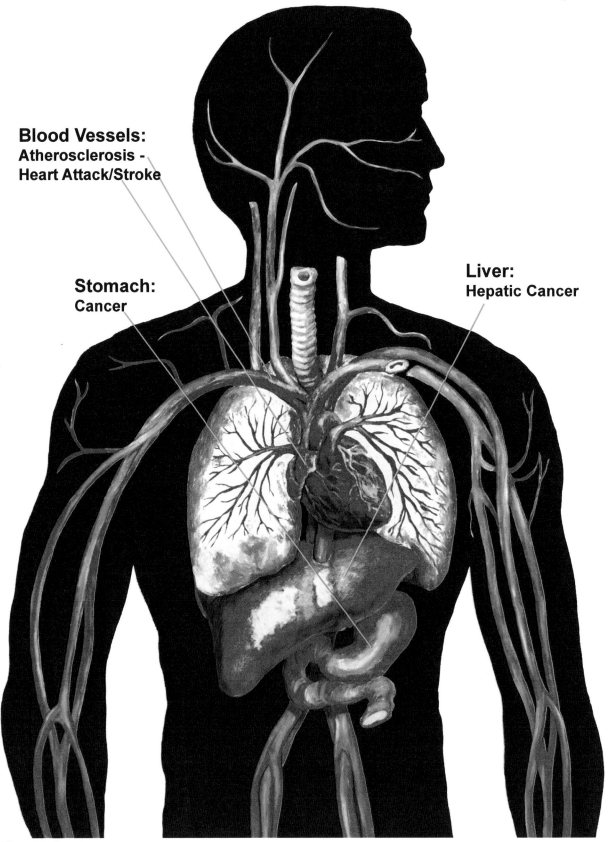

Blood Vessels:
Atherosclerosis -
Heart Attack/Stroke

Stomach:
Cancer

Liver:
Hepatic Cancer

Figure 5.2

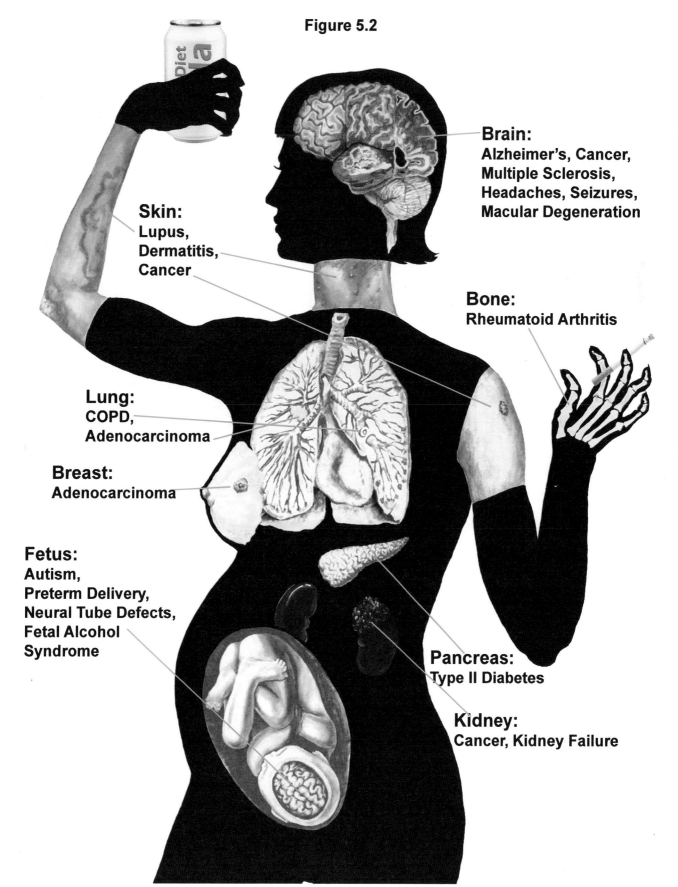

Brain:
Alzheimer's, Cancer,
Multiple Sclerosis,
Headaches, Seizures,
Macular Degeneration

Skin:
Lupus,
Dermatitis,
Cancer

Bone:
Rheumatoid Arthritis

Lung:
COPD,
Adenocarcinoma

Breast:
Adenocarcinoma

Fetus:
Autism,
Preterm Delivery,
Neural Tube Defects,
Fetal Alcohol
Syndrome

Pancreas:
Type II Diabetes

Kidney:
Cancer, Kidney Failure

Chapter 5

Chapter 6
How Methanol Kills

Acute Methanol Poisoning

All poisons can kill with the consumption of one large single dose, called an acute dose, or over a longer period of time, with a series of smaller doses, called a chronic dose. Often the results and symptoms of the two types of dosing can be quite different. Methanol is the only poison that has both a high and low acute dose that will both kill humans. The large dose causes death by the "solvent effect," and a very much lower acute dose causes a disaster that we will discuss below. The details of the mechanism which methanol uses to kill following the consumption of a single lethal dose will make it easier to understand how it may cause disease over a lifetime of chronic poisoning. We will explore the puzzle of why the symptoms of both acute and chronic poisoning are often the same, yet the visible damage done to tissue may vary considerably over time. It all boils down to common sense. You already know enough methanol chemistry at this point in the book to be able to follow the logic of how methanol harms human tissue.

Learning from the evolution of the unfortunate outcome of someone who has died from a single dose of methanol will allow you to garner some important insights into the power of this highly unusual poison. In Chapter Three, I described the last breath of an acutely poisoned victim, but a great deal occurs in the days leading up to that tragic ending. An "intercranial catastrophe" is what Dr. Stuart Schneck of the Department of Neurology of the University of Colorado Medical Center calls acute methyl alcohol poisoning.[21] He proceeds to explain how methanol attacks the visual apparatus, the central nervous system, the gastrointestinal and circulatory systems, and the respiratory tract. You can understand the logic behind this because these are where we find ADH – and, after a methanol poisoning, formaldehyde.

An Experiment to Help Understand Methanol Poisoning

Methanol and ethanol have a great deal in common. If you always keep in mind our bird counterparts of these two alcohols it will be a lot easier for you to visualize the *what* and *where* of methanol poisoning. Remember, ethanol is the big New Zealand pigeon and methanol is the New York City pigeon. You might be thinking the difference is negligible, and if the two were not side by side you might even be hard-pressed to tell one from the other. That is, in fact, exactly the way they behave within your body. The natures of both, except for their eventual toxicity, are really *almost* identical, save for size, and even that does not become important until the two compete for ADH. In fact, the average person would not know the difference between the two if he or she drank a shot glass of either – at least not for the first 24 hours.

A regulation shot glass of either alcohol contains 1.5 ounces. That's exactly three tablespoons, or nine teaspoons. The methanol literature that was written before the advent of the Methanol Institute tells us that one teaspoon of methanol has caused permanent blindness. If you recall, the young black girl from Chapter Three died within days after consumption of only one tablespoon of a 40% methanol solution. Most vodka, brandy and Scotch are 40% ethanol, which would give them a proof value of double that, namely, 80 proof. This is why those unscrupulous scoundrels who counterfeit them using methanol will use the same percentage. Later on when we hear about the advantages of taking one alcoholic drink a day, keep in mind that the literature is talking about the equivalent of one regulation shot glass of a 40% ethanol product.

If you are reading this book in the privacy of your own home and are neither an alcoholic nor pregnant, nor have any other reason not to drink alcohol, I invite you to perform the following little experiment with me now, unless you've eaten in the past two hours (this experiment is best performed on an empty stomach). When you're ready to start, grab a kitchen timer or some other timing device and set it where you can see it while you are reading. Now, find yourself a regulation shot glass or something that will let you measure out 1.5 ounces of an 80 proof alcoholic beverage of choice. I'm choosing brandy myself, but vodka, gin, scotch, or other selection will do just fine. I will wait here while you round up the necessary supplies. Don't worry – this won't hurt one bit!

You're back? We are now going to "toss down" our shot and then start the timer. Yes, yes – something right out of an old western saloon scene. Here goes: swallow, cough, cough! Now, on with the timer. It has been 40 seconds and I don't feel anything but a tickle going slowly down my throat. Some of the alcohol is already beginning to be metabolized by the ADH in my stomach lining. Being a man, I have considerably more ADH than most women, yet the fact is that because of the very high dose, only a small percentage of ethanol will be lost to my stomach lining.

It has been four minutes now and I feel no different than I did before this started, except for a warm feeling in the stomach area caused by the slight irritation of the high concentration of alcohol.

By seven minutes, I am starting to feel just a little light headed, and while the warm feeling is still in my stomach it also feels like it is traveling down my digestive tract.

At eight minutes I can tell you for sure that ethanol has made it into my brain. Had the alcohol I consumed been methanol, the travel time would have been a little less, and the lightheadedness would likely be less as well. I do not plan on testing that, but in general, the differences would be very minor.

It has been 12 minutes now, and I am definitely on the way to feeling the full solvent effect of the ethanol. Why am I feeling lightheaded? This is a very important question, and the answer will probably surprise you. It is not because the alcohol is being metabolized, not at all. The solvent effect causes the euphoria by the alcohol interfering with how some of my brain cells interact, and it will last as long as the concentration of the ethanol is maintained in my bloodstream.

Fourteen minutes, and now my typing is getting really bad. How do those cowboys in the westerns do it? I would be on the floor after five or six of these.

The important thing that we are learning is that these little alcohol molecules get into the bloodstream and past the liver in a very short period of time. Though the literature tells us the liver has a large supply of ADH, these enzymes have very little initial impact on the alcohol that passes through the liver the first time. Essentially all of the ethanol in that shot glass is now past my liver and wandering around my body on a route that will take it through all of my organs and back to my heart every ten minutes or so.

At the 20 minute mark, every cell in my body now contains some of the ethanol from that shot. Had we consumed methanol it would now be on the lookout for unoccupied ADH, and a deadly game of musical chairs would have already begun.[586] Some of the alcohol is already leaving my body via my breath, which is where I might get into trouble if stopped by the police and am required to take a breathalyzer test.

What is important to understand here is that at every location in my body where a supply of ADH can be found, the ethanol is now being metabolized into acetaldehyde. By the end of the day, it will be the liver that most likely will remove the majority of ethanol from my blood, and in doing so, it will produce nothing from the ethanol that will damage the other organs of my body. Dr. Majchrowicz showed this in his study.[134] Alcoholics consuming over a quart of ethanol a day had very little acetaldehyde put back into their bloodstreams. We might expect exactly the same result had the alcohol I consumed been methanol. The formaldehyde produced when methanol is metabolized by ADH in my liver would never have made it out of my liver, and even if it had, it would never have made it to my brain. The danger, however, comes when the ADH located within the various *other* organs of the body metabolize methanol in locations where the resulting formaldehyde has the opportunity to inflict tissue damage.

Both these aldehydes can be turned into acids by the liver. In the case of acetaldehyde, that acid would be vinegar. Vinegar is not harmful. Every cell in the human body very easily metabolizes vinegar into energy, and its toxicity is very low, much like the formic acid made by the liver from formaldehyde. Our concern about damage to the brain and the other organs, resulting in the various DOC, need not extend to the liver. While the liver can be damaged by both ethanol and methanol, its entire purpose is to give its all to defend the rest of the body. In short, nothing comes from the liver that can cause the DOC.

The damage that leads to the DOC comes from the methanol that is metabolized by the ADH located within the other organs. Significantly, the damage only occurs when no ethanol can be found in the bloodstream – a situation which, by the way, won't be happening in my brain or yours for at least six hours now. The ADH is being kept busy metabolizing the ethanol, which it prefers, and ignoring the methanol, which is harmless when left alone. Finally, after 45 minutes, I can feel the euphoria beginning to wear off. That means the ADH throughout my body is removing ethanol from my bloodstream and metabolizing it to acetaldehyde, and in so doing is reducing the concentration of ethanol in my blood, lowering the magnitude of the solvent effect on my brain.

Using Ethanol to Protect from Methanol

Ethanol is methanol's only antidote. When a modern emergency room admits an individual who is even suspected of consuming methanol, the first order of business it to get the individual intoxicated.[141] Fortunately, most of you will never suffer from acute methanol poisoning. You do, however, take in methanol whenever you smoke, consume a product containing aspartame, eat canned vegetables and fruits, or otherwise ingest those products listed in Chapter Two. Methanol presents the toxin; ethanol provides the antidote.

Only a very low level of ethanol can provide the protection you need against methanol, a level so low as to cause no feeling of intoxication at all. The regulation shot of brandy that we downed contained 14 grams of pure ethanol. The question is just how long will that ethanol remain in our bloodstream and protect us from methanol's conversion to formaldehyde? The general rule of thumb, in case you wonder how long you should avoid driving without risking arrest for driving while intoxicated, is that your body can process about one regulation shot of alcohol an hour. In reality, that 14 gram dose of alcohol remains in the blood stream longer than one hour, and in fact, you can actually stretch it to last all day.

Alcohol metabolism follows one of the most basic rules of chemistry, first put to pen by the chemist Henry Le Châtelier. Le Châtelier's principle tells us that any change in the status quo will produce an opposite reaction in the system so changed. So the more ethanol you put into your bloodstream, the faster the rate at which your body will metabolize it. If you consume five or six regulation shots of brandy, for example, then the concentration of ethanol in your blood stream will be high enough that you will burn about a shot an hour. The one shot that constituted our experiment would give us a much lower starting concentration, thus elevating the level of alcohol in our bloodstream for 4 to 6 hours, and perhaps even more. We know this because of the good work done by a man who at first didn't believe that ethanol could be manufactured in the human gut naturally by bacteria.

David Lester was a biochemist whose specialty was the study of alcoholism. He was frustrated by the fact that often patients who claimed not to consume alcohol (teetotalers) would be found to have small amounts of ethanol in their bloodstream. He performed experiments to determine the rate that the body metabolizes small amounts of ethanol such as found in a teaspoon of brandy. We now know that not only can the gut manufacture ethanol but that it can proceed so quickly as to cause the rare auto-brewery syndrome,[186] in which the gut turns dietary carbohydrate into enough ethanol to inebriate. Try to explain that one to your boss! Lester's work showed that if ethanol is introduced into the body slowly instead of throwing it down in shots, an average adult male weighing 154 pounds (70 kg.) would burn ethanol off at a rate as low as 0.79 grams and hour.[173] This could conceivably stretch out the 14 grams of ethanol in one regulation shot as protection from methanol metabolism for over 17 hours.

Now we probably can't stretch it out all that far because that would require a very slow alcohol drip into our veins or, ideally, a perfect micro flora in our guts that would produce a little ethanol all through the day and night. Some people may indeed have this perfect micro flora, but no one has studied this. In my article in the journal *Medical Hypothesis* I suggest that ethanol vapor in the air is very quickly absorbed into the blood by the lungs. We can make use of a vaporizer that would carefully and very accurately put ethanol into the room air in such a way as to keep a consistent level of ethanol in the bloodstream of those breathing that air day and night.[586] That probably sounds strange, but someday when the importance of ethanol is more generally recognized, such a thing will be practical. For now, there is a more practical way that you can get the most protection from methanol from your one alcoholic drink a day.

Thanks to Dr. Lester, here is what I do to help stretch the protection from that one alcoholic drink the U-shaped curve suggests we have each day. Every morning when I wake up I fill a container with the best water I can find. For every quart or liter of water I add a standard tablespoon of 80 proof vodka. I drink this water throughout the day. If I know that I am going out to a party or for some other reason I will be having an alcoholic beverage that day I drink water without the alcohol. I try to consume three liters of water a day, which provides my one standard alcoholic drink a day dosed in such a way as to keep the level of alcohol in the blood as long as possible. I have done this for the last ten years or so and have had no negative results.

You must never ever drink more than one standard alcoholic drink a day if you are a woman and two for men without risking putting yourself squarely on the wrong side of the U-shaped curve. If you become pregnant or are younger than the minimum drinking age of your country of residence and, therefore, can have no ethanol then you must try as best you can to completely avoid methanol (see Chapter 2). In case you are concerned about the cost of this ethanol supplementation, at one drink a day, a 1.75 liter bottle of 80 proof vodka will last one person more than a month. This shouldn't cause your neighbors to talk.

Let's use what we have learned from the above experiment to run through the entire course of an acute fatal overdose of methanol. What happens on a molecular level that can take a single dose of methanol and turn it into a homicide? Once finished, we will review a real methanol homicide. ADH is very reluctant to metabolize methanol into formaldehyde even under the most favorable of conditions, methanol takes over five times longer to be metabolized by ADH than ethanol;[122] therefore, a dose of methanol can be expected to stay in the bloodstream longer than an equal dose of ethanol.

The Lethal Dose of Methanol

The consumption of one regulation shot of a 40% solution of methanol by almost anyone would guarantee a slow and painful death that might take days or even weeks. At about three times the minimum lethal dose for a 150 pound man, the only way to save your life would be a combination of ethanol and dialysis to suck the methanol from your bloodstream. What would be the sequence of events if there were no treatment? Recall our experiment above with the regulation shot of brandy. For the first 8 to 48 hours the outward effect on your body would be exactly the same for either alcohol. A mysterious latent period follows the consumption of methanol, a time ranging between 8 and 48 hours when no symptoms of the poisoning are evident.[171] The scientific literature is at a loss when it comes to explaining this latent period, and so much else about methanol. But let me try to explain why I believe this happens.

Gut fermentation would never produce enough ethanol to prevent this large dose of methanol from immediately being serviced by every ADH enzyme in the entire body. You remember how quickly the ethanol got into our brain. We began to feel its solvent effect in less than 8 minutes. If we had instead ingested methanol, formaldehyde would have begun being produced almost immediately in the liver, the brain, the arteries and the veins of all of the organ systems containing ADH, and yet we would have experienced absolutely no symptoms for another eight to 48 hours. Why? The answer lies in what formaldehyde must do to kill. The symptoms of methanol poisoning will help us understand the process. But first we must explain why all attempts to reproduce the symptoms of methanol poisoning (except for the acidification of the blood called acidosis) by administration of formaldehyde have been unsuccessful.[458] The simple answer is that these other symptoms are primarily caused by brain damage. The only way to get formaldehyde past the blood brain barrier and into the brain is by the use of the Trojan horse, methanol. Formaldehyde is far too reactive, by itself, to enter a living brain with an intact blood brain barrier.

Table 6.1
General Symptoms of Methanol Poisoning

Headache [21]
Epigastric pain [211]
Memory loss and amnesia [21]
Excruciating upper abdominal pain [16]
Pain in the limbs [122]
Severe apprehension [21]
Massive cerebral damage [16]
Edema of the brain [444]
Elevations of lactate acid and pyruvic acid in blood [21]
Most had acidosis [414]
Shortness of breath even with minimal exertion [670]
Most had labored breathing [414]
Respiratory failure while severely acidotic [414]
Complaint of breathlessness even if acidosis is not pronounced. [215]
Blurred vision [444]
Damage around the macular area. [416]
Vision diminished over six to eight weeks. [416]
Tingling and paresthesia in the extremities. [21]
Mental confusion [21]
Hallucinations, delirium and maniacal behavior [444]

Being a very reactive molecule, formaldehyde cannot travel far from the ADH where it is produced. If it is to cause the demise of a full grown human with an exquisite immune system and substantial biomass it must be able to leverage what power it does have to disable enzymes and garner the unwitting assistance of the victim's own immune response. This takes time. Determining culpability as to which of these modalities was finally responsible for death would be much like determining the exact cause of an elephant dying from the onslaught of a cadre of army ants; too much is going at one time to make that precise a determination. Since formaldehyde itself disappears, it is to the symptoms we must look for clues to the *how* of methanol poisoning.

Hospital Admission

Admission to a hospital after consumption of the above toxic dose of methyl alcohol would be a cause for great concern. Even today, the prognosis for methanol alcohol poisoning is not encouraging, with a mortality expectation of between twenty and fifty percent[122] in even the most advanced medical facility.[672] The long term sequelae (pathological condition resulting from poisoning) is also grim, with one recent report of a patient dying from cerebral brain damage fully one year after initial recovery from his other symptoms following a single toxic methanol encounter.[673] Permanent motor dysfunction[137] and lifelong visual sequelae are quite common from methanol poisoning.[680] A recent six year follow-up study of a large methanol poisoning outbreak revealed that not only did all the patients who left hospital with sequelae still have neurological and visual complications, but of those who were originally released without sequelae, 36% went on to develop serious visual complications and another 36% were diagnosed with polyneuropathy, unstable walking, sensory loss, and other neurological disorders. The most significant findings were optical nerve atrophy, temporal pallor of the optic nerve head, concentrical reduction of the visual field, and loss of visual acuity.[672]

The Symptoms of Acute Methanol Poisoning

It is important that we take the time to explain every symptom of methanol poisoning even though not every individual who is poisoned will report having experienced all of these symptoms or outcomes. Each symptom mentioned here is referenced to a reliable scientific source. I will begin with the major classes of symptoms now, and explore others later on in the book when they can be used in context. I want to encourage you to pursue any you don't understand at greater depth in a medical dictionary or textbook.

Methanol poisoning is indistinguishable from the severe alcohol withdrawal suffered by alcoholics, which includes vomiting, delirium, various degrees of vision loss,[415] and occasionally maniacal behavior, convulsions, coma for several days, and death from respiratory collapse.[444] The tables that follow provide a good cross section of the symptoms that are important indications of the underlying tissue damage associated with methanol poisoning. I have listed commonly reported general symptoms in Table 6.1. The visual symptoms, all of which on occasion have been reported in association with the onset of multiple sclerosis, are presented in Table 6.2. Other specific symptoms that methanol poisoning shares with multiple sclerosis are listed in Table 6.3. I have devoted an entire chapter to MS and believe that when you have finished reading it, you will be convinced that MS, like so many other DOC, is a result of chronic methanol poisoning. Finally, Table 6.4 shows the common organ damage found during autopsies of ones who died from acute methanol poisoning. If you desire a more in-depth knowledge of these outcomes, please refer to the original articles. All are found on my website (http://whilesciencesleeps.com) using the reference number provided.

Table 6.2
Visual symptoms of acute methanol poisoning

Permanent blindness [3]
Temporary blindness [163]
Blindness of only one eye [674]
Multiple transient blindness over months [163]
Blurred or indistinct vision [16]
Loss green color sense, red, yellow and blue successively [416]
A play of scintillating colors before the eyes [414]
Flashes of grayness whitish or yellow [11]
Perception of dancing spots, vision as in a snow storm [21]
"Like stepping out into a snow field" [670]
Seeing the wind. [16]
Skim over the eyes [16]
Brightness [16]
A snowstorm [16]
Flashes of grayness whitish or yellow [11]

How does Methanol's Formaldehyde Kill?

The scientific paper concerning the couple who committed suicide by drinking pure formaldehyde solution will now resonate with some impact.

Those poor souls averaged over a month to die from just one dose of formaldehyde. The damage done by a little formaldehyde molecule attaching to a protein or DNA molecule is subtle and often requires time to eventually cause death. When a person drinks a lethal dose of methanol, it is the formaldehyde produced in the brain that will eventually cause death. The damage caused by the formaldehyde produced from methanol within the body is potentially much greater than the damage caused by formaldehyde that is swallowed because it is produced deeper within the tissues of the body, especially the brain. Pure formaldehyde that was swallowed could not possibly travel to the deep tissues before being blocked by the body's natural defense mechanisms. The only way formaldehyde can penetrate the defenses of the human body is if it is manufactured from a seemingly safe substance after having already passed through those defenses. Methanol metabolized in the liver will do some damage there, with excess formaldehyde being converted primarily into formic acid, which would be the very best outcome for the rest of the body.

The scientific literature recounts the results of numerous autopsies done on individuals who have died from acute methanol poisoning. The findings invariably show damage to the same group of organs: the brain and eyes, followed by the lungs, stomach, liver, kidneys, circulatory system, and occasionally the pancreas.[4153] We now know that all of these organs contain stores of ADH, which is required to produce formaldehyde from methanol. It is always, however, damage to the brain to which we can ultimately contribute the death of the individual. None of the damage reported to these other organs at autopsy appears sufficient to cause death.

Only two mechanisms act to kill an individual poisoned by a single large dose of methanol: the deactivation of the brain's

Table 6.3
Symptoms of Methanol Poisoning Shared with Multiple Sclerosis

Myelin damage sparing axons [148]
Temporary Blindness [163]
Astroglial hyperplasia [119]
Shooting pains [122]
Paresthesia [21]
Vertigo [16]
Unsteady Gait [672]
Tremulousness [119]
Blindness in one eye [674]
Dizziness [16]
Optic Neuritis [148]
Amblyopia [453]
Scotoma (loss of central vision) [37]
Headache [21]
Insomnia [59]
Spasticity [384]
Urticaria (skin) [228]
Weakness [16]
Seizures [148]
Retrolaminar demyelinating optic neuropathy [226]

Table 6.4
Symptoms of methanol poisoning found at autopsy

Cerebral edema with hemorrhages [16]
Extensive perivascular edema [416]
Epicardial hemorrhages [16]
Vascular injury [16]
Marked increase of the connective tissue around the blood vessels [15]
Pancreatic necrosis [16]
Small hemorrhages in most pancreatic tissue [16]
Congestion of lungs [16]
Lungs showed marginal emphysema with petechial hemorrhages [416]
Stomach exhibited hemorrhages [416]
Kidneys were uniformly increased in size [416]
Most of the tubules of the kidney revealed extensive degeneration [416]
Generalized and intensified postmortem rigidity and cyanosis [416]

power supply by formaldehyde and the swelling of the brain caused by the individual's own immune system.

Death by Power Outage: Formaldehyde Goes in, the Lights Go out, the Acidity Goes UP

Those who recover from methanol poisoning always complain of marked fatigue and malaise, pain in the limbs, and visual disturbances that may persist for some time afterward.[122] These are all symptoms caused by formaldehyde's direct attack on the enzymes that make life possible by allowing us to turn food into ATP. Adenosine-triphosphate (ATP) is the major energy source for every mechanical function of the body. No movement, nerve impulse or thought process can go on without having ATP to fuel the biochemical machine that makes it work. When the ATP content of brain cells go below a certain minimum the individual goes into a coma and some time after this bodily functions cease to the point where life is impossible.

The labels of all methanol-containing consumer products in the civilized world, with the unconscionable exception of foods and drugs, are required to have a warning that the contents can cause permanent blindness. Blindness is the condition for which methanol is most known. The term "blind drunk" refers to the down-and-out alcoholic who takes his life in his own hands and mixes in a little methanol to help "stretch" his expensive ethanol supplies. The ones who live will often experience many of the visual symptoms reported earlier in Table 5.2 and, as noted, some will succumb to blindness.

Another symptom, less well known to the public but equal in importance to emergency room physicians, is acidosis, a condition in which the acidity of the blood increases and its pH drops. If you have ever read the book *Andromeda Strain*, a science fiction account of an experimental virus that escapes from a research laboratory and seems destined to destroy the human race, you might recall the opening scene. An expedition of fully protected scientists comes upon a town where the virus has killed the entire population, save two survivors – a drunk going through alcoholic withdrawal and an infant who just won't stop screaming. To make a very long story short, this virus turns out to be sensitive to acid, and the only way to kill it is to lower the pH of the blood. The alcoholic survived because he was going through alcohol withdrawal, and the methanol toxicity was putting him into acidosis. The infant was terrified and hyperventilating, which also causes acidosis.

Recall from Chapter Three that the University of Iowa team used this approach, namely, imposing conditions that would induce severe stress and fear, to produce acidosis in the blood of their experimental monkeys.[132] Outside of such imposed conditions, acidosis is extremely rare in animal methanol poisoning.

These two symptoms are inseparable and are caused by the direct action of formaldehyde attaching to and damaging a group of enzymes that allow individual cells to produce life-giving energy. Here is exactly how it works. When formaldehyde attaches to enzymes it changes them – not by much, just an added carbon here and there – but the change is always destructive, and if the enzyme is a very important one that the body calls upon to do a very specific job, then these changes may make it impossible for the enzyme to serve that function. This is exactly the case for some of the key enzymes that are responsible for respiration. Respiration charges up our ATP batteries and gives us the energy to live and breathe. In Chapter Three I discussed the importance of the mitochondria as the source of life-giving energy to every cell in your body. Rather than send you back to review, here again, in abbreviated form, is the description.

The furnace that all living things use to produce the energy of life is the mitochondria. The mitochondria act just like a powerhouse attached to a big factory or city. They absorb oxygen and use it to burn fuel (glucose) to produce useful energy. Some of this energy is heat, which we can use to keep up our body temperature, but the lion's share is used to charge a very small biological battery, enabling easy distribution and utilization of the energy by any molecule in our body that needs it to perform a function. The fully charged battery is called adenosine triphosphate (ATP).

To avoid chemistry that you won't need, I will put it simply and say that the TP stands for three phosphates. When one of the phosphates is removed the result is the uncharged version of the battery, adenosine diphosphate (ADP). After the battery has been discharged by a protein molecule that needs the energy to do useful work, the undamaged phosphate and ADP are attracted back to a compartment of the mitochondria where they can be reassembled (a process called phosphorylation) and recharged with the energy produced from combining the oxygen and glucose. This conversion from ATP to ADP is extremely crucial and is the basis of all human life. Formaldehyde has the ability, even in extremely small concentrations, to prevent phosphate from attaching to ADP.[113]

The article I reference, *Biochemistry of methanol poisoning. 4. The effect of methanol and its metabolites on retinal metabolism,*[113] reports research performed in 1960 at the Department of Pharmacology of Yale University School of Medicine. To this day these results have never been refuted, but much like other good science proving formaldehyde dangerous, it has been ignored. The authors, Kini and Cooper, begin by stating, "It is generally accepted that formaldehyde is the toxic agent in methanol poisoning." The article proceeds to provide evidence in support of that proposition. If you are a scientist, this paper is a must read.

While the brain is dependent on oxygen and without it will die within a short period of time, cells have alternative methods for generating ATP that require no oxygen. Both of these forms of energy production are sensitive to – and can be stopped by – varying but extremely low levels of formaldehyde. Kini and Cooper establish that formaldehyde, in very low concentrations, can cause considerable damage to key enzymes required by cellular respiration. They also tested, in an identical manner, formic acid and acetaldehyde, demonstrating that between ten and one hundred times higher concentration level would be required to get the same results. It would be physically impossible to shove enough formic acid (formates) down the throat of a living organism to match the effects of formaldehyde. Kini and Cooper conclude by noting that present evidence shows "support for the contention that formaldehyde is responsible for all the manifestations of methanol poisoning." They continue, "It is our observation that formaldehyde is an extremely potent inhibitor of respiration and glycolysis; formate exercises only weak respiratory inhibition, and methanol itself has no effect."

Now, just what does this all mean? Most significantly, formaldehyde has the power to severely hamper aerobic respiration and, in so doing, cause cells that can switch to anaerobic respiration to do so. In turn, this causes a buildup of lactic acid within the cell, which quickly leaks into the blood. This partly explains the quick development of acidosis in the blood of methanol poisoning victims, a development that occurs long before the liver has a chance to produce detectable levels of formic acid in the bloodstream.[400] This also explains the symptoms of shortness of breath, fatigue, and muscle pains in the limbs and elsewhere, even before acidosis develops in the bloodstream.

The runners and other athletically inclined among you have likely experienced this phenomenon. While running or swimming hard, the proteins in your muscles were asking for ATP much faster than your mitochondria could produce it because you couldn't breathe in enough oxygen. Your muscles switched to anaerobic respiration, and you experienced catching your second wind. The downside is that this anaerobic respiration produces a large amount of lactic acid, and as it builds up in your muscles, so does the acidity within your legs. You perhaps felt the pain during the exercise, and it might even last for hours or days afterward, depending on just how much lactic acid was produced.

The formaldehyde produced at ADH sites throughout the body has the ability to turn off oxidative respiration within any cells that it penetrates. If this occurs in the liver, muscle cells, brain, or any other high-energy cell type, the affected cells will immediately begin the change over to anaerobic respiration and lactic acid levels will surge in the blood, eventually overpowering the body's ability to neutralize the acid – and ultimately resulting in full blown acidosis. Formaldehyde will also react directly proteins in the blood making them more acidic which will compound the acidity. Acidosis itself is never deadly, but it is symptomatic of insufficient respiration.

How does this type of reaction affect one's vision? Visual symptoms of methanol poisoning and acidosis are related in a very interesting way. One of the most energy intensive organs of the body is the retina, which requires a very large amount of ATP to make vision work. The rod and cone cells of the retina, which respectively are responsible for black and white and color vision, contain large numbers of mitochondria. The cone cells have higher mitochondria counts than the rods, indicating that color vision is a higher energy process. Cone cells come in three types: red, green and blue, each with a different energy requirement.

The retina is an ADH site that, during methanol poisoning, acts as a formaldehyde generator. Imagine the ADH of the retina generating formaldehyde molecules that disperse throughout the retina. Those that make it to the mitochondria will act to turn off the flow of vital ATP to support vision. The effect is different for each type of cell, thus explaining the sequencing of color changes and some of the other bizarre color vision distortions reported by those poisoned by methanol. The highest concentration of cones occurs in the macula of the retina, which is responsible for the sharpest vision. The high density of ADH explains the blurring of vision and, eventually, when the formaldehyde levels rise to a high enough level, the death of the rod and cone cells, resulting in permanent blindness. Even if the cells were not killed outright, enough mitochondria could be disabled to require their replacement – a very time consuming process. This type of interaction between the molecular and cellular processes will be featured prominently when I address the chemical basis of the DOC.

Death by the Immune Response

I wrote earlier regarding the effect that formaldehyde tagging can have on the activation of the immune system. Many of these tagged proteins act as beacons to the body's innate immune system, indicating the existence of a formaldehyde modified protein that needs to be eaten by a macrophage. If macrophages are close at hand, they will commence the process. Once they see the magnitude of the job ahead, they can become activated and respond by releasing into the bloodstream chemical substances that are essentially a call for reinforcements.

I won't go into the full detail that this issue deserves, particularly when we are dealing with the brain. But I will generalize by saying that when the macrophage calls for help, the monocyte, a small white blood cell that usually resides in the spleen, is dispatched to answer the call. The monocyte is actually an immature macrophage that is small enough to get just about anywhere within the body including the brain and can convert into a full-sized macrophage cell, causing swelling or edema. This process is quite fast as the immune system goes, but it still takes approximately eight to twelve hours for the monocyte to reach the site to which it has been summoned. Interestingly, this corresponds perfectly to the time delay of methanol symptoms (the latent period) after methanol is consumed.

You might ask, which of the methanol symptoms could these migrating macrophages be causing? This is an important question. Let's go back to my encounter with formaldehyde gas from that hand warmer when I was a child. It had been producing pure formaldehyde gas in my pants pocket for a good two hours during my walk. My doctor's appointment for my asthmatic attack was early in the afternoon of the next day. It was about 16 hours after my walk that the itching started and my doctor asked to see what was causing me pain. The tissue was, by then, red and swollen. The swelling was caused by the above inflammation response caused by the monocyte migration to the site of formaldehyde poisoning and formaldehyde modified protein.

This response to the formaldehyde in the skin of my thigh was uncomfortable, but quite bearable.

What would be the result of such a migration and swelling in the brain? It would begin as an excruciating headache caused by the pressure of an expanding brain pushing against the confines of the skull. Such headaches are the symptom generating the most complaints from victims of methanol poisoning,[16] but the problem doesn't stop there. The swelling, medically known as edema, can become extremely serious, causing the onset of coma and eventually, if enough pressure damage is done to the brain, death. At autopsy, it is a universal sign of acute methanol poisoning that the cadaver's brain shows such extreme edema that when the skull cap is sawn off, the tension on the dura (a layer of skin-like material that covers the brain) is severe, as if the brain is literally trying to pop out of the skull.

This is one way that acute methanol poisoning differs from chronic methanol poisoning. Headaches are present in both conditions, but in the case of an acute poisoning, the extreme nature of the swelling caused by the large amount of formaldehyde produced in a short period of time causes other damage that slow poisoning could not. The suffering brain has no control over innate immunity; the immune system is a completely autonomous mechanism developed to protect us even if we are born without a brain.

If you have a chance to view a skull in a science class, take off the skull cap and look straight down into the part of the skull that lines the very bottom of the brain. This area is not smooth like the skull cap; it has protuberances that are, in some instances, quite sharp. You can imagine the severely swelling brain expanding into these obstructions, crushing and slicing the tender brain tissue found on the lower portion of the brain, such as the putamen (a peach pit shaped structure located at the base of the forebrain), which is often found hemorrhaging in magnetic resonance imaging (MRI) of methanol poisoning victims, along with herniation of the cerebellum.[270] This damage is caused by the physical manifestations of severe edema. Autopsy of the methanol poisoned brain, when it is finally cut into sections, will always find edema, swelling, and congestion throughout the entire brain and brain stem.[416]

The proof of monocyte infiltration and the direct involvement of the macrophage during acute methanol poisoning is well documented.[148] In 1982 at the University of Toronto, an excellent pathological study was conducted that examined tissues from four patients who died in a hospital from severe acute methanol poisoning after stays as short as 30 hours and as long as 18 days. The brains of these patients were shown to have considerable infiltration by macrophages, along with associated myelin loss. The loss of myelin was interesting, inasmuch as all four patients had considerable instance of myelin having been eaten from around the axons in their brains, leaving the axons themselves intact.[148] This is a common occurrence in multiple sclerosis. The four patients also suffered from demyelination of the nerve cells in the cerebellum, which would easily account for the symptoms they suffered, such as tingling of the extremities (paresthesia), convulsions,[16] mental confusion, memory loss and amnesia,[21] all of which are also shared by those suffering from MS. The patient with the longest survival suffered the greatest macrophage-caused damage.[148] Much of this damage is associated with the optic nerve and may also account, in part, for the bizarre nature of some, but by no means all, of the visual symptoms reported by methanol poisoning patients.

Hallucinations, Delirium and Maniacal Behavior

Occasionally, methanol poisoning can result in hallucinations, delirium and maniacal behavior. These rare but interesting symptoms that relate to an altered state of the brain's perception of reality are difficult to pin on the demyelination and extreme pressure on the brain associated with the immune response of the brain to formaldehyde production. Possibly the lowered energy level brought about by the deactivation of the respiratory enzymes in certain areas of the brain may be capable of inducing a temporary hallucinatory state with a concomitant delirious or maniacal response. Dr. Majchrowicz theorized that the formaldehyde produced from the methanol buildup during withdrawal from an alcoholic binge could react with natural amino acid-like compounds in the body, called biogenic amines, and result in the formation of "aberrant neurotransmitters," as well as other compounds. These might act like certain addictive alkaloids and react to produce altered states of consciousness and perhaps even addiction.[133]

Formic Acid Causes None of These Symptoms

Search for the symptoms of formic acid poisoning… PLEASE! Wherever you look, you will find that the acute symptoms are listed as SLIGHT. Yet the consensus in the scientific literature is that the liver is where all methanol is metabolized into formic acid and it is the formic acid that does all the damage.[273] Anyone who believes that the kind of damage we are discussing here can be caused by formic acid is seriously delusional. The absurdity of it is beyond overwhelming and speaks to the lack of chemical knowledge possessed by the medical community in general. What a bad idea it was to accept pre-med students that majored in philosophy and to allow the medical schools to teach them the chemistry "they needed." Okay, I will not go there…

The bad news is that the "general consensus" is a daunting foe. I could very well be the only scientist on planet Earth that worries about the formaldehyde produced by methanol within the body. This does not make me feel smug or holier-than-thou; it honestly just makes me sad. The thought that monied interests can control scientific thought and perpetuate a blatant lie, putting a large percentage of the population in harm's way and killing many in the process, bodes badly for the future of the truth. It is fortunate that you can personally act on this matter and spread the word as you see fit. The purpose of this book is to educate the average person to protect themselves and their families. I have no faith either in my peers or in any government agency. I know enough and have been through enough to understand that this last lunge is aimed at a very substantial windmill.

The truth is that the other side of this issue has never proven beyond a reasonable doubt that formaldehyde is not involved in methanol poisoning. To the contrary, irrefutable evidence exists that the methyl alcohol from the aspartame molecule turns into formaldehyde within living tissue.[7] Arguments from the dark side of this issue refuting the outcome of this study are meaningless gibberish.[40] Many of the symptoms of acute methanol poisoning[3] are identical to those of alcohol withdrawal,[385] and not one of them has ever been associated with formic acid toxicity.[365] Most convincing of all is that even though formic acid is found in the blood of those who consume large quantities of methanol, the levels are extremely variable – but never high enough to inflict harm or to account for any of the major symptoms of methanol poisoning, including the increased acidity of the blood that has been shown to be caused by lactic acid, not formic acid.[3,400]

The older and more reliable research in this area has time and again established that the maximum amount of formic acid that can be produced from methanol in cases of poisonings is "without question"[16] far too small to account for the acidity of the plasma in actual poisoning cases.[498] As early as 1922 it was suggested correctly that our acidic Crazy Hawks could be directly responsible for acidosis by neutralizing the amino acids of protein through the formation of methylene derivatives.[108,443] Professor Roe, the father of the ethanol cure for methanol poisoning, did the calculations to prove with certainty that nowhere near enough formic acid was produced during methanol poisoning to cause the recorded acidosis.[3]

The fact is that every molecule of formic acid found in the bloodstream is a blessing, inasmuch as it accounts for one less molecule of formaldehyde attaching to an enzyme and causing problems. In a recent study of the biggest methanol outbreak (51 hospital admissions) for which serum formate was measured, the patients were divided into three groups: Group I survived without problems, Group II survived with long term problems, and Group III died. The highest blood formate levels measured in each group, expressed in mmole/L, were Group I: **27**, group II: **8** and group III: **6**. This indicates that the higher the level of formate the more likely the survival of the patient.[673] Remember also that although it may be almost impossible to test for formaldehyde in a hospital setting, the odor of formalin on the breath or in the urine of poisoned individuals has been reported.[670] This will be the last I have to say about the folly of blaming formic acid for the sins of formaldehyde.

Murder by Methanol

I was asked by individuals directly involved in the case of the death of a young man who was killed by methanol to review the details of that case. I have served as an expert witness on a number of food related deaths and have always donated my time on the side of the plaintiff. This was my first time on the side of the defense, but the circumstances were such that I could not in good conscience refuse. In this case the man's wife was accused of murdering him by adding methanol-containing car windshield cleaning fluid to his favorite re-hydration drink. She claimed that the deadly dose of methanol actually came from his consumption of diet soda over an extended period of time. I will only reveal the details of the victim's dying, as that is all that is pertinent here. As I write this, I have before me the 16 pages of hospital and pathological reports that constitute the details of the last two days of this healthy, non-smoking, athletic young man's life. The evening of day one he presented himself to the emergency room of a well-equipped modern US hospital complaining of a recent history of nausea without vomiting, shortness of breath, and change of mental status. He was classified by the physician on duty as being mildly to moderately confused. Blood tests showed his blood was highly acidic (acidosis). He was immediately put under hemodialysis.

Additional blood tests returned 5 hours after admission indicated that on admission his blood contained the equivalent of a dose of 58 grams of pure methanol. An ethanol drip directly into his vein was begun to counteract the methanol. The hospital took further precaution to prevent any additional conversion of methanol to formaldehyde by administering Fomepizole, which is 4-MP or 4-methylpyraxole, a competitive inhibitor of ADH that is now gaining favor for use instead of ethanol in methanol poisoning.* Concurrently, a CAT scan was performed on his brain that showed nothing unusual and, in particular, none of the hemorrhaging associated with high doses of methanol poisoning; specifically, "no necrosis of the putamens was seen."

The next morning he fell into a deep coma from which he did not recover. His respiration was seriously affected and a tube had to be placed into his lungs to assist breathing. That afternoon his respiration ceased and his life was maintained by mechanical means. At that time another CAT scan was performed and reported considerable brain edema, hemorrhaging and other intracranial damage reminiscent of methanol poisoning. I quote the radiologist report:

"Comparison is made with the previous examination of June 12. Bilateral large basal gangliar hemorrhages have developed measuring 5 x 3 cm. on the right and 5.2 cm. on the left. There is compression of the ventricles and there is 8 mm. right to left shift of the septum pellucidum. There is blood within the temporal horns and left occipital horn. There is edema and there is compression of the cisterns around the brain stem consistent with transtentorial herniation and uncal herniation. Cerebellar edema is also noted." That evening he went progressively downhill into a deeply comatose state and died, two days after admission.

Here we have a case of a very large dose of methanol killing a healthy individual in 48 hours. The autopsy report and testing while the patient was alive showed clearly that the liver was working well throughout the course, never showing the signs of injury that one would expect if it were responding negatively to formaldehyde or formate. This is the normal response to acute methanol poisoning. Historically, it is the down-and-out alcoholic that succumbs to accidental methanol poisoning. Their lifetime of alcoholism presents a liver at autopsy as profoundly unhealthy, probably more a reflection of a lifetime of poor diet and incessant binging.

This man died from both the respiratory and the immune response of formaldehyde. The formaldehyde produced within his brain tagged sufficient protein to elicit a delayed immune response (edema), which was severe enough to squeeze his brain like an orange against the rough bottom of his skull. It took only 24 hours during treatment for the development of all the visible damage noted in the CAT scan and subsequent autopsy. The fact that no signs were found of edema brain damage just before the dialysis began is key. Dialysis quickly removed any formic acid, along with most of the methanol. For the brain to suffer such a considerable insult during dialysis and ethanol treatment makes sense only if it was a delayed response to formaldehyde produced in the brain prior to hospital admission.

Respiratory failure, which is indicative of considerable formaldehyde production, was one of the reasons he sought help at the local hospital. His inability to catch his breath and his loss of stamina were keys to his physical complaints. These symptoms preceded visualization of any physical brain damage by his first CAT scan. In my discussion of respiration, I go into detail about the work done at Yale using levels of formaldehyde to stop respiration. These levels reflect methanol doses similar to those apparently administered to this patient.[113]

This tragic death ends our discussion of acute methanol poisoning. It is my contention that the study of chronic methanol poisoning would best be undertaken by studying the major diseases of civilization, which constitute the end result of the interaction of environmental methanol poisoning, endogenous ethanol and an individual's genetic constitution.

The DOC: the Result of Nature and Nurture Working over the Course of a Lifetime

The development in an individual of one of the diseases of methanol poisoning is much like a ceramic art cameo carefully painted in great detail onto a white porcelain blank. The final image remains invisible, a mystery, until the piece is put to the kiln and fully fired. It is only then that both we and the artist can understand the significance of the work. Consider the DOC working on a canvas that is the human body, and the two pigments on the pallet of heredity are the enzymes ADH I and ADH III. The brush is genetics, and the strokes reflect a code of Nature's design that may always elude us. The resulting delicate painting remains invisible, harmless… until a lifetime of consumption bathes the constitution in a developing solution consisting of a mixture of ethanol and methanol. The final picture that emerges reflects the nature, the details and the magnitude of a unique presentation of good health or disease. Such is the slow birth of the Diseases of Civilization. No matter what your innate genetic pattern of enzyme distribution or the level of compromise of your organs at birth, all of the DOC can be prevented by simply removing only the methanol from this scenario.

Let me reword the above analogy, as this concept is vital to your understanding of the fascinating process that moves a healthy person toward disease. The distribution of the bad and good ADH enzymes in your body is your birthright. If you have excellent distribution of the good ADH III to cover locations of the bad ADH I, then you will be naturally free from suffering any of the DOC. If only one of your organs lacks protection, then you might only be susceptible to one or two of the DOC. We don't know much about the distribution of these enzymes, nor do we know why Nature sees fit to distribute them as it does. We are, however, beginning to become more aware of the importance of these enzymes and their relevance to disease origination.[216]

I do not consider it vital to learn more than we now know before we use what we do know to expunge these diseases from this planet. Since approximately twenty five percent of the population of the *civilized world* does not have one of these diseases emblazoned on their death certificates, then we might guess that one in four of the population is so protected. If your mother has not consumed sufficient methanol to damage you as a fetus, and you are born DOC-free, then even though you may have many unprotected locations throughout your body that would make you vulnerable to the damage from the formaldehyde produced by methanol, you can still maintain freedom from DOC. The caveat is that you must avoid methanol or alternatively be plied with the perfect amount of its antidote, ethanol, to keep you from harm. Freedom from methanol is what blesses women who are far too poor to buy their infants expensive jars and aseptic pouches of carrots, peas and other such *baby foods* which, after a perfect birth, would begin their child's travel down the road of chronic methanol poisoning and the DOC. Such encounters eventually lead to the full development and expression of the weakness of their genetic countenance and risk an early death from one of the DOC.

Where Do the DOC Fit? Categories of Disease

There are many diseases that science distributes into a number of different categories. We mentioned this in the first chapter but, now that we will be getting down to the business of proposing a unique cause for some well known diseases, we need to think about the reason that diseases exist in the first place and reclassify them in a more natural order that suits our discussion. We have no interest in the diseases that are caused by inborn errors of metabolism or other purely genetic diseases such as muscular dystrophy. Generally, the causes of diseases may be categorized in one of three ways: parasitism, opportunism, and nutrition.

Parasitism

Many human diseases are the direct result of parasitism, in which bacteria, protozoa, or worms find the human body irresistibly tasty and put themselves in a position to feast on the many organic molecules that we contain. In some cases this goes on for just a short period of time until either our innate defenses or the foreign intruder gets the upper hand. In some of these diseases, such as trichinosis, the feasting goes on for a lifetime with the invading organism forming a defensive cyst to protect it from the macrophage while absorbing enough nutriment to keep itself alive until our death. It escapes only after our bodies are consumed by a new organism for it to ravish. Our immune system is at its best defending against these parasitic organisms, with the macrophage being the first line of defense, orchestrating the production of antibodies to more quickly mark the offending organism should it attempt additional attacks at another time.

Opportunism

Other diseases are caused by opportunistic organisms that have no taste for us, per se, but merely have perceived a better use for our biochemistry. These independent hostile organisms, such as virus, prion or politician, feel they have a better use for our bodies than we do and commence to ply us as a means of their own reproduction, satisfaction or other gratification. The duration and symptoms of these diseases can vary dramatically depending on the tactics used or the term of occupation by the offending creature. The immune system is not always successful against the craftier of these offending organisms. The virus will succumb to the macrophage or other of the innate immune warriors until it takes refuge deep inside a living cell, outside the range of the detective mechanisms of the white blood cells. (This, by the way, is exactly how formaldehyde from methanol produces Alzheimer's disease, by traveling well inside the living cell and attacking the memory protein outside the detection range of the macrophage.)

Within the cell, the virus is in a perfect position to convert the cell into a factory capable reproducing millions of clones of itself. Some viruses have the ability to evolve an outer coat that changes so frequently that the production of antibodies becomes fruitless, thereby avoiding being marked immediately as they enter the body, when they are the most vulnerable. The flu and the HIV viruses are two of the many that have this capability, which allows them great advantage.

Nutritional Diseases

Occasionally, two very different diseases can be caused by the same substance, and such cases are critical to our understanding of nutritional disease. In fact, an essential nutrient can cause either a poisoning disease, in which too much of it is ingested, or a deficiency disease, in which too little of the same exact substance is consumed. The truth is that the science of nutrition is the study of just these two expressions of the same substances. All nutrients have an essential level which must be met to achieve optimum health, as well as a consumption level that can cause a poisoning or disease. Nutrition provides us with the first expression of a U-shaped dose response, with a different set of diseases on either side of the curve.

Rickets, for example, a disease that marked my early childhood, is caused by vitamin D deficiency. I can still taste the doses of cod liver oil that were forced down my throat to keep my young bones from further malformation. Science learned the use of cod liver oil as a cure for vitamin D deficiency from the Inuit. The Inuit, or Eskimo people, are an ancient culture who, much like the Aztec, developed a superb practical toxicology long before the birth of Christ and the evolution of the null hypothesis. The Inuit enjoy a culture that survived in a hostile Arctic environment for many thousands of years. Their reverence for nature that provided their sustenance is exemplified in this customary Inuit saying, which hints of their attention to the details of nutrition and toxicology:

"The great peril of our existence lies in the fact that our diet consists entirely of souls."

As their saying suggests, in the winter the traditional Inuit consumed a diet consisting entirely of animal flesh, free from plant material and, therefore, lethally deficient in Vitamin C. Yet scurvy (the deadly disease of vitamin C deficiency) has never been observed or recorded in the traditional Inuit people. Scurvy was, however, the cause of much suffering and death among the Arctic explorers and scientists who wintered in the same environment.[629] The Inuit developed, over the eons, a dietary tradition and taste for unusual dishes composed of rotted animal flesh which, through fermentation, supplied more than ample ascorbic acid to keep the Inuit free from scurvy.[629] One can only imagine how this intriguing toxicological solution evolved in such a seemingly primitive culture.

Of equal complexity and importance to our discussion here is the Inuit people's unique answer to the dichotomy of rickets (vitamin D deficiency) and the very real danger of the often terminal disease of vitamin D toxicity (hypervitaminosis D). The touch of sunshine produces vitamin D in the naked skin of humans. Rickets is normally considered a disease of sunshine deficiency. Untreated, it can kill, and by all rights it should have decimated the Inuit civilization long before it ever gained a foothold in the Arctic zone, where winter brings a solar angle that prevents the well-covered Inuit skin from producing any vitamin D for four months every year. Inuit culture, however, treasures the nutritional qualities of the livers of the fish they use for food, the very best dietary source of Vitamin D. When the Inuit sacrifice an animal for food, the first organ consumed is the hot liver fresh out of the carcass. Interestingly, though polar bear flesh has always been one of their staple foods, they have a taboo against eating this one animal's liver, a taboo considered nonsense at first by visiting explorers and scientists before the Age of Enlightenment. As early as 1596, arctic expeditions returned to Europe with accounts of a horrible new disease of the Arctic that typically included severe headache, bone pain, blurred vision and vomiting, along with the loss of hair and involvement of the skin, sometimes leading to full-body skin loss, leaving the underlying flesh bloody and causing excruciating pain. These are the symptoms of Hypervitaminosis D – the disease caused by an overdose of Vitamin D, which occurred after explorers ignored the Inuit and consumed the livers of freshly killed polar bears.

Vitamin D, therefore, has a classic U-shaped curve of disease outcome. The consumption of too little causes a deficiency (Rickets), while consuming too much induces a strange and painful death. Most important of all is that at some dose, vitamin D is not only beneficial but essential for life. Many of the essential nutrients present us with such U-shaped consumption curves, but universally they have very different disease outcomes at each side of that curve.

Is Ethanol an Essential Nutrient?

Ethanol is a dietary substance unique from any other inasmuch as it presents us with a U-shaped consumption curve that has the same diseases on either side. The breathtaking part of this unique outcome, now proved in numerous incidences of DOC,[279] is that apparently, a dose of ethanol exists which is essential for optimal lifetime protection from these very same diseases.

We technically should classify chronic methanol poisoning as a nutritional disease; after all, we have been told by a chief toxicologist of the FDA that methanol is a food. The evidence is clear that no matter how much methanol is consumed, it can be successfully countered by sufficient consumption of ethanol to protect us from harm. Under these circumstances, do we call ethanol an antidote or an essential nutrient?

I told you that for ten years I have been consuming ethanol in my drinking water in quantity sufficient to guarantee I receive one standard alcoholic drink a day. I try not to consume methanol-containing foods and probably do not need to consume this ethanol. I have done this as an experiment to see if such a regime can do any harm. I have subjected myself to blood testing and physical examinations, which recently included a full body MRI examination. The results of this testing prompted me to share with you my personal experiment. The fact is, I would much rather remove methanol from our food supply than recommend ethanol supplementation. It is always better to stop a poison from entering the body than to constantly try to guess at the proper dose of the antidote. What of those people who cannot consume ethanol, particularly pregnant women and young children? I will not now take the stance that ethanol is essential, but instead will join most ancient cultures in my reverence for it as a powerful and useful medicine to be used judiciously. If in the future we discover that endogenous ethanol production in the gut by fermentation is indeed essential then I will be convinced otherwise and add a new topic to my vitamin lectures.

What Are the DOC?

The diseases of civilization are all the result of chronic poisoning by methanol, due to a deficiency of ethanol. It is a phenomenon unique to humans. The numerous symptoms reflect the assortment of things that can go wrong when formaldehyde is released within various biochemical compartments of the human anatomy. These are exotic places where Nature never usually allows formaldehyde to go unescorted. DOC are the reflection of the nature of various organs as they respond with every tool they can summon to our defense. It is Life attempting to regain order and preserve itself at all costs, against an immune system incapable of compromise. The disease that finally prevails after the interaction of all these variables is what is eventually written on the death certificate, but in the end, only one real cause remains: chronic methanol poisoning. It is as simple as that.

The first DOC we will discuss in detail in the next chapter is also the first disease discovered to conform to the U-shaped curve of alcohol consumption: Atherosclerosis.

Chapter 7

Atherosclerotic Cardiovascular Disease (Heart Disease)

It has been thirty years since the U-shaped curve of alcohol consumption was trepidatiously berthed and set afloat in the backwaters of the river of collective scientific knowledge. To this day the healing power of ethanol has yet to find either explanation or, more importantly, exploitation. The most significant curative force to come from over a hundred years of scientific investigation of the horror of heart disease has taken a back seat to a taboo born of temperance, prohibition and the need to protect the unprotectable from their own destinies. This is an impossible scenario and will stand in the eyes of history as an inexcusable blunder done in the name of God by those who practice medicine... while science sleeps.

The major causes of death in the developed world [682] are the diseases that we will be discussing in this chapter, commonly called the atherosclerotic cardiovascular diseases (ACD). The ACD all derive from one identical cause: the remarkable migration of macrophages, microsomes and low density lipoproteins (LDL) to a sweet spot lying between two very thin layers of the human arterial wall. Our compelling interest here is the little known fact that this area of the arterial lining is where over 97% of all the ADH in the circulatory system of the human body can be found,[220] making these sites capable of producing formaldehyde from methanol. The U-shaped curve of alcohol consumption tells us that the incidence of atherosclerosis often doubles in populations who refrain from consuming any alcohol, which could have prevented this conversion. Cigarette smoking, a major source of methanol, is one of the established major risk factors for coronary heart disease. "Unequivocal proof has been provided for the important role of smoking in the etiology of premature severe atherosclerotic disease and its clinical sequelae."[470] Add to this the proven fact that methanol's only antidote is ethanol, and the thoughtful mind is drawn to the obvious.

At this point, those of you who have read this book carefully will be able, on your own, to piece together the cause of atherosclerotic cardiovascular disease (ACD), with the exception of the involvement of the LDL. But please read on, as the LDL issue will be a fascinating addition to your growing knowledge of how methanol kills while science slumbers.

The One Unifying Factor of All ACD

The atheroma (Greek for "lump of gruel") is both the namesake and the mother of those diseases which make up the ACD which include atherosclerosis, coronary heart disease, stroke and heart attack. The atheroma is best described as a pus- and cholesterol-filled pimple of the artery wall that requires many years to develop. Its presence initiates an easily understood group of catastrophic events, ultimately causing damage through the obstruction and blockage of the arterial plumbing that is the direct source of the life-giving blood flow to the body. We will go over the nomenclature of these closely related phenomena so that you can more easily read the vast literature of this disorder if you so chose.

The following terms can be confusing: *arteriosclerosis* is a general term describing hardening of the arteries (from the Greek arteria, meaning artery, and sclerosis, meaning hardening); *atherosclerosis* is a hardening of an artery specifically due to an atheroma. The term *atherogenic* is used for substances or processes that cause atherosclerosis.

The atheroma is a swelling within the artery walls that is made up of an accumulation of macrophage cells (white blood cells) that have consumed too many LDLs, turned into foam cells and died. The swelling is found between the endothelium intima lining and the media of the artery. While the early stages have traditionally been called fatty streaks by pathologists, they are actually accumulations of macrophages that have taken up oxidized low-density lipoprotein (LDL). When foam cells die, their contents are released, which attracts more microsomes, which then turn into macrophages and make things worse. Over time, this process results in a thick core made up of the cholesterol from the LDLs in the center of each atheroma. The outer, older portions of the atheroma become calcified and more physically stiff over time, producing what is called atherosclerotic plaque. This plaque is reminiscent of the perivascular plaque of the brain found in the brain during multiple sclerosis.

The process of atheroma development within an individual is called *atherogenesis*. Macrophages are well known to cause swelling and inflammation in response to a bacterial infection however atherosclerosis is a germ-free inflammation that develops within the walls of an artery with no invading microorganism present. What makes the atheroma even more unusual is the presence of large numbers of LDLs.[682] Coronary heart disease (CHD) is atherosclerosis specifically of the coronary arteries that supply blood to the heart muscle itself. CHD is the underlying cause of both heart attacks and stroke. When an atheroma blocks blood flow to the heart muscle, the result is a heart attack. When an atheroma from anywhere in the circulatory system becomes too big it can rupture, acting to block blood flow when its contents spill out and travel to the brain. This rupture can generate blood clots that stop blood flow to the brain, thereby causing a stroke. These four manifestations of atheroma production are responsible for more deaths than any other human disease. Atheroma continues to be the number one underlying basis for all civilized human disability and death.[683]

The Long Slow Progression from Atheroma to Full-Blown Heart Disease

Atherosclerosis can show absolutely no symptoms for decades. As the atheroma slowly increases in size within the artery it produces no discomfort or pain. Its growth will eventually cause two serious problems. First, artery enlargement, called an aneurysm, compensates for the extra wall thickness without reducing the flow of blood. Eventually, however, atheroma grows large enough to limit blood flow. This narrowing is then made much worse as the result of a rupture of the atheroma and the formation of blood clots within the artery. The clots that don't kill eventually heal and usually shrink, but leave behind a permanent narrowing of the artery, or worse, complete closure and, therefore, an insufficient blood supply to the tissues and organ it feeds.

These complications of advanced atherosclerosis are chronic, slowly progressive and cumulative. Most commonly, a soft plaque pimple (atheroma) suddenly ruptures, causing the formation of a clog (thrombus) that will rapidly slow or stop blood flow, leading to death of the tissues fed by the artery within minutes. This catastrophic event is called an infarction. One of the most common scenarios is called coronary thrombosis of a heart artery, causing myocardial infarction (a heart attack). Even worse is the same process in an artery to the brain, commonly called a stroke.

Another common scenario in very advanced disease is insufficient blood supply to the legs, typically due to a combination of both atheroma growth and arteries narrowed with clots. Since atherosclerosis is a body-wide process, similar events occur also in the arteries to the brain, intestines, kidneys, legs, etc.

Some Necessary Background

How the Circulation Works

Laboratory supply houses of all sorts were my favorite mail order venue when I was a teenager. They were my Amazon.com of that day and it was through them that I would purchase the chemicals and other supplies that I needed to stock my laboratory. The lab consisted of a sturdy little building that my father built for me among the trees far enough from our home to prevent any of my experiments from disrupting the peace, quiet and smell of the household. My favorite catalogues were from the Carolina Biological Supply Company and Wards Natural Science Establishment. I would read through them as if they were science texts with prices attached.

One of the fascinating items they offered for sale was frogs that had been injected directly into the heart with blue and red latex to fill and color their veins and arteries. The dead frogs were then dissolved away with acid, leaving behind the perfect three dimensional outline of the entire circulatory system. It was an excellent learning tool to help understand the workings of the circulation and how nature gets oxygen and food to every part of the body and drains away waste products. It was easy to see that the entire system was really just one organ; the heart was merely a wide part with valves that facilitated it acting like a pump that sucked the blood from the blue venous side and pushed it back into the red arteries.

Looking at the circulatory system exposed in that way teaches a lesson that will never be forgotten. It is patently obvious that a blood clot or clog of cholesterol breaking off from an atheroma of an artery is going to quickly get stuck in the system as it travels up to the brain or back to the lungs or down to the extremities. Once the blood flow has stopped, sensitive tissue will be cut off from its oxygen and food supply, killing tissue and causing stroke, myocardial infarction, pulmonary embolism, or gangrene, depending on exactly where the clot lodges.

The biggest vein in the body (inferior vena cava) returns blood back to the heart. It is here, just inches from the entrance to the heart itself, where the hepatic vein coming from the liver connects to the primary circulatory system. This vein dumps the entire residue from digestion, including methanol and the full gamut of nutrient byproducts, just inches away from where the lymphatic system dumps the fat particles from your most recent meal into the same blood supply headed toward the heart. This heavily-laden blood enters the heart and is pumped directly to the lungs, where it is well mixed. There it picks up oxygen, along with fresh methanol from a puff of cigarette smoke, and then reenters the heart, where it is brought up to a pressure high enough to open the valve and force this interesting concentrated mixture directly into the aorta. The physical appearance of blood after a meal of moderate fat content is that of a pink cream, due to its burden of fat. This is why you are always asked to refrain from eating anything for at least eight hours before they take your blood to determine your blood lipids.

Where Do LDLs Originate?

When you put food into your mouth you begin a process that is considerably more complex and interesting than most imagine. The living thing that has been sacrificed for your dining pleasure, be it plant or animal, is a very complex mixture of nutrients and toxins. When you eat it, you make a commitment to process it in such a way as to use the good stuff to replace the losses that burden your body as a result of the act of living, and to render the poisons harmless. Few foods that enter your stomach can be absorbed as is, directly through your digestive system, and flow into your hepatic portal vein to your liver. Glucose solution, ethanol and methanol are the exceptions; even sucrose (table sugar), which is made up of just two simple sugars bound together, must first be broken apart into glucose and fructose before the body will allow it to flow into the circulation.

The body treats the entire length of the digestive system as hostile space. Whatever passes through that long tube is kept separate from your circulation, although at times the barrier is only a cell or two thick. The intimate yet separate relationship is vital to allow the closeness necessary to successfully extract ninety eight percent of the useable nutrition from the food we eat, yet the distance is absolutely required to protect us from those many things we eat that would be offensive to our innate immune system. It is not just the bacteria that we harbor in such high concentrations in our colon, but also the protein molecules of the plants and animals that we consume that would be our downfall if they were to enter our circulatory system without being first broken down into individual amino acids that are then indiscernible from our own amino acids. Foreign proteins in our blood would cause the innate immune system to respond with such violence that even a few drops of egg white injected into our veins would cause our bodies to explode into anaphylactic shock and we would most surely perish within minutes.

It is the fats that we eat that present, by far, the most complex challenge and considerable problem to the digestive process. Simple sugars, amino acids, salt and such are all quite soluble in the blood and, unless their concentrations get too high, they will cause no difficulty while traveling through the circulatory system to the cells that can use them. This is not the case with fats. Fats are not at all soluble in the plasma of the blood, and although some are liquid at body temperature, they still pose a considerable physical problem. This inability to dissolve into the bloodstream makes the presence of natural fat and oil in the circulation an extremely grave danger. Fat has a way of coalescing into larger and larger droplets as time goes on, much like what happens after you shake a jar of oil and vinegar salad dressing. A droplet of oil or cholesterol caught in the arterial system can cause the flow of blood to back up behind it, inducing a stroke, embolism or tissue death as easily as a blood clot or ruptured atheroma would.

Because of this, the cells that line the small intestines have the responsibility to change all of the fat from the food we eat and combine it with cholesterol and package it with an outer membrane rich in protein called a chylomicron. These tidy packages are soluble in the blood and can travel harmlessly throughout the body. It is interesting to note that the body does not trust these fat particles enough to send them directly through the hepatic portal vein to the liver. Instead, the chylomicrons are released into the lymphatic system and allowed to more slowly flow toward the heart. Along the way, a percentage of them are picked off at will by hungry cells with appropriate receptor sites. These cells use the fat contained in the chylomicrons for energy and use the cholesterol to rebuild cell membranes. Eventually, by way of a complicated interaction with the liver and other tissues, these comparatively large chylomicrons are converted into the other fat-containing structures that we typically associate with heart disease.

Several different types of these lipoproteins circulate through the body – HDL, VLDL and LDL – but we will concern ourselves just with LDL (low density lipoprotein). We pick this particular lipoprotein because we know that it is the one most responsible for the fat and cholesterol content of the atheroma.[690] You know from your doctor that the LDL is the source of "bad" cholesterol and it is universally associated with heart disease. LDL particles come in various sizes from small to very large. The small particles are denser due to their higher ratio of outer shell (which contains protein) to content (which is all fat). That is the reason their movement through the blood stream is more sluggish. The larger particles contain more fat and, therefore, are more buoyant, somewhat like balloons filled with oil floating in water, and the more oil they contain the better they float. High blood LDL levels, especially higher concentrations of the smaller size LDL particles, contribute to heart disease. Studies show that people whose LDL cholesterol is predominantly made up of smaller dense particles have a threefold greater risk of coronary heart disease. [687] For this reason, the number of small, dense LDL particles in the blood is a more accurate predictor of the risk of heart disease than is a simple measurement of the total LDL cholesterol.[687] We will examine this more closely as we get closer to the truth of heart disease.

The Scene of the Crime

The entire circulatory system is composed of layers of tissue that give it structure, strength and just the right amount of porosity to allow for the free flow of the plasma of the blood to every living cell of the body. The lining of the inside of all the vessels is called the *endothelium*. It is composed of two distinct layers. The innermost layer is a smooth layer of cells that are spaced very closely, forming a glassy surface that offers little resistance to the flow of blood. This layer is only one cell thick and would remind you of that thin, nearly transparent layer just beneath the dry outer layer of an onion peel. Under this is the *intima*, a thicker layer of support cells for the thin outer layer. Under the endothelium is the *media*, a thick layer of muscle cells and elastic fibers that give strength and durability to the vessels. We have talked about the intima and media layers previously because they contain the vast majority of the ADH to be found in the circulatory system. The very outer layer is the *adventitia*, which is composed of collagen fibers that make the vessel cohesive and elastic.

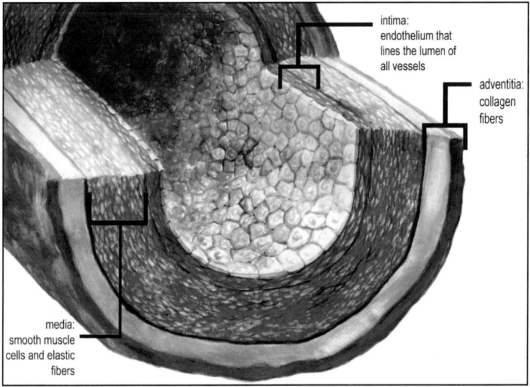

intima:
endothelium that
lines the lumen of
all vessels

adventitia:
collagen
fibers

media:
smooth muscle
cells and elastic
fibers

Figure 7.1

Atheroma: Acne of the Artery

I am using the word "acne" here because it is something that is a personal experience for many and relates very closely to the physical and anatomical actuality of what goes on in the arteries of those who have atherosclerosis. Atheroma can indeed be better represented as what it really is: granulomatous eruptions of the artery. The body's response to a skin pore that is infected from bacteria is quite similar to atheroma evolution, and the end result – a swelling filled with the carcasses of sacrificed innate immune cells and other debris that is prone to rupture if the pressure becomes too great – is a good one. We call the swelling produced in the artery, the atheroma, a "sterile eruption," which signifies that the foreign object being attacked is not a bacterium nor are bacteria present among the other debris. What I want to get down to now is the exact nature of the offending "foreign" entity that the macrophages are attacking.

If the foreign entity that the innate immune system is attacking is not a bacteria or virus, then what could it be and how did it get sandwiched in between two layers of the artery? My contention is that methanol is transformed into formaldehyde within the intima of the artery by the ADH present there. The formaldehyde reacts with some of our own protein that makes up the cells of the intima. This formaldehyde modified protein is identified as foreign protein by macrophages, which then push their way through the endothelium of the artery and into the intima to devour and remove these sterile invaders.

Here is a quick run through of how the entire process probably works. You will need to read this more than once to get it and the proof will come later... trust me! Here we go! Methanol from a puff of cigarette smoke has been absorbed into the artery wall encountering ADH there and no ethanol to prevent it from becoming formaldehyde within the intima lining. Protein will be modified by the formaldehyde, and a macrophage traveling in the bloodstream will seek out that modified protein (called antigen). If it cannot remove all of it by itself, it will send out a chemical signal to call for microsomes, which will migrate to the site to help out by maturing themselves into macrophages. All this is happening in between narrow layers of the artery, which will begin swelling from the influx

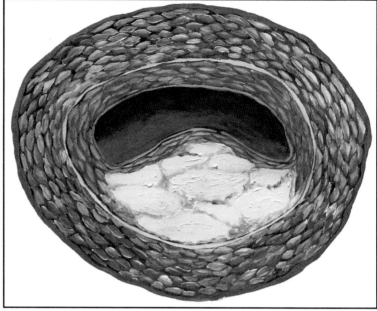

Figure 7.2

of developing microsomes. The swelling will put pressure on the layer of endothelium cells that line the artery, causing increased spacing, or fissures, between the cells making up this thin lining. Eventually, the increased fissures will allow sufficient space to permit the smaller of the LDL cells to be pushed between the endothelial cells and enter into the intima. Once this happens, excess formaldehyde is free to attack the protein lining the outside of the native LDLs, converting them also into a formaldehyde modified – or more specifically an oxidized – LDL that may activate the scavenger sites on the macrophage and induce its conversion into a foam cell. As the foam cells devour the formaldehyde modified LDLs, they will transform its cargo of cholesterol into the esterified form always found in atheroma. I like this story and I am sticking with it! However, it would be important for me to have some corroborating evidence to substantiate the premise. Have patience!

I know you remember my story about the hand warmer that poisoned my thigh with formaldehyde and produced a serious case of granulomatous eruptions (macrophage- and foam cell-filled swellings) on my leg. These eruptions, by the way, are identical to the atheromas we are talking about here. My purpose in telling that story was to lay out the process by which formaldehyde can react with our own self protein and induce a macrophage uprising against what *appears* microscopically to be, but no longer is, our own tissue, having been virtually imperceptibly changed by the formaldehyde. You should also recall from that story that the skin harbors important structures called fibroblasts, which contain considerable ADH capable of turning methanol into formaldehyde. I told you that drinking diet soda containing aspartame was capable of causing granulomatous eruptions identical to those caused directly from the pure formaldehyde from my hand warmer. It is time now to go more deeply into how methanol can incite the immune system against us.

The Approach that Modern Science Takes to Atherosclerotic Cardiovascular Disease

You know enough of the basics and the terminology now to do some reading in the scientific literature. A good place to start is an excellent review article out of the Harvard Medical School that speaks directly to the mechanism by which the innate immune system (macrophages) acts during atheroma formation.[682] For the benefit of the majority of my readers, I will translate and paraphrase the essence of this important recent article below. Those who are up to the science will find reading the original quite rewarding. I underline those items that are vital.

Atherosclerosis is an inflammatory disease. The current paradigm suggests that LDLs cross the endothelial cell layer and accumulate in the intima, where they are subject to modification by oxidation. Although the precise nature of the LDL modifications remains a matter of debate, it is believed that these modified LDLs provoke an innate immune reaction that kindles inflammation in the artery wall and drives plaque formation. This evolutionarily ancient host defense system is the body's first line of defense against invading pathogens and modified host proteins.

The macrophage, a major cellular component of the innate immune response, is the predominant cell type in the early atherosclerotic lesion. This gives the macrophage a unique and primal role in the development and progression of atherosclerosis. Macrophages recognize and consume modified lipoproteins, leading to cellular cholesterol accumulation. This protective response appears to become overwhelmed, leading to massive cellular cholesterol accumulation and the trapping of over-fed macrophages in the intima. These cholesterol-laden macrophage "foam cells" define the early atherosclerotic lesion pathologically and form what is known as fatty streak lesions. The release of chemical signals by these accumulated macrophage foam cells modulates the progression of atherosclerotic lesions, including the recruitment of microsomes, the deposition/degradation of extracellular material, necrotic core formation and plaque rupture. Thus, the recruitment of macrophages to the artery wall is a key event of the innate immune response in early atheroma formation, and recent studies have shed new light on that process.

Central to the development of atherosclerotic lesions is the influx of monocytes into the arterial intima. The conversion of macrophages into cholesterol-laden foam cells is believed to constitute the foundation of the atherosclerotic lesion. Native LDL has traditionally not been considered capable of generating foam cells. Modification of the LDL is, therefore, required to drive massive lipid uptake by macrophages. Over the past thirty years, multiple means have been identified to alter the LDL chemical structure to facilitate its consumption by macrophages and conversion into lipid-laden foam cells. The widely accepted paradigm for the modification responsible has been the oxidative modification hypothesis. This theory posits that a heightened oxidative stress in the vascular wall of yet unknown origin gives rise to oxidized forms of LDL that are recognized by scavenger receptors on the macrophage.

While the evidence implicating the activation of innate immunity pathways in atherosclerosis is strong, the challenges of creating new therapeutics directed at these pathways are formidable. The role of innate immunity in protecting against microbial pathogens raises the specter of rendering hosts susceptible to a multitude of infectious agents when these pathways are interrupted for therapeutic benefit. Many of the mice that have been genetically engineered to lack components of the innate immune system are capable of surviving into adulthood without apparent major infection susceptibility, but when they are challenged with specific infectious agents, they are clearly impaired in their host defense mechanisms. Any attempt to weaken these defense systems for therapeutic benefit would, therefore, have to carefully examine the issue of infection susceptibility in humans.

A growing body of science has implicated innate immunity in the development and progression of atherosclerosis. These pathways result in the establishment of a sterile, chronic inflammation in the artery wall that ultimately leads to the narrowing of the artery and the subsequent rupture of plaques, which are the critical underpinnings of clinical coronary artery disease events. While our knowledge of the receptors involved in innate immunity has expanded rapidly in the past decade, <u>the precise molecular structures that trigger their engagement in atherosclerosis remain unknown.</u> Drugs are currently in development that could inhibit the innate immune pathways. In the meantime, progress in the development of more predictive animal models of atherosclerosis and the imaging of atherosclerotic lesions is urgently needed, if these innate immunity pathways are to be targeted directly for <u>the treatment of the major cause of human morbidity and mortality in the developed world.</u>[682]

For any number of reasons, the medical community is floundering in its efforts to cure and treat the many diseases of civilization. Drug companies have discovered a distinct financial advantage to treating a disease rather than curing it. Furthermore, a drug company scientist is always at a distinct disadvantage when beginning to treat diseases before knowing their exact cause; when you put the cure before the cause then your only recourse is the "let's fix nature" approach. At this time, all the DOC, such as atherosclerosis and, in particular, MS, have many drug companies and cadres of their paid medical people recommending far-fetched remedies with an efficacy that is so marginal it would make a witch doctor blush.[615] In fact, it makes me uneasy to see embedded within the fine review article above the insinuation that it is the exquisitely honed "ancient innate immune system" that is at fault and needs to be "blocked." In this age the use of the word "ancient" implies that we need a new one. Nature, on the other hand, must cherish the testing and tweaking that time can do to her workings.

If there is one thing we don't want, it is a pharmaceutical company "inventing" another expensive new drug for daily administration that will "inhibit the innate immune pathway," slowing atheroma growth slightly but, in the end, causing more harm than good. A much more trustworthy, but obviously less profitable approach would be to stop this problem before it starts – to find out what causes the oxidation of the LDL that makes it so appetizing to the macrophage which, after all, is simply doing the ancient job that never seemed to cause a problem in the Pleistocene era. Let's not allow Big Pharma to kill off our macrophages. (You will see also in the treatment of MS that it is the macrophages they have targeted.) The macrophage takes very seriously its job of eating formaldehyde modified protein. Our job in preventing all these diseases is seeing to it that the proteins don't get modified in the first place.

Formaldehyde from Methanol is the Cause of ACD

I agree wholeheartedly with the current paradigm for the development of atheroma as expressed in the review article above. I wish only to fill in the one missing piece of the puzzle, thus completing the paradigm nicely and turning it into a useful tool for prevention. You know where I am going with this! The formaldehyde produced from methanol by the ADH within the intima is what attaches to the protein coating on the outside of the LDL, changing it sufficiently to activate the macrophage. The macrophage starts devouring these formaldehyde-modified LDLs, turning itself into ravenous foam cells that can't stop eating as long as the LDLs are tagged by formaldehyde. This hypothesis helps explain why cigarette smoke, which is rich in methanol, is the most notorious of the atherogenic agents.[345]

It has been shown experimentally that when macrophages are removed from the human blood by centrifugation, concentrated and placed in a test tube overnight with native LDLs from the same individual, the macrophages will not eat any of the LDLs. Take those same LDLs and place them in contact with small aldehydes like formaldehyde for a few hours to allow the aldehyde to react naturally with the LDL, and then place them in with the same macrophages and by the next morning all the LDLs will have been consumed by the macrophages, many of which will have already been converted to foam cells.[507]

This is extremely important, so bear with me while I explain the above to my scientist friends in their language. You should try and follow this explanation; the language is not very stilted and I render in parentheses some assistance.

I imagine that you are having a difficult time understanding why, with all the science in place to make formaldehyde from methanol a clear contender, the current theory of atheroma development does not include methanol's formaldehyde as a causative agent of atheroma? One possible reason could be that if it were, some very unhappy pharmaceutical houses out there would find themselves peddling a number of ostensibly useless products. I will give my colleagues the benefit of the doubt, however, take the high road, and blame the oversight on formaldehyde itself. Formaldehyde, as you now know, is one difficult bird to find.

The simple statement above that formaldehyde is acting as an oxidizing agent speaks to formaldehyde when it is found in a water solution (you remember the Crazy Hawk). Well, trust me when I say that only a handful of physicians in the United States have had sufficient chemical training be able to understand the full significance of that statement. Add to that the enthusiastically disseminated lie that formaldehyde is not a noteworthy byproduct of methanol breakdown in human methanol poisoning, and perhaps we can explain the medical profession's ignorance of formaldehyde in general. In this particular case, where the scientific community has to be shown that they have no clothes, I will have to take things to a higher level and introduce several other lines of circumstantial evidence that will make my argument irrefutable. Of course, I have no guarantee of acceptance by the mainstream, but it will serve my most important purpose of convincing my readers and friends that they should avoid methanol. But first, let's see the theory in action and take some time to visualize exactly how our theory fits in with the general paradigm. Let's get back to the basics.

> **Scientific Aside**
>
> Formaldehyde in water solution acts as an oxidizer that modifies the LDL protein by inducing a negative charge.[689] This chemical modification, which abolishes positive lysine residues and increases the LDL's net negative charge, has been shown to convert the LDL into a ligand (something worthy of binding to) for the macrophage's acetyl LDL receptor.[156] This receptor is one of the well-defined binding sites (scavenger receptors) on macrophages that activate them when they encounter either LDLs treated with small aldehydes[507] or other formaldehyde modified proteins.[691] The activation of this site has been demonstrated to initiate the innate immune response of the macrophage sufficiently to encourage overwhelming foam cell production in the presence of sufficient modified LDLs.[507] Not only can the cholesterol from the LDL be found within the macrophage, but also it will have already been converted to the esterified cholesterol always associated with atheroma plaque formation.

How Methanol Causes Atheroma

I have had the pleasure of working with a gifted artist, Becky Miller, who is illustrating this book for me. Becky was able to visualize and put to paper the concept of the Crazy Hawk and all of the other characters that I wanted to use to bring life, color and personality to what otherwise would be a rather boring essay. I will never forget the day she asked me to visit her studio and see if what she was doing with the illustrations for this chapter were on the right track. When I arrived she uncovered the storyboards in sequence. What I saw brought tears to my eyes and the sudden realization that this match of illustrator and scientist was going to make a difference. Let's use Becky's illustrations and tell the story of how your body's response to a puff of a cigarette or sip of diet soda may add up and proceed slowly to a lifetime of disease.

It is important when visualizing molecular interactions to put things into perspective, and for that reason the diagrams here fit the same scale as those in previous chapters. Remember Venus and her brain cell, which is the size of Manhattan Island? We are now adding a new component. Just where does an LDL fit into the mix? When Becky asked me this question I answered that using our Venus scale, the average LDL would be about the size of the Goodyear Blimp. Well little did I know that she would take me for my word and incorporate this image into our model, and as you will see, it works well. Size is critically important when it comes to this particular lipoprotein. As mentioned earlier, it has been shown very convincingly that if your blood contains a larger percentage of the smaller LDLs you will, all else being equal, have a much greater chance of developing an atheroma. A close look at Figure 7.3 might help you understand why.

This is probably not the illustration that Becky thought I would use to start, but it makes a very important statement. What appears to be a large number of blimps competing to squeeze between two sandstone cliffs is meant to represent small denser LDLs easily being swept by the flow of arterial blood plasma into the

Figure 7.3

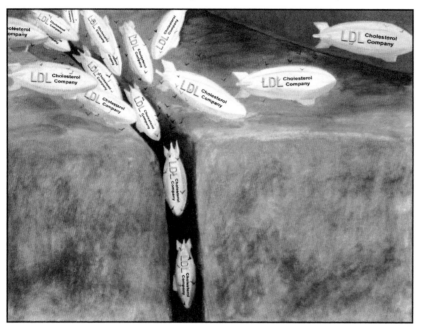

narrow space between two adjacent epithelial cells that are lining an artery. These spaces vary, and you would expect them to be bigger as the artery experiences more swelling and damage due to formaldehyde production and atheroma evolution. Nevertheless, you can see the larger, more buoyant LDLs haven't had much chance to enter into the intima of this artery where the formaldehyde is being produced. How do I know formaldehyde is being produced? Take a very close look at what are in perfect scale circling around those smaller blimps as they are pushed down into the media: pigeons, the small ones that

Figure 7.4

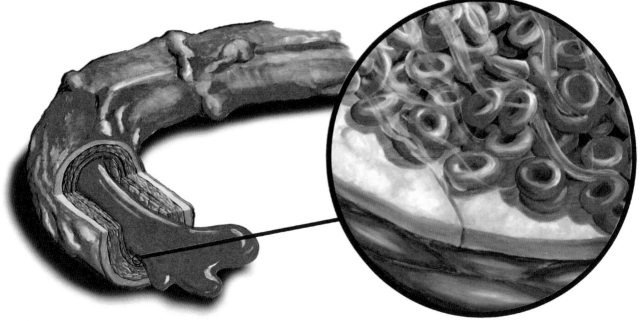

represent methanol. Remember the last time we saw Venus; she was smoking a cigarette and sipping a can of diet cola to wash it down.

Let's back off a bit so we can grasp the scale shown in this illustration. Figure 7.4 takes us back far enough to see the artery itself. The circular window highlights a small segment of the cross section of the artery wall, with the single-cell-thick outer endothelium fully exposed, and the ADH-rich intima directly under it giving it support. You recognize the red blood cells being swept along by the flow of plasma. The fine mist represents the LDLs, now almost invisible at this magnification.

Closer now and something of great importance becomes patently obvious (see Figure 7.5). LDLs are not living things and have no means of locomotion. Unlike the Goodyear Blimp, the LDLs are at the mercy of the media, in which they float, and are swept to wherever the constantly flowing plasma of the blood sweeps them. The lighter and more buoyant LDLs are more likely to be pushed away from the wall of the arteries and eventually make it all the way to the end of the arterial system to the capillaries, where they will have direct contact with the muscle cells for which they become a perfect food.

This graphically explains why it is the arterial system that is exclusively prone to atheroma production. Although veins are made up of exactly the same layers of tissue (with different thicknesses) and comparable ADH concentrations within the intima and media,[220] they never exhibit atheroma. The venous system is meant to drain blood from the organs and the general flow of plasma is out of the tissue. Without a constant influx of LDLs, the formaldehyde produced by the ADH in the venous system must leave the vessels to find other proteins with which to react and other mischief to perpetrate.

One exception to this rule proves the point. Veins do not develop atheroma unless they are surgically moved to function as arteries, as occurs in bypass surgery when a vein is taken from the leg of a patient and used to replace an atheroma-clogged artery to the heart.

Figure 7.6 shows the normal behavior of the LDL without methanol. You would be interested in what happens to the LDL that is pushed into the intima and media of the artery when no formaldehyde is waiting to oxidize it and set it up for removal by the macrophages. LDLs that are not oxidized are called native LDLs and many tests have shown conclusively that they are not at all attractive to the macrophage in that form as food.[507]

Figure 7.5

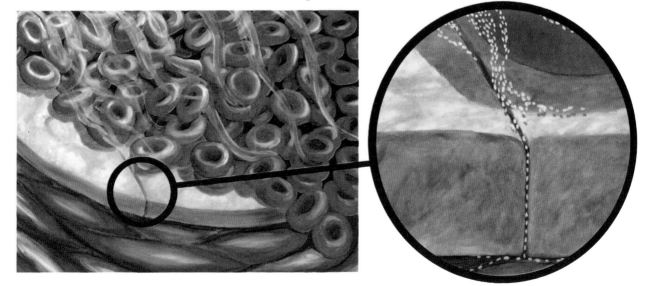

The LDL is an important food source for muscle cells, which have receptor cites that are specific for them (we call them "ports" here). The many smooth muscle cells of the media would make short work of the daily input of LDLs.

Figure 7.7 provides a good close-up of LDLs being accompanied into the interstitial space between endothelium cells by flocks of pigeons. I can only see two ethanol pigeons in the mix, so that means that very little resistance will be available to stop the methanol pigeons

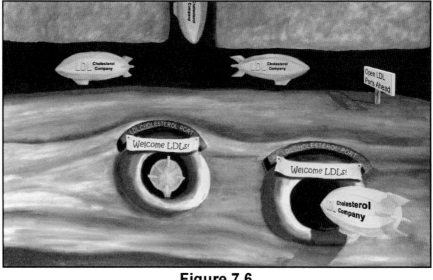

Figure 7.6

from turning into Crazy Hawks as soon as they reach the ADH of the intima and media. Figures 7.8 and 7.9 will show the aftermath up close and personal.

Mayhem is the result among the macrophages and their LDL food. Once the methanol is turned into formaldehyde the Crazy Hawks make a mad dash for the nearest LDL blimp and tag it. This is all that is required to attract the attention of the macrophage. You will note the tremendous size difference between the LDL and the Macrophage. That large blue orb on the right of the picture represents some poetic license with the persona of the macrophage. Macrophages do not, of course, have eyes; eyes wouldn't do much good where they spend most of their time, but in giving them a personality Becky does us a favor and helps us with comprehending the size difference between the players in this biologic drama. You might wonder how on earth something so very large can efficiently capture and consume something so very small. The tentacles are a great artistic touch but the fact is that the entire surface of the macrophage has on it these scavenger receptors that can bind to and internalize formaldehyde-modified LDL and other proteins. The exact process is described beautifully in a wonderful article by Brown and Goldstein.[156] If you are a scientist I suggest you have a read. I would do most of my readers no service at all by confusing them with the details.

The scale here is perfect; the cute-looking macrophages are hanging out where they do not belong, and

Figure 7.7

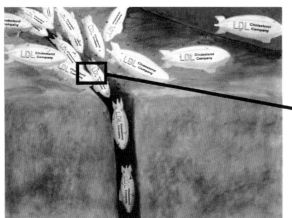
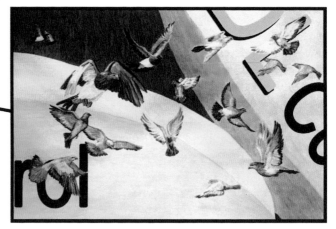

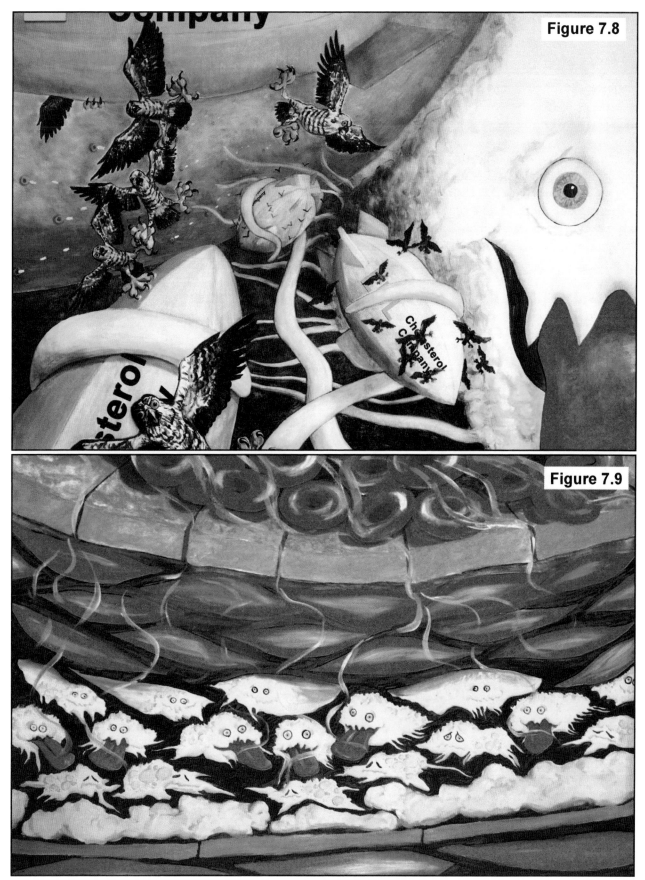

Figure 7.8

Figure 7.9

the LDLs appear as a mist seeping through the single layer of endothelium into the intima, where the macrophages can eat beyond their fill, turning into unhappy-looking foam cells and eventually dying and spilling their contents of partially-digested LDL parts and cholesterol. The cholesterol and other cellular bits and pieces will mound up after years, applying pressure on the walls of the artery, causing swelling, and beginning the production of a full-blown atheroma.

In the civilized world the earliest detectable presentation of atheroma is often found in toddlers and looks very much like what you see in this illustration. At that early age it is called "fatty streaks" and is comprised of thin layers of macrophages and foam cells from recruited monocytes.[610] This early presentation should be no surprise to us, with the popularity of canned pureed fruits and vegetables as baby foods. The ability of formaldehyde produced from dietary methanol by the ADH sites within the wall of the artery to modify LDLs and other protein and, in doing so, to attract macrophages with subsequent recruitment of monocytes has never been considered as an initiating cause for this, the most common of the DOC. That oversight ends here.

Where to Now?

It is unusual to have to apply additional proof to a scientific argument after having presented the molecular basis and third party laboratory substantiation of an intuitively obvious biological outcome as I have above. One's first question would be: have I missed something?

I have carefully searched the scientific literature in order to determine if perhaps some study might be found that would cause a researcher to think that formaldehyde would *not* induce changes in the LDL that would cause activation of the macrophage and, hence, atherogenesis. I found only one article whose misinterpretation might indeed be seen as that missing link. Its elucidation will make it an excellent example of the importance of understanding the complex nature of formaldehyde bonding.

In 1975 a group of researchers was looking for ways to make LDLs radioactive to simplify their detection when they are released in the body. They reacted radioactive formaldehyde with human LDL; however, they used formaldehyde in conjunction with a powerful chemical called sodium borohydride to guarantee that the only type of bond that would be produced between the formaldehyde and the LDL would be a methylation bond.[693] But the key here is that a methylation bond is the wrong bond. If you review Chapter 3, you will recognize this type of bond as the transformation of the Crazy Hawk into the peaceful nesting dove. Remember, it is the temporary "Tag You're It" bonding that activates the macrophage, not the permanent methylation bond. In short, some might mistakenly interpret the result of this experimental work as evidence that formaldehyde does not react with LDLs in such a way as to activate macrophages. You must, however, understand the sparrow hawk and the Crazy Hawk, as well as the bonds that they are capable of producing,

Scientific Aside

If you want to learn a more natural way to treat LDLs with formaldehyde to test for macrophage activation potential, follow the method of Harrach and Robenek.[692] Their method was applied to human LDLs, from which was produced polyclonal antibodies to the formaldehyde-reacted human LDL. When electron photomicrographs of arteriosclerotic plaque tissues from human femoral arteries were treated with a label developed from the above formaldehyde fixed LDL antibody, a marked increase was noted between intensities produced by it, as compared to identical markers produced from non-formaldehyde treated LDL.[690] My interpretation of this is that the formaldehyde treated LDL is what caused the process in the first place and, therefore, is what was being detected by the perfect marker. You may not agree.

before you begin trying to interpret the scientific literature.

Let me put this into a more naturalistic scenario. Remember that Nature has a use for formaldehyde. What Nature does with formaldehyde is produce methylations. Nature does not have to use sodium borohydride; she has some very efficient enzymes that will turn the Crazy Hawk into a nesting dove much more efficiently than that. The methylation reaction is what Nature uses to regulate your genome, turning genes off. Remember the new science of epigenomics, whose practitioners insist upon calling formaldehyde the "methyl molecule," is based on studying how and for what reason the body performs its methylations.

Nature would have no reason to want her methylations to be undone by activated macrophages, which is, most likely, why macrophages have no interest in the detection or destruction of methylation bonds. It is interesting to note that this inability of macrophages to undo unwanted methylations might actually work against us. During chronic methanol poisoning, nothing can prevent excess formaldehyde or "methyl molecules" from wandering into the nucleus of a cell and attaching to DNA. Once this occurs, all that would be necessary is the appearance of the appropriate enzyme to finish the methylation and turn that gene off.

We know that along with the other changes we discussed in atherosclerosis, often the number of smooth muscle cells is increased within the intima. This causes a thickening of the arterial wall that is also found in methanol poisoning (see below). It has recently been shown that methylation of the DNA of the proliferating cells increases markedly compared with that of normal artery muscle cells.[567] Hypermethylation of the DNA is being linked to more and more disease states as we begin to learn about the interaction of the epigenome and disease.[560] Unwanted excess formaldehyde evolved from dietary methanol is the only way to easily explain this phenomena.[586]

Does Diet Soda Cause Coronary Heart Disease?

I received a gift from a friend while I was working on this chapter. He emailed a copy of a report just presented at the American Stroke Association's International Stroke Conference in Los Angeles. While analyzing data from the Northern Manhattan Study (NOMAS), a long-term study of about 2500 individuals over 40 years of age that has been ongoing for about 9 years, it was discovered that those who consumed diet soda every day had a fifty percent greater chance of suffering a myocardial infarction, stroke or vascular death than those who consume sugar sweetened soda.[686] During the time period of the study the great preponderance of diet sodas available contained aspartame, which contains 11% methanol by weight. A cardiologist from the University of North Carolina, when asked about the presentation, was quoted as saying that the study "adds to the growing evidence of an association between diet sodas and cardiovascular disease."[686]

Over the last 30 years, we have witnessed a global epidemic of atherosclerotic cardiovascular disease (ACD).[532] As we discuss the various DOC in other chapters, you will repeatedly notice a thirty-year epidemic theme. All of the other diseases of civilization, with the exception of ACD, have increased dramatically in incidence in the United States, with an apparent origin of change at or about the early 1980s.[586] As you well know by now, I believe the primary reason for this is that the US food supply has, since the summer of 1981,[472] experienced a literal flooding with hundreds of tons of additional methanol from a single source: aspartame.[1]

You may wonder why in the United States the incidence of heart disease has gone down during that same period. The reason is that over the last 50 years cigarette smoking by men has plummeted, and with it the incidence of ACD. Since the mortality rates of ACD are far greater in males than in females,[684] this has complicated our ability to determine the overall influence of the dietary change on ACD since the introduction of aspartame, which occurred during an overlapping time period. One has to keep in mind that men are considerably more vulnerable to the absorption of methanol via the lungs and have much greater protection from dietary methanol than women because of the higher concentration of ADH in their stomach lining. The real question that must be asked is whether the incidence of ACD has declined as much as it might have over the last thirty years if it were not for the introduction of another major source of methanol… aspartame.

It is clear that methanol poisoning from aspartame can damage the circulatory system. After all, significant amounts of the bad ADH enzyme can be found sandwiched within the lining of human blood vessels.[220] The pathology literature very clearly shows that the circulatory system is a direct target of methanol poisoning in both humans and some experimental animals. It is vital to understand that full-blown atherosclerosis takes decades to develop; it is a true chronic manifestation of methanol poisoning and we will need to interpret the literature with care.

The Proper Interpretation of Animal Experiments to Test Methanol's Safety

No perfect animal model for atherosclerosis can be found that will duplicate exactly what happens in humans. You now know enough to expect this of a methanol-related disease. The fact is that while the human aorta has the highest concentration of ADH of any human vessel, the rat aorta has absolutely no detectable ADH.[220] Such discrepancies, along with the ability of animal catalase to protect them from methanol poisoning, makes all laboratory animals extremely insensitive models. This does not, however, mean that we cannot learn something if methanol is applied intelligently to an animal that has some similarities to man under high dosage conditions.

I have been very critical about using animal models for testing methanol toxicity. It may make you think that I am a hypocrite when I occasionally bring up some research done on animals to help support my argument of methanol's danger to humans. The truth is that if you look at my own work I have used rats as a model for testing methanol for both Multiple Sclerosis[2] and birth defects.[177] Why on Earth would I do that?

Many scientists who test the safety of chemicals on animals do not have the proper training to fully understand that animals can only be used for testing if the systems of the animals are legitimate models of the corresponding human system. On occasion, when a difference exists, one may compensate for problems in some way. This is the case with methanol poisoning. In reading bad work, I am often reminded of a contractor friend of mine named Bill who did a lot of construction work for me when I lived on a farm in Arizona. I would sometimes take a break from the university and join Bill to help out with building projects. He would give me this or that project to do, thinking I would have the skills to do the task correctly. His favorite saying to me, accompanied with a deep sad sigh was, "Woodrow… you gotta be smarter than what you're working with."

As you know, all animals, save for the human, have a powerful detoxification mechanism called catalase enzyme that protects them from the lion's share of methanol that they consume. But one method allows scientists to fool this system so that whatever stores of ADH do exist in the animal can be allowed to begin converting methanol to formaldehyde, thus mimicking the human experience.

This was discovered by coincidence over a hundred years ago. It was during the time when it was being proved over and over again that, for all laboratory animals, Richardson's Rule applied and the acute dose of ethanol required to kill was far lower than that of methanol. Several laboratories were doing chronic toxicity studies that showed something quite remarkable.[125] While ethanol could be fed to animals at high doses, even close to the acute lethal dose, on a daily basis for months at a time with no mortality, the same experiment with methanol would always cause death within a few weeks. When the methanol was reduced somewhat the deaths stopped. This demonstrates that at some dosage the catalase of the animal is saturated with methanol and can no longer keep the methanol away from the animal's extra hepatic stores of ADH.

The tremendous lack of sensitivity of animals to methanol (a factor of 100) makes them a very bad model for methanol poisoning. Using them for toxicity testing would more than likely hide most, if not all of the potential toxic outcomes experienced by humans. However, and this is something you must understand, if they do show "any" negative response, this response becomes exceedingly important and must be taken very seriously indeed. When Donald Rumsfeld's company was told by its independent testing laboratories that aspartame was causing birth defects in the brains of rabbits, its only legitimate response should have been clear.[677] Instead of hiding the information from the public, researchers should have applied a factor to the dosage to make up for the insensitivity of the animal model. This would have shown that they were putting in harm's way a much greater percentage of the human population than should ever have been allowed. Aspartame should have been abandoned right then and there.

In the proper hands and heart the result of animal studies can save human lives and prevent human suffering in a way that no other research can. It is Big Pharma that wants to stop animal testing. Such testing has often exposed side effects of their ill-conceived concoctions long before humans are exposed. It is unfortunate that organizations such as PETA and similar more radical organizations unwittingly play into the hands of the pharmaceutical giants and put animal testing and those who must perform it in harm's way.[550]

The Circulatory System is a Target of Methanol Poisoning

Two major issues point to methanol poisoning as the cause of atherosclerotic cardiovascular diseases. The first is habitual cigarette smoking,[345] a known rich source of methanol.[62] Smoking is responsible for as much as tripling of the likelihood of ACD and doubling the chance of stroke. A recent policy statement of the American Heart Association (2011) puts smoking into perspective: "Cigarettes are the most important preventable cause of premature death in the United States. Most of those deaths are from heart *disease, not cancer.*" The second issue is the U-shaped curve of alcohol consumption. ACD was the first of the diseases of civilization whose incidence was conclusively proven to be dramatically reduced by a small daily dose of methanol's only cure – ethanol.[176] The only plausible explanation for these outcomes is that ACD is a disease of chronic methanol poisoning.[586]

The autopsies of those who suffered prolonged deaths from methanol poisoning consistently show signs of circulatory disturbance,[37] with numerous hemorrhages in the brain and digestive system lining[110] and petechial hemorrhages (tiny dot bleeding) in all the organs throughout the body.[414] When rabbits, one of the few animals used successfully to study some aspects of atherosclerosis in man, were forced to breathe methanol fumes for 8 hours a day for several months, all developed a marked increase in the thickness of their blood vessels. Dr Eisenberg's microscopic examination of the rabbits' circulatory tissues attributed the changes to "the actual proliferation of the fixed tissue cells, as seen by the very marked thickening of the adventitia and media of the blood-vessels."[15]

Most telling of all is one of Oluf Roe's ground-breaking articles, published in the early 1940s investigating a massive outbreak of methanol poisoning that killed and blinded numerous of his countrymen. Roe made a profound observation while investigating the optic discs of several of his poisoned patients. These men, one of whose age was only 32 years, had survived between 6 and 12 weeks after their acute methanol poisoning. Dr. Roe, the father of the use of ethanol to treat methanol poisoning, states:

> *"There was at the same time marked irregularity of the caliber of the large blood vessels with thickening of their walls. These changes resemble those seen in the blood vessels of the retina in arteriosclerosis."[49]*

It cannot be overlooked that even relatively low-level contact with methanol can induce the type of change that a lifetime can magnify into ADC.

An Alcoholic's Arteries

At some point in my very early days at Arizona State University I remember calling up the office of the Maricopa County Medical Examiner looking for help. I needed some human tissue for a study I wanted to begin on the residual mercury of those individuals who had mercury amalgam fillings. I talked to the medical examiner himself and explained exactly what I required. He listened quite courteously, waited until I was finished, and then asked, "How many autopsies have you assisted at?"

I was silent for a moment, and then stuttered that I had never even attended an autopsy, although I had done some extensive animal dissections. "Fine," he said. "I need a hand down here. When can I expect you?"

By the time I reached the morgue and suited up, he had three bodies in queue. Maricopa is a very big county that includes the entire Phoenix metropolitan area. It is the job of the medical examiner to perform autopsies on any death that is not attended or is of a suspicious nature. The three poor souls that lay before me on gurneys covered by opaque plastic sheets were to change my life and help ground this book in stark reality.

As it turned out, the Medical Examiner was a consummate teacher and when he heard that a young Nutritional Science faculty member had never been to a proper autopsy he took it upon himself to both see what I knew and to show me a thing or two about what made the human body stop working. His first lesson consisted of a gentleman of about sixty years of age who had smoked most of his adult years and now lay dead of an extreme case of atherosclerosis. The exact cause of death was severe internal bleeding while in the recovery room after a valiant attempt at replacing a portion of his savaged aorta had failed due to the lack of sufficient healthy arterial tissue to suture the replacement tube into place.

After the Y incision was made into the man's chest it took some time to remove leaked blood from his chest cavity. This gave me a chance to regain my composure. The shock of watching someone cutting violently into a human body was almost too much for my nervous system to handle, and large sections of my visual field were disappearing into a hazy mist as my face must have completely drained of blood. The Examiner looked up at me and kindly asked if I needed a break. It took every bit of strength I could muster to say, in a shaky and insincere, barely audible whisper, "No thank you."

This reaction is common, I hear, and for me it lasted only as long as it took my eye to find something of interest inside the cadaver. The examiner reached in and carefully removed an adrenal gland. As he held the glands to measure their size I could see that they had an appearance like no other adrenal glands that I had ever seen. This man had been dead only a few hours, yet the color of the glands was not the light glistening pink that I was accustomed to seeing when dissecting fresh animal tissue. This specimen was a sickly brown color and looked as if it were dissolving into a puddle as the examiner attempted to weigh it. I asked why the organ appeared so unhealthy. "Smoker," was all the examiner said. That was all he had to say.

I now recalled at the opening of the corpse that I had braced myself for the odor that I had come to expect when first opening an animal's body cavity. It is a smell hard to describe, but reminiscent of a cross between barnyard and fecal matter. This cadaver's smell was different, and the reason didn't hit me until the examiner's enlightenment: what made this cadaver smell even more repulsive than usual was the added strong note of ashtray. This man's carcass was severely marked by his habitual smoking. Not one of his organs was free from either the odor or the deterioration caused by the combination of methanol and tar that make cigarettes so toxic.

The arteries themselves were to be the lesson taken away from this autopsy session – the tough, fibrous leathery texture of the arteries themselves and, in various stages of development, those fascinating atheroma. The atheroma took me by surprise. They were nothing like what I had pictured after reading about them in textbooks. I asked if I could take off my gloves and the pathologist joked that he would have to ask the patient. The squishy feel of the fat and dead macrophage-filled cysts had me mesmerized. I put additional pressure on one large atheroma which at first moved around under the endothelium but then it ruptured as it would have on its own prior to an infarction. They strongly reminded me of the swellings that developed on my thigh after my encounter with the formaldehyde from that hand warmer.

We spent a great deal of time examining the arteries and then moved on to the heart itself, which had a number of discolorations that, when sliced through, revealed areas of partially healed-over infarctions. These were places where, when an atheroma broke open, the blood flow to that part of the heart was cut off and heart tissue had died. The medical examiner said that such occurrences could have been felt as severe chest pain without even being reported as actual heart attacks. None of them involved enough heart tissue to cause death, but most likely cut down considerably on the man's stamina while he lived.

In stark contrast to the first autopsy, the last one of the day was of a man in his 70s who would have, when I was a child, been classified as a derelict alcoholic or "Bowery Bum." He was a person who had spent his life working menial jobs or just panhandling or begging for enough money to constantly stay drunk. The part of Phoenix where the morgue was located is just the part of town where these individuals would hang out forty years ago when this death occurred. The body was brought in by the police the previous evening with no signs of foul play, but it took an autopsy to determine that he had fallen asleep dead drunk and belched up part of his last meal, aspirating it into his lungs for a fatal outcome while sleeping.

I was by now an old hand as an autopsy assistant and had no trepidations about what might lie inside this third carcass of the day. The previous cadaver had been a gentleman of about the same age as this alcoholic who had bumped his head against his windshield during a minor traffic accident. His sudden death four days after the accident turned out to have been caused by an interaction of his brain with one of the sharp protrusions at the base of his skull when the brain shifted slightly during impact. The medical examiner took the time to lay out the exact details of this interaction after he carefully removed the brain and exposed a part of the skull to which I had never given any thought. This was a great help in understanding the pressure damage to the brain done by methanol that I was to see again thirty five years later when I reviewed the case of murder by methanol that I described in the previous chapter.

This third autopsy was the biggest surprise of the day. By now I was used to seeing atheroma, which had made dramatic presentation in the first autopsy of the heavy smoker, whose cause of death was, in reality, atherosclerosis. The second gentleman had been in his late sixties and, although in much healthier condition than the first, was still of the age where the examiner could easily find some small atheroma and thickening of the arteries that he confirmed goes along with aging in our civilized culture. The third gentleman – the alcoholic – had a large fatty and unhealthy-looking liver, but his circulatory system was flawless. Looking in all the usual places within the full length of the aorta and slicing his heart completely into half inch thick slices we could find nothing that even looked like he might have ever had an atheroma or an infarction. The lining of the aorta was smooth and glistening, with no bumps or even the fatty streaks that the examiner had grown accustomed to seeing appearing as early as preteens. None of the arterial hardening that was so prominent in the first two examinations was present in the alcoholic. This man's circulatory system was faultless and might well have served him for another 70 years. I was stunned by this and asked the examiner just what made this man stand out. The medical examiner said that this was indeed the norm. It was rare indeed for him to find any serious atherosclerotic plaque formation on any hard core alcoholic derelict. The exceptions were what he called "part timers" or binge alcoholics. This is the group that often has the worst of circulatory outcomes.

As it turns out, for half a century medical examiners like my teacher in Phoenix and others throughout the world had been reporting on a number of occasions that an obvious inverse relationship existed between chronic substantial alcohol abuse and atherosclerotic disease, including coronary disease.[87] In 1995, the University Institute of Forensic Medicine in Denmark published a study that confirmed over a five year study period that particularly alcoholic men had a significantly lower degree of atherosclerosis in the coronary arteries than normal controls.[296] In other words, those who consistently and heavily abused alcohol were spared both atherosclerosis and coronary heart disease. I am not talking here occasional drinkers, nor am I talking about the U-shaped curve. I am referring to drunks who stay drunk. This particular group is spared the ravages of atherosclerotic cardiovascular diseases (ACD).

Has your doctor ever mentioned this to you? Of course not. Yes, alcoholics do have other serious health problems; but the very individuals dying from alcoholism and alcoholic cirrhosis have far less evidence of coronary heart disease and atherosclerosis than the average person.[87] It is the other complications they experience that preclude us from suggesting alcoholism as a healthy lifestyle. But if we truly want to find the answer to the cause and prevention of the DOC, we must not pay any heed to the religious or ethical implications of alcohol consumption. The only considerations that should interest us here is the science behind why stone-hard drunks are protected from the ACD. Answer this question and you will unlock the secret of all the diseases of civilization.

The Girl Who Switched to Aspartame

The name of the scientific article in the prestigious Annals of internal Medicine is "Aspartame-Induced Granulomatous Panniculitis."[228] It tells of an otherwise healthy 22-year old girl who had consumed between three and four cans of aspartame-containing diet soda each day for a period of about two weeks before she began developing deep granulomatous panniculitis nodules between 0.5 and 5 cm in diameter on her thighs and calves. After two months without resolution, she was examined by Dr. Nelson Novick, a board certified dermatologist working at the Mt. Sinai Medical Center in New York City and author of the article. The descriptions of the lesions were physically indistinguishable from those I experienced on my thigh from my direct formaldehyde gas exposure. Dr. Novick reported the nodules were freely moveable and, on occasion, coalesced to form larger plaques exactly like mine did. The atheroma nodules I was able to examine with my bare hands on the aorta of the cadaver in Phoenix had the same unusual behavior and consistency.

Dr. Novick's patient had habitually consumed a daily equivalent amount of a popular saccharin-containing diet drink for six years, but switched to the same manufacturer's aspartame-sweetened diet drink two weeks before symptom onset. She had made no other changes to her diet. Dr Novick suspected the involvement of the recently introduced aspartame sweetened diet soda. He advised his patient to stop consuming the aspartame drink. During the next four weeks, no new lesions appeared and all previous lesions spontaneously disappeared. He then asked her to renew her daily consumption of the aspartame-sweetened diet drink; ten days later she again developed the nodular lesions on both legs, but this time in greater quantity.

Most doctors would have stopped at this point, but Dr. Novick wanted to dispel all doubt. He acquired pure aspartame and produced capsules containing 50 milligrams of aspartame. He asked his patient to take four of these a day at even intervals. Aspartame cannot be absorbed directly into the bloodstream and is broken down into the individual amino acids and methanol, which is absorbed separately. The total dose of methanol would have been 22 milligrams a day. For a girl of 45 kilograms in weight this would be about one 200th of the lethal dose, or just about one 80th of the dose of methanol that Majchrowicz found could cause severe alcoholic withdrawal symptoms.

After ten days of pure aspartame consumption again the granulomatous panniculitis returned. Doctor Novick was able to confirm during consultation with the FDA that aspartame had been linked on previous occasions with unconfirmed "dermal eruptions," urticaria (often found in MS) and even a similar macular eruption on the retina in individuals consuming aspartame sweetened products.

This is where my friend Bill would be a good tutor. As he would say, "You have to be smarter than what you are working with."

What is it about aspartame that could possibly cause your macrophages to attack you? A molecule of aspartame is composed of two amino acids and a molecule of methanol. We rule out the amino acids, and that leaves only methanol. Methanol itself will not induce macrophage attack; the only possible way that aspartame could induce granulomatous panniculitis in the human body would be by first converting it into formaldehyde and then for the formaldehyde to produce a formaldehyde modified protein (antigen) capable of inducing a macrophage attack. By proving that aspartame produces such an immune response Dr. Novick, in one fell swoop, proved that not only does methanol turn into formaldehyde, but also that enough methanol is found in an average dose of a diet food product to induce a serious physiological change in the human body.

Here is a very important issue. If a few cans of diet coke can produce enough formaldehyde in the skin of an individual to induce a full-blown granulomatous eruption, then how would that differ from producing an atheroma or any other type of auto immune reaction that springs forth from the same type of formaldehyde interaction?

Do you understand now how diet soda could easily be responsible for causing an increase in coronary heart disease?

The U-Shaped Curve in Depth and Beyond… Far, Far Beyond

Without a doubt, the business of the U-shaped curve of ethanol consumption has been a great embarrassment to the medical community as a whole. From its quite accidental and apparently unwanted discovery to this day, excuses are rampant throughout the literature and physicians gossip among themselves incessantly that this information will somehow be harmful to mankind. The taboo against drinking runs deep in western society and those of us who cherish ethanol as a useful drug have a nearly impossible row to hoe. Because of this, the full meaning and true consequence of this startling discovery of the beneficial face of ethanol has been neglected, if not de-facto hidden from the general population. Perhaps most embarrassing of all to the medical profession is its total inability to explain this phenomena. They have no idea as to what causes this apparent need for ethanol.

We know the cause and will use their research to prove our point. You and I will not concern ourselves with the apparent moral reservations expressed by the medical community, by the religious community, and – amusingly enough – by Big Pharma, relative to the dangers of implying a beneficial effect of ethanol consumption. What the U-shaped curve represents to us is confirming evidence that methanol is a disease-causing agent and the root cause of many chronic human diseases. Logic compels us to the conclusion that the only reason that abstinence from ethanol could possibly be a causative factor in disease development would be if the basis of the disease in question was caused by methanol turning into formaldehyde in the absence of ethanol. Ethanol is, in fact, the *only* cure for methanol poisoning, both acute and chronic.

Avoid Ethanol and Risk Disease.

Whatever mechanism acts to maintain a small amount of ethanol in the bloodstream for the longest possible time will be protective from disease.

It is vital that you understand the full ramifications of this important statement. We are going to discuss the so called U-shaped curve in detail now, and then I will explain how a very important genetically endowed difference in the actual structure of human ADH, which changes the rate that ethanol is lost from the bloodstream, adds considerably to our evidence that methanol poisoning is indeed the root cause of many diseases. Go have a cup of coffee and put your brain in learning mode… this is important stuff!

The All-Important U-Shaped Curve

We are told that the vital lesson from the U-shaped curve is that those who don't drink alcohol (teetotalers) are more susceptible to disease than those who consume a moderate amount. Cardiovascular diseases were among the first whose prevention was found to respond positively to alcohol consumption.[176] This accidentally discovered favorable response to ethanol was, in fact, so powerful as to outweigh the response to any known preventative drug therapy. This outcome has engendered considerable pharmaceutical company funding of studies that attempt to disprove the relationship. Under this considerable pressure the protective effect of ethanol has persevered and been expanded to encompass other diseases and mortality in general.[279]

Few realize that the original research that uncovered the beneficial effect of ethanol consumption on heart disease was much more powerful than is generally known and did not show only a U-shaped curve. The curve for cardiovascular deaths revealed by the thoughtful interpretation of the drinking habits and ten year mortality distribution of over 85 thousand patients of the Kaiser-Permanente Medical Care Program is stated best by the authors as follows:

> *Cardiovascular disease was the most frequent cause of death (41.7% of all deaths). The cardiovascular deaths were most numerous among nondrinkers and least numerous among those who drank one or two drinks a day, a difference largely reflecting a significant excess in coronary mortality among nondrinkers. Among all deaths attributed to acute myocardial infarction, those who drank more than six or between one and two drinks a day had the lowest mortality from this cause.*[176]

Step 1

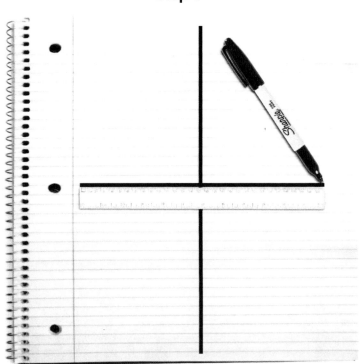

In other words, alcohol consumption, no matter at what level, protects those who drink from all the cardiovascular diseases.

For the sake of those who don't know what a U-shaped or any other curve is all about, let me just take a paragraph or two of your time and start with the very basics. The truth is that data from significant natural events expressed in graphic form is all a good scientist needs to make conclusions. If the data talks to you in a strong enough voice visually, then statistics are a waste of time and can even obfuscate Nature's true meaning. We will see a handful of plotted data during the telling of this story. It is important that you not only understand the basic process, but also grasp the importance of what you are viewing. Please do me a favor and grab a ruler and a sheet of white paper, or heck, open this book up to one

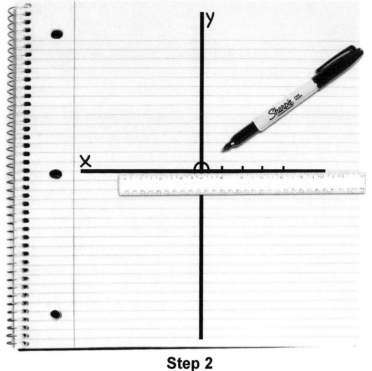

Step 2

of the blank pages in the back and have at it. Learn this little trick and no data can hide from you ever again.

Draw a vertical line right down the middle of the page and then draw a horizontal line to make a perfect cross in the center of the page. We have important names for these lines: the one that goes with the horizon is always the x-axis and the one that goes up and down is the y-axis. Remember this and you might be mistaken for a scientist someday.

We are now going to do some very exciting graphing of our own. We will take the data from the first study that defined the U-shaped curve of alcohol consumption and plot it for ourselves.[176] Take your cross and, at the very spot where the x and y axis touch in the middle of the sheet, write the number zero so that a quarter of the zero lies in each of the four portions of your graph (like this: ⊕). Next, lay down your ruler along the x-axis and put a mark every inch to the right of the zero. You only will need 3 dots, but you have room for four with a little room left over. Each dot will represent a different group of alcohol drinkers that took part in this famous study. Let's label them: we already have the 0. This will represent those who do not drink any alcohol (abstainers). One inch to the right we will label with a 2 to represent two drinks or less

a day. The next mark we will call 3-5 and the third we will call 6+ drinks a day. These are the groups that the researchers used in their study.

You are thinking that it would have been better if they would have just done it one drink at a time. Well sometimes people just don't respond well to such precise questions. How many drinks do you average a day? See what I mean!

We are halfway done already. Next we have to represent the death rate of the people in each group. The y-axis will represent the death rate. There are several ways of doing this. Since the article is an exceptionally good one and gives us the number of deaths for each disease within each group during the period of the study we could actually plot this raw data. However, the authors also present

Step 3

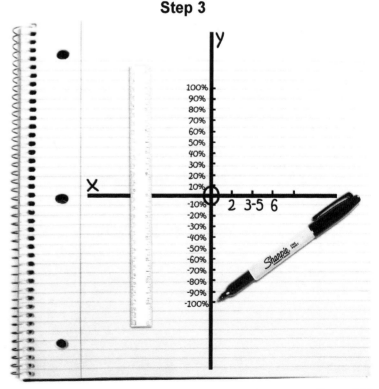

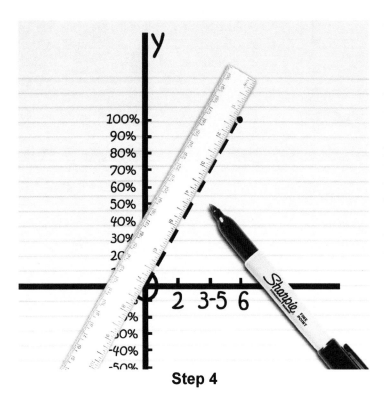

Step 4

us in the text of the article the percentage change in the death rate for each drinking group using those who don't drink as the standard. I have decided to use that form of the data, which would be easier for us all to understand. We will, therefore, mark the y-axis into percentage change markings. Take your ruler and put marks up and down the vertical axis every half inch from the zero in the center. Now we label these marks from the zero up, starting with 10% for the first, 20% for the second, and so on, all the way up to 100% at the top. Now going down we do the same thing, but start the first one as -10% and so on down to -100%. So you see how it will work, we already have the teetotalers marked as zero because they are going to be our control and no matter what their death rate is we are more concerned with how much the drinking groups change from that number as a percent.

As an example we start with the curve of "death for any reason" that made this article famous. It turns out that over the ten years of the study, the rate of death for all reasons (even those shot for trespassing) among participants that fit into the highest drinking category of over 6 alcoholic beverages a day was twice the rate of the abstainers. We now have two very important points for our plot. The zero at the point of origin represents the death rate of the abstainers and will be our first data point; the second we have to draw ourselves. Go to the mark on the x-axis that represents the 6+ drinking category and use your ruler to measure straight up a full five inches, which would be parallel to the top of the y axis, and put a dot right there. That point says that those people who drank six drinks a day had a death rate that was twice that of the abstainers, or 100% higher. Well we have two dots now, the one at the origin and the one high above the 6+ mark.

Step 5

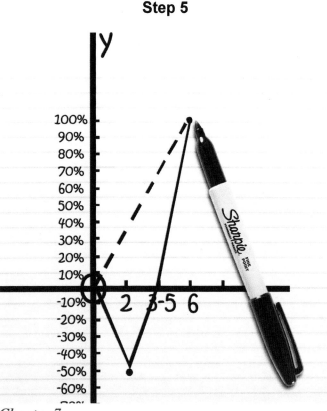

Next, I want you to take your ruler and place one end on the zero origin of our graph and the other on the data point we just placed and draw a dotted line between the two. This is a learning tool. It represents what everyone was expecting the curve from this experiment was going to look like. It is no secret that the authors of this study were expecting a linear effect of alcohol on death. In other words, they were expecting that the more alcohol one consumed, the higher the mortality. Well, were they surprised!

Let's fill in the two missing data points and see what really happened. It turns out that those who drank two or fewer drinks a day had the lowest death rate of any group, and it happened to be 50% less than the abstainers. Put in that data point by placing a dot under the 2 drink a day category by measuring down to the level of the -50% mark (2.5 inches below the x-axis). As for the 3-5 drink category, their death rate was the same as the abstainers, so just put our last data point right there directly on the x-axis where the 3-5 mark is. Now use your ruler and draw solid line and connect

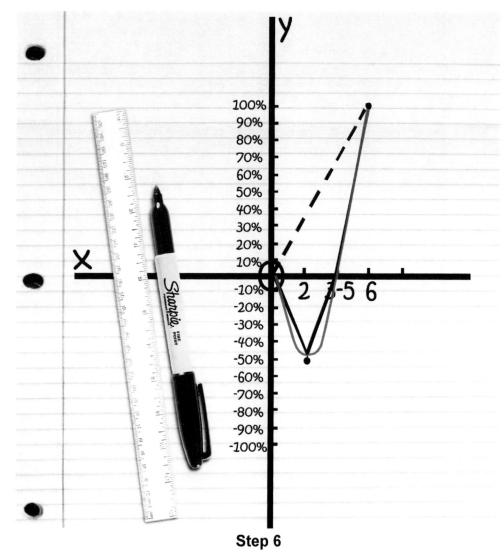

Step 6

the dots together in sequence from left to right. What you wind up with is a V-shaped curve. If you did a little freehand drawing to connect the dots you would have rounded things off a little and produced the famous U-shaped curve that changed the way the world thinks about alcohol.

The U-shaped curve of total mortality acts as the public face of this now famous article. Even though it shows that alcohol has a protective effect, it is clear that drinking too much ethanol also has a down side that plays to the "wages of sin" morality bent of American society toward hard drink. It is important that you understand what causes all those extra deaths in the individuals who consume over six alcoholic drinks a day. These are, for the most part, alcoholics and they are prone to dying much more frequently from such things as accidents and all manner of liver disorders, such as cirrhosis. However, as we saw above in the same study, when looking only at cardiovascular deaths the picture changes and in a way that helps reinforce what we have learned about ACD.

The curve that we are really interested in is the one that shows mortalities of all four drinking groups in the "cardiovascular causes of death." This curve is drawn the very same way as the one above but using data showing the death rate from heart diseases only. This curve is very much different. The greatest number of deaths in any of the four groups occurred among those who abstained from alcohol completely. The death rate goes back down to the lowest level among those who had one or two drinks a day. It then climbs back up in the 3-5 drink a day group but not as high as the abstainers. The U-shape curve holds to this point but then to everyone's surprise it drops again in those consuming more than six drinks of alcohol a day. So instead of a U-shaped curve, in reality we have more like a sine wave shaped curve, forming a U at first but then coming back down again. This shows that any alcohol consumption, even in excess, protects from heart disease. Since this study was done, other studies have verified the definite and statistically significant trend of the protective effect of alcohol consumption from all cardiovascular diseases, myocardial infarction, coronary heart disease and angina pectoris.[172] The question is, WHY?

The Details of the U-Shaped Curve Explained

Lack of ethanol in the blood exposes the human body to the danger of methanol converting to formaldehyde. Without ethanol, the human body is prey to the uncontrolled conversion of methanol into formaldehyde at a number of ADH sites after exposure to methanol from the civilized diet, the environment and smoking. Atheroma, the root cause of all cardiovascular disease, is born of the interaction of formaldehyde, LDL and the macrophage at just such a location within the wall of the artery. Only the constant presence of ethanol at the ADH sites can prevent all formaldehyde production and the disease it brings.

While good evidence exists that ethanol can be produced in the gut from fermentation, the supplementation of this unreliable source through the daily consumption of ethanol drink would increase the statistical probability that the concentration of ethanol in the blood might never be reduced to zero, a state which would guarantee formaldehyde production. As the amount of ethanol in the diet increases beyond some point above two drinks a day, however, the human liver begins perceiving ethanol itself as a chemical threat and it activates the cytochrome P-450 microsomal enzyme system that helps remove ethanol from the bloodstream at twice the rate as before activation.[392] The activation of this powerful system in the liver can linger for months after ethanol consumption has abated. Once the P-450 system is activated, the individual is removing ethanol from the bloodstream at a rate which makes is difficult to maintain ethanol in the blood, particularly through the overnight fasting hours. This explains the greater protection afforded by two drinks or less a day, as opposed to the risk engendered as we approach five drinks a day and risk ethanol depletion by activated liver action.

It will be obvious that at some point an individual can maintain ethanol in his or her bloodstream at all times by consuming ethanol at a rate which, even with P-450 activation, exceeds the body's ability to metabolize it. These are some of the individuals who fit into the category of exceeding six alcoholic drinks a day. This further explains the dip in death rate in the curve for the "all cardiovascular causes of death" for drinkers consuming more than six drinks a day. The revelation that was so clear to me during the autopsy of the atheroma-free arteries of the aged alcoholic validates the truth of this final consumption category.

Keeping Ethanol in the Blood: The Genetic Bombshell

If you have learned anything from this chapter it is that maintenance of low levels of ethanol in your bloodstream at all times will protect you from methanol's conversion to formaldehyde. One way to do this is to prudently consume alcoholic beverages. The U-shaped curve presents powerful evidence that the consumption of one or two alcoholic beverages on a daily basis protects better than any known prophylactic medication against cardiovascular diseases,[176] myocardial infarction,[485] coronary heart disease, angina pectoris,[172] dementia,[534] and lupus SLE.[73] The list grows as other accidental discoveries of the U-shaped curve response are revealed through the analysis of dietary population studies of other diseases.

The major drawback with alcohol consumption is that at some point above 3 or more drinks a day ethanol becomes a trigger for the liver to increase its rate of removal of ethanol from the bloodstream (P-450). This

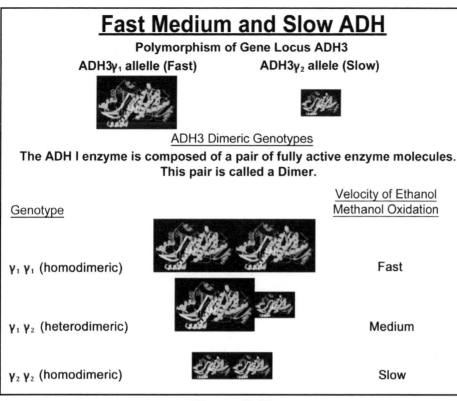

Fast Medium and Slow ADH

Polymorphism of Gene Locus ADH3

ADH3γ₁ allele (Fast)   **ADH3γ₂ allele (Slow)**

ADH3 Dimeric Genotypes

**The ADH I enzyme is composed of a pair of fully active enzyme molecules.
This pair is called a Dimer.**

Genotype		Velocity of Ethanol Methanol Oxidation
γ₁ γ₁ (homodimeric)		Fast
γ₁ γ₂ (heterodimeric)		Medium
γ₂ γ₂ (homodimeric)		Slow

Figure 7.10

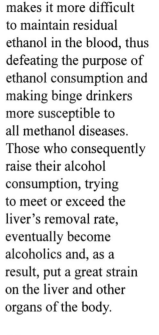

makes it more difficult to maintain residual ethanol in the blood, thus defeating the purpose of ethanol consumption and making binge drinkers more susceptible to all methanol diseases. Those who consequently raise their alcohol consumption, trying to meet or exceed the liver's removal rate, eventually become alcoholics and, as a result, put a great strain on the liver and other organs of the body.

A better way to accomplish the desired result of maintaining ethanol in the bloodstream would be to reduce the rate at which the enzyme ADH metabolizes ethanol and removes it. I know this might sound like some harebrained scheme from the addled mind of an industry scientist, but no, this is not something from Big Pharma. Genetic variations in the structure of alcohol dehydrogenase (ADH) can be found as a genetic trait in some individuals. These structural variations are called genotypes and are responsible for considerable differences in the rate at which each version of ADH can metabolize ethanol. Since the ADH molecule is made up of two molecules of ADH bound together (dimer) the way the fast and slow versions pair up can make a considerable difference in the final outcome of any particular individuals inherited ability to metabolize ethanol (see Figure 7.10).

To put it all very simply, the truly amazing outcome of this is that individuals who are genetically endowed with the configuration of ADH that metabolizes ethanol 2.5 times more slowly than the normal version of the enzyme have an 86% reduction in risk of developing myocardial infarction – but only if they consume ethanol on a daily basis.[483] Other laboratories have begun to investigate the role of variants of ADH in the evolution of other important diseases.[216] This is very powerful and convincing evidence that it is the maintenance of ethanol in the blood for the longest period of time that is responsible for the protective effect of the U-shaped curve? The only conceivable benefit of ethanol consumption would be the prevention of conversion of methanol into formaldehyde.

A Review

You must understand by now that if the immune system is mandated to do something, it will accomplish that function in very short order. If it was the mission of the immune system to produce a lump of dead macrophages and cholesterol between two layers of the lining of your aorta, it is perfectly reasonable to believe that your death from such an atheroma blockage would not take very long at all. It should be obvious that the reason it takes twenty years or more to develop symptoms from atheroma production in the arteries is that this result is not natural, but is something you might expect from an intermittent poisoning rather than the result of an error in the innate immune system itself, which would manifest much more quickly.

Clear your minds for a moment and together let us take inventory of the considerable evidence that posits methanol as the cause of heart disease.

The Molecular Evidence

In the absence of ethanol in the bloodstream, the enzyme alcohol dehydrogenase (ADH) found in the intima of the human artery wall turns methanol ingested from cigarette smoke and diet soda into formaldehyde. As the small reactive formaldehyde molecule diffuses from its ADH genesis it makes contact and oxidizes native LDLs, turning them into bait that attracts the macrophage. The formaldehyde modified protein from the oxidized LDL does something strange to the macrophage – it turns off the mechanism that controls the macrophage's appetite and allows it to continue eating modified LDLs to its heart's content, all the time converting the cholesterol they contain into the esterified form always found in atheroma. This is called activation. If the supply of formaldehyde-treated LDL does not end, the macrophage will stuff itself until it turns into a foam cell, eventually eating so much it explodes. The exploding foam cell releases its contents into the intima, this process releases a substance that attracts microsomes from the bloodstream that will evolve shortly into macrophages, continuing the process which eventually produces an eruption – called an atheroma – on the artery wall.

The Toxicological Evidence

The circulatory system is a known target of methanol poisoning, with short term exposure causing thickening of the intima of the artery walls as seen in *arteriosclerosis*. There are few sources of dietary or environmental methanol poisoning. Cigarette smoking is the most reliable and is universally considered the major cause of coronary heart disease, stroke and the other atherosclerotic cardiovascular diseases.[345] Aspartame is another known source of methanol whose daily consumption has recently been linked to a fifty percent increase in death from heart disease and stroke.[686]

Epidemiological Evidence

Hunter-gatherer populations have little or no contact with methanol and enjoy an extremely low incidence of atherosclerotic cardiovascular disease. Exposure to methanol, as in cigarette smoking, has been proven to increase all the cardiovascular diseases and stroke.[345] Ethanol is the only cure for methanol poisoning and intuition tells us that continuous safe exposure to a known antidote to a poison should help protect us from the destructive effect of that poison. The discovery of the so called U-shaped curve of ethanol consumption shows the power of maintaining a low level of ethanol in the blood supply to prevent any instance of methanol being metabolized into formaldehyde and thus eliminating macrophage activation and disease development. Recent studies of individuals who consumed at least one alcoholic drink per day show subjects had an additional 86% percent reduction in risk of myocardial infarction if they were genetically endowed with a type of ADH I that was 2.5 times slower to remove ethanol from their bloodstream than those who were born with normal ADH. These findings show that whatever it takes to keep ethanol in the bloodstream for as long as possible will protect us from cardiovascular disease.[483] This was the ultimate discovery of the startlingly powerful protective effect of ethanol.

Chapter 8
Alzheimer's Disease and Its Perivascular Nature

Short History of Alzheimer's

Alzheimer's disease was first described by the German neurologist Alois Alzheimer in 1907. This was early into the century that marked the purposeful adulteration of food and drugs with methanol as a replacement for ethanol. Alzheimer's is a disease that takes time to develop, with a mean life expectancy of seven years following diagnosis.[704] Though deterioration of memory is the major symptom of the disease it does share some symptomology with the other major perivascular disease of the brain – multiple sclerosis. Both diseases are characterized by difficulty in speaking and walking, incontinence, and confusion, all of which are also symptoms of methanol poisoning.

Thirty years ago it was suggested in a review article by the respected neurologist Frederick Wolfgram that because multiple sclerosis and Alzheimer's are perivenular in nature, starting and evolving around the small veins of the brain, the culprit might be "a simple molecule of low molecular weight which arrives at the brain via the blood supply."[153] He further mused, "It is interesting that the damage is often perivenular because the flow of blood is slowest in the venules, and this may provide an optimal situation for the toxin to escape from the vascular system."[153]

Another feature that these two diseases share is they are both presently experiencing "epidemics." Alzheimer's scholars admit that although the disease is presently one of the most common diseases of the elderly, very little mention of it can be found in the world's scientific literature before the 1960s.[533]

There is very good reason to believe that Alzheimer's disease is caused by a poison. I will provide the facts and a logical argument to support that possibility. I will also present methanol as the culprit. Whether I am right or wrong about the specific cause of this affliction, you must come away from this chapter with some considerable concern that the public agencies charged with protecting your health and the health of your children are not working properly and are, in fact, broken. You are not being properly warned or protected by government agencies that the public supports and should control. In this maturing age of democracy, no bureaucracy ought to exist for any reason other than to protect and serve. A government that dominates for the benefit of the regal few is a paradigm of the Dark Ages and must not be tolerated.

I have spent my career fighting government employees over food safety issues in public agencies in the United States and to some small extent in New Zealand. I have consistently confronted salaried individuals in leadership positions whose scripted purpose was to maintain the health of all people, but who instead, with every act and deed, supported the interests of big business while giving only lip service and the very minimum effort to their sacred duty to protect the common man. It is beyond my power to change this – I have tried. It is fortunate that all the issues that I deal with in this book require fixes that are within your personal control. These are all diet modifications that are easily manageable. I will be the first to admit that all of the diseases we discuss here have eluded science for many years, but recent developments make their cause inescapable and their prevention trivial and elective.

Alzheimer's deceives by advancing slowly, with much similarity to what we are told is the natural outcome of aging. We expect to lose memory as we grow older so the harsh reality of its steady progression is buffered by our expectations. At some point the conscious brain is lost to the disease and self is gone long before death ensues. This is not a natural outcome and, as you are, by now, used to hearing of methanol diseases, Alzheimer's research has no suitable animal model. The uneven worldwide distribution and recent astronomical increase in its death rate, particularly in the United States, is substantial proof that this is a man made phenomenon. I believe we are dealing with a food poisoning, and like all poisonings it has cause and culprit. Let us investigate this hypothesis and attempt an elucidation using the knowledge and tools learned in previous chapters. We will stand on the shoulders of the ancient Aztec and Inuit who solved complex health conundrums with simple logic, instinct and much less information than we have at our disposal.

I remember clearly the sympathy I felt while reading Ronald Reagan's heart wrenching letter revealing his Alzheimer's disease diagnosis. It began with "I have recently been told that I am one of the millions of Americans who will be afflicted with Alzheimer's disease." I was saddened by the thought of countless souls witnessing their brains being turned off, not knowing what treasured memory, what loved one, they would forget next. Reagan was a man with a legendary memory that was considered by some to be photographic during his years as an actor. In contrast, as his presidency progressed, stories of forgetting the names of officials, cabinet members and important press personas became legion.

Ironically, it was just prior to the inauguration date of his first presidency – January 20, 1981 – that a personal friend of Reagan's, Donald Rumsfeld, the president of the company that invented aspartame and a member of the Reagan Presidential Transition Team, did what he could to see to it that the sitting FDA would be unable to act on its substantial opposition to, and intention to prevent, aspartame's use in foods. The summer of that same year aspartame was approved by the new FDA after 15 years of bitter controversy over its safety. It quickly became the major source of methanol in the human diet. Ironically, all through his years in office Reagan was known to carry on his person little blue packets of aspartame sweetener. They were as visible to his presidency as the little jelly beans that he insisted be made available at every cabinet meeting. He, like so many others, developed a taste for Rumsfeld's aspartame and always made sure he had it close and available. It wasn't until the end of his presidency that a reporter allegedly asked Reagan whatever happened to his little blue sweetener packets, to which he is said to have replied, "Well, you just never know what might be in those sweeteners."

While I was at the center of the controversy over aspartame the two most frequent complaints to me from consumers were headaches and memory loss. Amnesia is also a common complaint from those accidently poisoned with methanol.[49]

The Ignored Epidemic of Alzheimer's

While atherosclerosis is fresh on your mind from the last chapter it would be a good time to have a look at a review article published a few years ago in the prestigious medical journal *Lancet*, entitled "Convergence of Atherosclerosis and Alzheimer's Disease."[540] This fascinating paper reveals that increasing evidence suggests a link between Alzheimer's and atherosclerosis. The article suggests that Alzheimer's arises as a secondary event related to atherosclerosis – a "toxic effect of vascular factors." It also reveals that over the past five decades researchers have observed a sharp rise in the death rate from Alzheimer's. Their graph (Figure 8.1) is taken from one published by the United States Centers for Disease Control and Prevention (CDC)[325] and shows more specifically that the lion's share of the increased death rate in the US from Alzheimer's has occurred since the introduction of aspartame. We will now make it clear exactly where that connection is and the molecular basis for the link of the two most deadly of the DOC.

Figure 8.1 is overburdened with information about the lethality of a number of diseases with very diverse death rates in the US population. It is all data collected by the CDC. The CDC is tasked by the US government to collect statistical information on the causes of death and disease of the citizens of the USA and see to their prevention. As a bureaucratic governmental agency, it is prone to political manipulation and, therefore, capable of both some very good and some very bad work. Generally speaking, its data collecting is impeccable; the trick seems to be getting the agency to share it all with you. This is particularly problematic when it comes to birth defects or anything else related to industrial poisonings. We will discuss this in the final chapter. Since the diseases with which we will concern ourselves in this chapter are not at this time politically charged, we can take the CDC's numbers on this chart, along with the others that I will present before this book is finished, as reliable.

Let's begin by examining the CDC data in Figure 1 as an epidemiologist should, with one eye on cause and the other on prevention. I have traced the Alzheimer's disease curve in red ink so that you could easily make it out from the other 14 diseases presented. Without a doubt, something very extraordinary has been going on with Alzheimer's over the last 20 years. The real truth of the matter, however, is being hidden by the type of graph used to present the death rates. The significance and, more importantly, the magnitude of the increase in Alzheimer's over the most recent years is charted, but the true nature of the information is obscured. I will give the CDC the benefit of the doubt. In order for them to get this number of vastly divergent diseases on the same chart they had to use an exponential or logametric scale on the y axis (vertical axis, remember?).

Figure 8.1

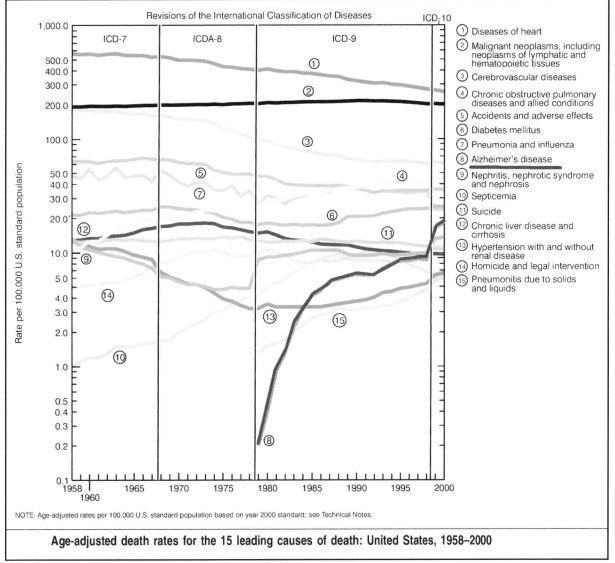

Age-adjusted death rates for the 15 leading causes of death: United States, 1958–2000

This scale is used to squeeze a great deal of information into a small space and, unfortunately, it has a way of distorting reality very much the way a wide angle lens distorts an image.

The death rate from Alzheimer's disease has changed over the last 20 years from 0.2 to over 20 per 100,000. To put this into proper perspective, if in 1980 you lived in a city of half a million people, only one of your townsfolk would be expected to die that year from Alzheimer's. The same community twenty years later would be losing over 100 souls a year to the disease. The change is breathtaking, but the graph is not.

I have taken the liberty of plotting the CDC Alzheimer's death rate data from Figure 8.1 onto an ordinary linear graph (Figure 8.2) very much like the one I showed you how to draw in the last chapter. You will notice that on this graph (and on all the graphs to follow) I use the horizontal or x axis as a place to show the progression of years from 1978 on. The only other change is that I have put the vertical or y axis, which shows the number of deaths per year from Alzheimer's, on the right side of the graph instead of on the left. I have done this because I want to do more with this graph than just show the death rate of Alzheimer's disease. I also want to plot, on the same graph, the consumption of aspartame in the US during the same period of time.

This is what epidemiologist do to correlate various environmental factors with the death or incidence rate of diseases, to look for clues to causation. For instance, this technique was utilized to prove that thalidomide was the cause of birth defects. The relative shape of the two lines on the graph, one representing disease rate and the other the rate of consumption of a suspected causative (etiologic) agent, can provide and indication and in some cases produce all the evidence necessary to prove a connection between, let's say, a new tranquilizer (thalidomide) and the sudden increase of a birth defect.

In order for us to evaluate the relationship between aspartame and Alzheimer's, therefore, we will plot aspartame consumption over the years on the same sheet of paper as Alzheimer's deaths during the very same period. The aspartame curve needs to have its own vertical axis that represents the amount of aspartame consumed. Before we do that bit of detective work let's learn what we can from the death rate of Alzheimer's plotted on a less distorting type of graph that I made from the original CDC data (Figure 8.2). I invite you to do this for yourself; it is simple and will make you feel a part of the discovery process.

Figure 8.2

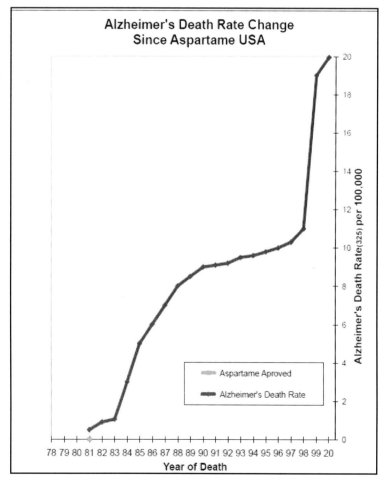

You can see how easily the data can now be read from our new graph and how different it appears from the CDC version. The most important difference between the two figures is the change in the shape of the death curve itself. We have teased out the breathtaking increase in Alzheimer's deaths at the very end of the 90s, the almost vertical line that shows a doubling of the death rate of the disease between 1998 and the year 2000. Once you get your breath back your first question will be, "How can such a thing happen?"

Alzheimer's is a slow disease that takes years to blossom. Something must have happened in the environment years before this explosion in Alzheimer's deaths that set in place the cause for the destruction of so many minds. How else can one explain an increase of 100 times in the death rate of a disease over a period of less than twenty years? How do we choose what to plot on this graph to test its veracity as an etiologic agent capable of causing this disease? Certainly, we don't want to waste our time plotting sunspots or high fructose corn syrup consumption. That would be silly. We need something that we know has a deleterious effect on the brain that might be increasing in the environment. I dare say that the first thing that comes to mind is methanol.

Methanol from Aspartame as a Cause of Alzheimer's

From chapter one and two we know that the dietary sources of methanol began increasing substantially 40 years or so ago. The increase in consumption of heavily processed fruit juices to replace carbonated beverages for the health conscious has increased steadily over that time period, with many vending machines being modified to accommodate both soda and juice products. If we had the resources of the CDC we could assign some staff to do a credible estimation of the average methanol content in these numerous juice drink products, but then we just might get in trouble with the agriculture lobby – or more likely the vending machine lobby.

You and I must keep in mind this juice factor, but it turns out to be trivial compared to the methanol from diet products and need not stop us from applying what we do know. We know that aspartame is by weight 11% methanol. We know that the average 12 ounce can of diet cola contains at least ten times more methanol than the average 12 ounce bottle of drink fortified with juice. We know that 100 times more diet cola is consumed by the US population than fruit and vegetable juice. Most important of all, we have exact figures on the consumption of aspartame by the population of the United States from 1981 until 1996, the years before Alzheimer's exploded.

I have chosen aspartame for my graph because I know it to be the major source of methanol in the human diet and methanol's primary poisonous effect on the brain sharing symptoms with the disease. The little blue dot on the x axis of Figure 8.2 indicates the first date that aspartame appeared in the general food supply six months after the Reagan inauguration.

The little box within the graph which contains the labeled colored lines is called the legend and it is where the identity of the plot lines is revealed. For the purpose of continuity we will

Figure 8.3

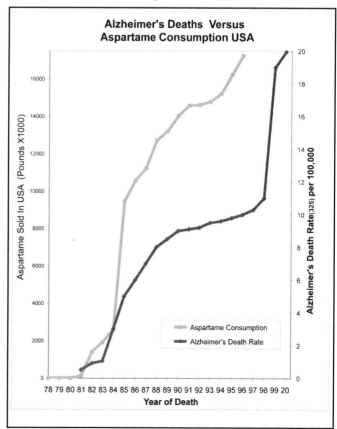

use this same labeling protocol throughout this book. The red line will always represent the disease statistics, be it death rate, as in this case, or incidence. The blue line will represent aspartame at the rate at which the unsuspecting public of the Unites States devoured it over the years. We are fortunate to have this valuable information available from day one of aspartame's appearance in the marketplace. I wish I had been able to continue receiving that consumption data up to the present day, but those who made it available to me were risking their careers and stopped before they were discovered. The CDC would have no problem obtaining that data using its subpoena power, and someday if CDC officials can summon the courage to retrieve it I would be glad to show them exactly what can be done with it.

I want to take a moment to impress upon you the significance of what is going on right now in the aspartame world. It was reported in the media on March 19, 2011 that a major soda company, to whose diet product we refer from time to time in this thesis, has had its diet cola drink "bubble up" to the second spot in the U.S. soft drink market. The company announced that in 2010 it had sold 927 million cases of that one carbonated diet drink in the US alone, which would require 9 million pounds of aspartame as an ingredient to sweeten it. The methanol in that much aspartame amounts to just about a million pounds, or more precisely, just over 73 million lethal doses of methanol. In the same story it was announced that 4 of the other top ten soft drinks sold in the US were also diet products.

Now our detective work begins. In Figure 3 we have applied another y axis on the left side of our Alzheimer's death graph that indicates the pounds of aspartame sold in the US in the years since 1981. The scale goes from zero to 18 million pounds a year. We could have used any other unit of weight – it really doesn't matter. What is vitally important is the relative change in consumption of the sweetener itself. You can easily see from the blue line on the chart that the consumption of aspartame rose gradually until it reached about two million pounds a year in 1983. 1983 was a year of great significance; it was the year that an emasculated FDA allowed aspartame's use to be expanded to include carbonated beverages and diet sodas. That was the year that I filed a petition to the FDA to stop this from happening. The FDA turned me down with no good scientific counter to my methanol argument. I went to court over the issue and eventually took them all the way to the Supreme Court of the United States – to no avail, I might add.

The ultimate result of adding this pleasant tasting sweetener to this very popular category of carbonated beverages was a drastic increase in aspartame's consumption rate over a very short period of time. Aspartame consumption increased by a factor of 5 the very next year – 1984. The explosion of consumption is ominously and tellingly matched 14 years later by a sympathetic explosion in deaths from Alzheimer's. In a tragic footnote, recent research shows that the mean life expectancy following diagnosis of Alzheimer's is seven years,[704] with fewer than 3% living longer than 14 years.[703] Under most circumstances this evidence alone should be enough to take the product off the market. But instead, the data is ignored. Why?

This tragic exercise in political food additive approval against the advice of the best informed of the scientific community turns out to have been an experiment of untold utility to those of us who have an interest in methanol toxicity. Throughout this book I have been lamenting that methanol toxicity can only be tested on humans. What better way to test methanol than to administer it secretly to an enormous human population over a long period of time and then look for changes in the disease distribution of that population – particularly the diseases that can be linked to the biochemical behavior of methanol? That is exactly what has occurred over the last 30 years.

This makes 1983 a date of the greatest importance to toxicologists. It is as if a starting gun went off and people of the US began consuming large amounts of methanol from that point forward. I know this because I was caught up in the politics of that time. It was well known that the fix was in and that aspartame would be allowed in carbonated beverages. The manufacture of the sweetener was already geared up for higher production and the soda companies had their new formulations ready to go. When the official word was released, the extremely popular diet drink that we discussed above with millions of consumers had its formula changed virtually overnight, with the effect of producing a spike of methanol consumption in a population that had not been previously exposed to that product… an epidemiologist's dream come true.

As good proof of the importance of such graphic correlations in the hands of concerned epidemiologists, let's look at the evidence that proved that cigarette smoking was an important cause of lung cancer. Sales statistics were available for cigarettes between the years 1900 and 1950. When this data was correlated to the number of lung cancer deaths starting twenty years later the resultant graph showed a story chillingly similar to our aspartame-to-Alzheimer's correlation. This curve acted as the primary evidence that turned the medical establishment against smoking. See Figure 8.4.

Figure 8.4

Remember the young girl from the last chapter with skin eruptions from aspartame? Her reaction only took a few weeks. Each methanol disease requires a different period of time to manifest itself. Granulomatous Panniculitis may take weeks, while Alzheimer's takes, based on an educated guess, an average of 7 years to evolve. I know it sounds just terrible for me to go on in this manner about an obvious crime against humanity, but ignoring this travesty and pretending that nothing ever happened would be worse than exploiting it and making some good of it. May we never again do what the world did with Josef Mangle after the Second World War – let him escape and live out his years unpunished while simultaneously destroying all of the records of his heartless experimentation. Surely, the many dead from both these atrocities would not want their suffering to go for naught.

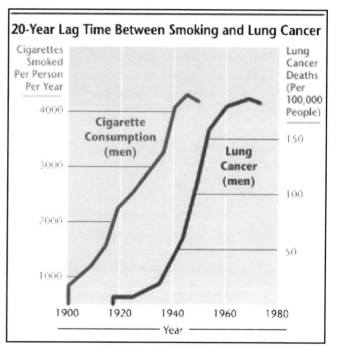

What Connects Methanol to Alzheimer's

Alzheimer's is clearly a prime candidate for consideration as a methanol disease. Aside from the fact that its incidence has risen dramatically during the age of aspartame it fits another of our criteria to be classed in the methanol disease category. Alzheimer's is more frequent in those who consume no ethanol and has been shown to respond in the U-shaped manor to ethanol consumption.[531] Here we have another case where the U-shaped relationship to ethanol consumption was discovered by accident during a study to determine if the herb Ginkgo was beneficial for memory. Self-reporting moderate drinkers had a 37% reduced risk of developing dementia over a period of 6 years. In another study similar results were reported during a 34-year follow-up study of women in Germany with a 40% reduced risk of Alzheimer's with moderate wine consumption.[535]

The disease also appears to be causatively linked to cigarette smoking,[696] though the data is compromised. This connection has allegedly been obscured for years by a concerted and expensive campaign by the tobacco industry to seed the medical literature with pro-tobacco misinformation.[249] All of the studies done to investigate the connection between smoking and Alzheimer's that were performed by laboratories affiliated in any way with, or funded by, the tobacco industry had to be removed from consideration before it could be shown that those who smoke have almost twice the chance of contracting Alzheimer's.[696] The research done by industry-connected laboratories was so skewed that some of the tobacco-funded studies actually showed that smoking protects from the disease. In the end, to be fair, tobacco smoke appears to contain something that is protective against Alzheimer's disease – nicotine is suggested in some articles – but overall, the negative effects of methanol on the brain far outweigh any possible benefits that might accrue from this undetermined ingredient.

Most important of all is the molecular details of the mechanism by which Alzheimer's can be induced with even very low levels of formaldehyde within the brain. In brief, Alzheimer's has been shown convincingly to be causable by intercranial formaldehyde, the source of which can only be methanol.[234] The story is considerably more intricate, but you need to learn a bit about the brain and the disease before you will understand its significance.

The Scene of the Crime

The brain and spinal cord are immunologically independent and separated from the rest of the body by the layer of endothelial cells that coat the intima of the blood vessels of the central nervous system. The endothelial cells of the vessels of the brain are more densely packed than those lining the rest of the circulatory system. This tight endothelium is, in fact, all that constitutes the much discussed "blood-brain barrier." This important layer of protection acts to largely prevent bacteria, viruses, antibodies, and reactive chemicals such as formaldehyde from reaching the brain. For this reason the central nervous system is often called "immune privileged."

Even macrophages and microsomes have difficulty penetrating this barrier, and for that reason the brain and spinal cord must have their own resident macrophages. These are called *microglia*, but they behave in all ways as macrophages and act as the innate immune defense of the central nervous system. Microglia are constantly scavenging for damaged neurons, infectious agents and formaldehyde modified protein. They must react quickly to recognize and swallow foreign bodies and to interact with T-cells to spawn antibody production (antibodies from the rest of the body are too large to cross the blood brain barrier).

Alzheimer's is a perivascular disease. This means that the damage it causes begins in extremely close proximity to – and directly surrounding – blood vessels of the brain, affecting primarily the axons of nerve cells passing through that area. Figure 8.5 shows cross sections of small blood vessels from the brains of Alzheimer's victims. The dark areas are plaque deposits. Alzheimer's shares this perivascular classification with only one other major disease – multiple sclerosis (MS), which we will discuss in the next chapter.

Alzheimer's disease has been identified as a protein misfolding disease, caused by the accumulation of abnormally folded and unnaturally bound together tau proteins that normally reside within the axon of nerve cells.[697] The unnatural bonding and aggregation of the proteins create tangles that continue to bind together and grow into senile plaque, which blocks and disintegrates the axon's transport system, eventually bursting through the cell's membrane and killing the nerve cell.[698] This behavior is very similar to what happens when we expose our limbs to very cold temperatures: ice crystals slowly increase in size within our muscle cells until they finally break through the cell membranes, killing the cell and causing frost bite. In Alzheimer's disease, the formaldehyde induces chemical changes in the tau protein that are similar to the changes made to the LDL prior to atheroma formation, as we discussed in the last chapter.[235]

Interestingly, Alzheimer's, unlike atherosclerosis (and MS), does not, in the very early stages of the disease, involve macrophages. This is probably due to the fact that the modified tau protein is initially located deep below the nerve cell surface, beyond detection by the scavenger sites of the macrophage. However, as the disease progresses and axons are broken open, exposing formaldehyde modified protein, the macrophages (microglia) become heavily involved. They increase in number and, most important of all, greatly increase the expression on their cell membranes of the identical scavenger receptor sites responsible for formaldehyde modified LDL detection. The macrophages located in close proximity to the senile plaques are activated, and some transform into foam cells like those found during atheroma production.[679] They are being activated, not by formaldehyde modified LDLs, but by some other formaldehyde modified protein (probably tau). Macrophages are intensively involved in the end stage of the disease where they are, as in MS, associated with considerable demyelination.[679]

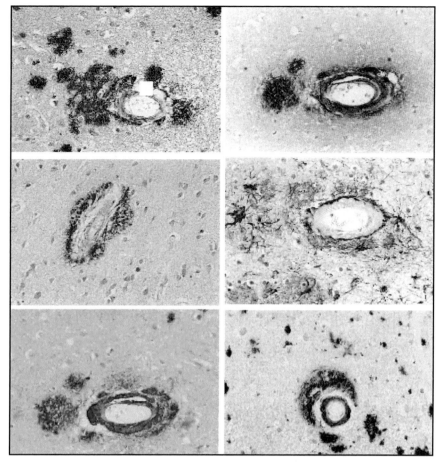

Figure 8.5

Location, Location, Location!

Human blood vessels are the location of much of the alcohol dehydrogenase class I outside of the liver (extra-hepatic ADH). The previous chapter discussed the damage done within the intima of the artery during the pathogenesis of atherosclerosis due to an inopportune interaction between formaldehyde, LDL and the macrophage at the very source of formaldehyde production. Both the vein and artery intima and media contain ADH[220] that is capable of formaldehyde production from methanol. What other mischief is this formaldehyde capable of causing, what other sensitive proteins can react with it?

The travel distance of formaldehyde within the human body is limited by its extreme reactivity. The formaldehyde hawks find much to keep them busy close to their point of origin and will not wander further than their nearest molecular prey. Yet it must always be remembered that formaldehyde is one of the smallest of molecules and is capable of going anywhere very quickly if not distracted. Much like a real hawk, formaldehyde that isn't reacting with something is always on the move. Once formaldehyde is produced from methanol it is diffused out into the watery world of human tissue hunting for prey in both its acid and basic forms.

What this all means it that much of the damage from methanol poisoning will be found close to home within tissue surrounding the blood vessels and in close proximity to other ADH sources of formaldehyde. Only a handful of diseases are well known to conform to this "perivascular" modus operandi, with most, if not all damage clustered in sites surrounding blood vessels, particularly small veins, with no other logical physiological boundary criteria. The reasons for this anatomically unexplainable behavior have always been elusive. Again, the two most important of these diseases are Alzheimer's disease[233] and multiple sclerosis.

The reason that the vascular sites of ADH formaldehyde production are so critical in the elucidation of these two diseases of the brain is that, other than these sites within the lining of the cerebral veins and arteries, the brain is completely free of Alcohol Dehydrogenase Class I.[218] The good news for many, but obviously not all, is that the brain does have very significant,[327] but genetically serendipitously endowed distributions[216] of the good enzyme ADH III (which destroys formaldehyde). Interestingly, a genetic deficiency in ADH III, detectable in mitochondria, has been shown to significantly increase the risk of Alzheimer's disease in Japanese individuals so disposed.[590] Given the nature of these diseases a very substantial epidemiologic significance must be given to their perivascular origin,[233] favoring methanol as their only logical cause.

Of particular importance is the fact that the ADH sites are located on the brain side of the blood brain barrier[218, 220] within the lining of the blood vessels which act as that barrier. Methanol has no difficulty diffusing across the blood brain barrier to reach the ADH located on the brain side of the barrier, but formaldehyde would find it difficult to pass through the barrier, which is why we know it must be produced on the brain side. Formaldehyde produced in this manner becomes trapped inside the brain. The cross-sections of "perivascular tissue" of Alzheimer's victims show clearly just how closely to the veins the plaque production starts (Figure 4).[233] The early Alzheimer's plaque is always found at the media of the vein or artery,[233] right at the point where the ADH acts on the methanol as it crosses the barrier into the brain.

How can formaldehyde produce such large plaque configurations that they break through cell membranes and myelin sheaths surrounding the axon? Under suitable conditions the molecules of many compounds can be linked together into giant molecules by methylene bridges when subject to the action of formaldehyde.[446] Remember our little Crazy Hawk with its large claws just waiting to grab onto anything it can?

I am reminded of when I lived in rural Canada for a three fantastic years in a place called Powell River just two ferry boat rides north of Vancouver. My home was down the beach from where a salmon spawning stream ran into the sea. I saw many birds of prey fishing in the abundant waters just off the coast and I remember once actually observing a bald eagle with a salmon in each claw. Well imagine our little Crazy Hawk with the equivalent of a small whale in each of its claws. This happens all the time in the amazing world of formaldehyde chemistry.

The exact molecular mechanism that initiates the transformation of tau protein into tangles and then plaque has been explained and experimentally demonstrated by the venerable Dr. Rong Giao He of the Chinese Academy of Sciences in conjunction with a group from the University of Nottingham. In a brilliant series of in vitro (in a test tube) and in vivo (in living tissue) experiments, Dr Giao He deduced how formaldehyde produced from methanol[235] might interact with tau protein, binding to it and producing tangles, as he depicts so elegantly in Figure 8.6, which he has kindly shared with us.[234]

Tau is a basic protein. It is a very soluble and open molecule, which makes it vulnerable to attack by the acid Crazy Hawk persona of formaldehyde. Dr Giao He's diagram is an example of formaldehyde chemistry at work. The red dots represent our hawks. The Crazy Hawks attack the tau protein with one claw and, as soon as a sparrow hawk comes close, grab hold with its other claw, thereby commencing the process of methylene bridge-making. On his diagram, he labels this first stage "formaldehyde polymerization." The tau protein so attacked becomes "sticky." When another tau protein comes into close proximity, the last Crazy Hawk on the methylene bridge grabs hold of it and off we go to make a tangle. Formaldehyde produced from the ADH within the lining of the veins and arteries of the brain eventually bonds the tau protein into aggregates, which then bond to other aggregates to produce the plaque of Alzheimer's.[234] Dr. He has recently discovered marked elevation of urine formaldehyde levels in patients with dementia.[591]

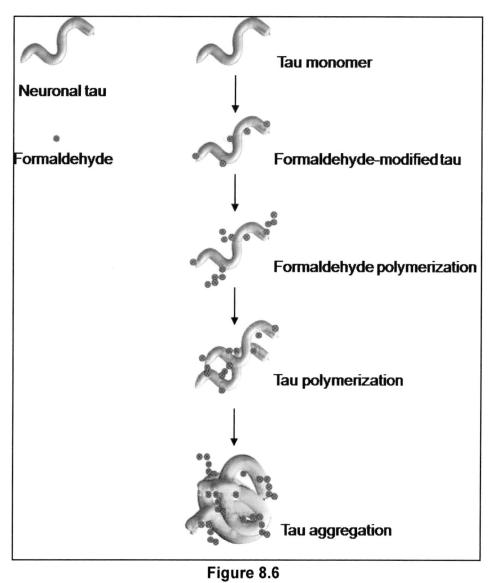

Figure 8.6

In the absence of ethanol, dietary methanol easily penetrates the blood brain barrier and passes into the intima and media of the veins and arteries of the brain, where it is transformed by ADH into formaldehyde. Formaldehyde diffuses into nearby nerve cell axons and penetrates until it locates tau protein, which is modified and polymerized to produce plaque. Once the plaque breaks through the cell membrane and myelin layers of the axon it is exposed to the brain's macrophages, which become activated, leading to the inflammation of Alzheimer's.

The Toxicological Evidence:

The brain is the target organ of methanol poisoning, and methanol's infliction of damage on the brain is the direct cause of all methanol mortalities. Amnesia and memory loss is a common symptom of methanol toxicity.

Epidemiological Evidence:

Alzheimer's is a disease whose incidence is reduced considerably by moderate ethanol consumption, with a classic U-shaped curve response. The curve of aspartame consumption over the last thirty years appears to track directly with the deaths caused by Alzheimer's disease, with a 14 year delayed response.

Again let me stress the importance of carefully reviewing the data provided by the US Centers for Disease Control presented in Figures 8.1-8.3. The death curves presented there show an absolutely alarming increase in deaths from Alzheimer's since the advent of aspartame in the early 1980s. Remember also what we have learned about the general increase in methanol consumption via processed fruit and vegetable drinks, which started some years before the introduction of aspartame into the American diet. Serious consideration must be given to the manmade origin of this epidemic and the real possibility that it results from methanol's conversion to formaldehyde.

Chapter 9
Multiple Sclerosis

Nature does not recognize disease; in her eyes, all has purpose, all is equal, and no one natural process is better than another. If you seek the cause of any unknown you are wise not to impede your vision by limiting your course of study. Learn about a natural mystery by taking it in completely; smell and taste it if you can. You must make close acquaintance with what you study before you can hope to see how it fits, discover its origin, and resolve how to make peace with it. View all of life's systems as timely events of a perfect interaction between equals – and you may begin to see their purpose. Let your prejudice be engaged only after the whole truth is plain to you and the course is clear.

The very brightest among you may be doubting me now. You know that the diseases of civilization are all due to a single mutation that changed the shape of our catalase enzyme at the most vulnerable time for our species. Yet how can a transcendental change in our genetic code fall into the same category as the diseases with which we are more familiar, where one life form appears to rage against another? My perception of Nature is perhaps different from yours and warrants explaining.

The notion that Nature's entire realm of life forms is extremely rare in the cosmos, confined to this and other similar lonely cold rocks floating in space, is a limiting confine that is, to my mind, unreasonable. Life as we know it here on Earth consists solely of molecular creations that glean their energy from the electrons of others, using the miracle of enzymes to lower the activation temperatures of various chemical reactions, then taking a share to run the mechanisms of life. All this happening because there is no other choice for our existence at temperatures so very close to absolute zero.

Yet to me, it seems the more logical places to look for life are where a preponderance of free energy may be found, places where the more bountiful power of the nucleus may be shared to raise life to levels heretofore unimagined by our own low energy biology. Perhaps in such circumstances, a less needy and predatory mode of living could evolve – one that strives for harmony, rather than dominance. Could stars such as our own sun be home to colonies of vibrant life that are so far removed from our own limited perception as to have eluded our direct observation for all these millennia? The mechanism that starts the fire of stars from the omnipotent cloud of hydrogen that is the origin of everything but time and space is, to me, a force of life. What else would explain the seemingly infinite number and variety of cosmic entities and events that surround us in every direction?

Why haven't we been able to decipher the communications between such energetic living things? The pulses are there, in many wavelengths and even particle streams. As compelling as they may be, they are yet constantly being screened as "interference" by SETI, our program designed to search for extra terrestrial life forms. Perhaps we set our sights too low looking solely for life that closely resembles our own. Frankly, I find the thought that we have the skills to detect intelligence from all but our own human schema to be laughable. What successes have we had deciphering the true depth of communications between and among the million or so other species with which we share not only the same little rock but the identical tricks of living? Do you dare to believe the whales' songs are but simplistic repetition? To me, Nature is the majority of all we see when looking up – and that opens all the permutations and possibilities of interactions extending far beyond even my wildest imaginings.

We all die. The sentence is imposed at the first beat of our anxious hearts. Few suffer a more prolonged passing than those who succumb to multiple sclerosis (MS). The symptoms, a constant reminder that the brain is losing control of the organism with which it was once master. The young women who are the primary target of this tragic disorder can only cling to hope of a misdiagnosis or the rare outcome of complete remission. We will in this chapter discuss this disease as if the cause has been discovered and relief is on the way. I will be ridiculed for this approach, but then abuse has been the burden of discovery since the beginning of thought.

The Conflagration that is Multiple Sclerosis

Multiple Sclerosis was on my mind when, at the dusk of a lovely summer day on a flight over California, I witnessed another of Nature's catastrophes – the unforgettable sight of a forest fire engulfing an entire mountainside. Thousands of acres of blackened bare tree trunks were outlined by a thin encircling ring of flame where the damage effectuated. It immediately occurred to me that this was a very powerful descriptor of MS plaque. Plaque is the anatomical equivalent of a slow forest fire, where nerve axons are being slowly stripped bare of their insulation. It is the defining feature for which the disease was first named by the French neurologist Jean-Martin Charcot in 1865.

I was in an introspective mood, and a stout drink or two later I began to daydream. What if, I imagined while reminiscing about the miles of desolation, an alien space ship were to land at the scene of this fire some time after the terrain had gone cold? What if these were brilliant alien scientists and explorers from a planet with little oxygen in the atmosphere and, therefore, no such phenomenon as fire? Surely their curiosity would draw them to this desolate spot that was so different from anything they had ever experienced on their own planet. Their cargo bay would soon be loaded with samples of all manner of charred remnants of plant and animal matter in various degrees of deterioration and decay, along with detailed pictures of the damage done to the terrain and life forms.

As a fellow scientist now caught in such a conundrum myself I imagined their fruitless search for the cause of this blight in the midst of a vibrant living forest, the endless rhetoric that would ensue during their long return flight home, the search for the invisible beasts responsible, the manuscripts of descriptive biology and

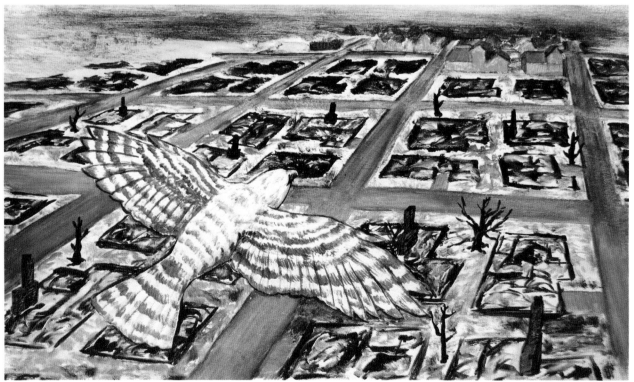

theoretical speculation written after years of study and debate back on the home planet that had no knowledge of flame.

As I write this, lying on my desk, long closed, is a damaged copy of just such a tome, the fourth edition of McAlpine's *Multiple Sclerosis,*[305] a fifteen pound, thousand page technical masterpiece done in six colors and a print far too small to be easily read by those visually impaired MS sufferers it purports to describe. The damage to my copy was caused by my ripping it in half to save postage between the two continents I call home. This publication would have much in common with the works produced by my imaginary visiting alien intellectuals. It contains a collection of hard won scientific data, factually correct but in the end, due to just one missing bit of knowledge, providing no help to the suffering and no answer to the most important question: *Why?*

McAlpine's is not listed among the handful of literature that I classify as "must reading" for someone who wishes to learn about multiple sclerosis. This compendium of the "present knowledge" belabors the trivia of the long history of medicine's failures with MS while incredibly failing to encourage in any way the compelling evidence that support the possibility that an environmental poison might just be its cause. Methanol and formaldehyde do not appear anywhere among its near million words. The bias of the chief editor is expressed in print[616] in his critical, unreferenced review of an article which I hold in great esteem, authored by a good scientist who steps back and takes a careful, thoughtful, yet critical view of his own discipline and how it connects with reality. His approach is rare, especially among the ranks of the Delphian medical sciences. If you have MS or love someone who does I encourage you to read the brutally honest and thought provoking twenty page review, *The Pathogenesis of Multiple Sclerosis Revisited,*[615] and while you are at it take a look at *What if Multiple Sclerosis isn't an Immunological or a Viral Disease? The Case for a Circulating Toxin.*[153] These articles will prepare you for what I have to say about the subject.

The hostility between the various factions of those who now study multiple sclerosis may actually be encouraged by the machinations of the major drug companies who sell extremely expensive competing palliatives for the disease, none of which cure it. The rivalry between these companies, who are responsible for directing most of the funding for the search for the "cure" of MS, is inspired by the fact that even the least effective of their concoctions have proven to be billion dollar product lines, due solely to the desperation of MS sufferers and their loved ones. To trust the cure of any disease to a group whose existence depends upon its perpetuation seems counterintuitive, if not outright stupid (by "group," I mean both the pharmaceutical companies and the various MS societies who encourage and support each other in, to my mind, unproductive ways).

The heated debate between the various competing groups of scientists studying MS is a debate between those who believe that MS is a defect in the immune system, those who think it is a viral disease, and those very few who believe that the disease is the direct result of a toxic agent from the environment. Though it is well known that animals do not develop MS, no consensus has been reached as to whether animals can be used as experimental models for the disease when artificial methods are used to induce them to lose myelin. These issues have been continually debated for over a hundred years with, up until now, each side presenting only enough evidence to show that they may be on the right track but not enough to assign culpability. Aside from what I will demonstrate to you in this chapter, few instances have ever been recorded where the incidence of MS has actually been manipulated. When Norway was occupied during World War II food was severely restricted for several years and the incidence of MS went down dramatically; unfortunately, this has been virtually ignored.[153]

I am not so very much interested in belaboring every detail of the slow, complex conflagration that is multiple sclerosis. My intention here is to give you what you need to know to prevent the fire from reaching the fuel.

Listening to Nature's Whispers

In June of 1550 the Spanish conquistador Cortez kidnapped and eventually killed the Aztec emperor Montezuma in a successful attempt to steal the golden treasures of the Aztec people. From the time of Columbus it was the admitted intent of European invaders to plunder the newly discovered territory of the Americas, no matter what the cost to the "savages." Among other bounty were the golden seeds of a plant unknown to the conquering rabble. This was to be the first of the corn seeds from the Americas to be received enthusiastically by the old world, but to have attached unforeseen dire consequences. The seeds did not come with instructions. Although the Aztec people had much they could teach the Spaniards, their traditions were not heeded. Perhaps these Europeans had such a high opinion of their own civilization that they could not easily accept cultural knowledge from those they so easily conquered. Whatever the case, unimaginable misery was the wage of implementing a new food without sufficient knowledge of its safety. Pellagra, the disease of corn, was to take European scientists over 400 years to rediscover and cost millions of innocent lives to a slow and agonizing death.

Eight thousand years before the Old World finally put an end to their culture, the Aztecs had begun experimenting with native grasses, turning them into something new to Nature. They persisted, and after generations of observation and painstaking manipulation, with careful crossing of strains, they produced a new life form that could have never evolved naturally. It was the birth of what appeared on first blush to be a valuable food crop – corn (maize). No record exists of who these individuals were, but without a doubt the work that they performed was a non-invasive genetic manipulation (GM). The most critical way that Aztec science differs from our modern GM is that the Aztecs took the ultimate responsibility for bringing their work to completion. Over a period of years, the dark side of their unnatural invention was to present as a plague of biblical proportions. Entire villages of corn eaters would succumb to symptoms of what must then have appeared to be many different diseases. Some individuals would develop devastating and painful skin lesions, while others would lose all semblance of civilization and go mad. Death would finally come to most when the heart would refuse the brain's signal to continue beating.

By observation, Aztec scientists were able to determine that it was the corn that was the cause of these apocalyptic outbreaks, and further – and of much greater significance – they observed that when corn was treated overnight with powdered limestone or the ash from a wood fire the suffering would not come. By pure and patient observation of Nature's response to their own unnatural product these ancient people solved the riddle of Pellagra and successfully implemented a reliable prevention. This complex conundrum that we know now was a nutritional deficiency of niacin was laid to rest by observation, intuition and intellect alone.

We have already discussed other ancient cultures that were adept at such research and developed traditional adaptations of the way they prepared food to ultimately prevent premature death and suffering caused by nutritional deficiencies and poisoning from naturally occurring toxic substances. With the exception of the accidental discovery of antibiotics by a university microbiologist and vaccination by a country physician who was really more of a naturalist, our modern medicine men are wretchedly inept at discovering the cause and prevention of disease. If only we could discover what is so very wrong with our scientific methods that makes it impossible for our researchers to tease such revelations from Nature's grasp! We can only guess that part of it may be that present-day medicine appears to have no stomach for the combination of observation, intuition and common sense that ancient peoples would have been forced to employ to come to their cures for food borne diseases. Modern medical researchers, particularly those funded by the pharmaceutical industry, often demean such observations by using the term "anecdotal" and employing an inflection and tenor as if they were uttering a curse.

My use of observation, intuition and common sense, combined with careful study of the research of many

Chapter 9

whose narrow perspectives prevented them from seeing the answers they sought, has led me to believe that diseases of civilization (DOC) and, in particular, multiple sclerosis, were originally caused by human meddling with the food supply. In this chapter I will apply both anecdotal observation and the more traditional methods of modern science to point to the cause and prevention of the poisoning that causes MS.

The Scene of the Crime

The brain, along with the rest of the central nervous system, is made up of about 50% neurons (nerve cells) that communicate with other cells of the body via long wire-like strands called axons. Multiple sclerosis results from the progressive deterioration of the protective myelin sheath surrounding the axons. Axons are in many ways similar to a telephone cord, which is made up of a conductive wire surrounded by a protective coating, without which the signal would be interrupted and muted as it travels from the mouthpiece to the phone line. The disappearance of myelin distorts nerve cell communication, leading to a long list of neurological symptoms including loss of sensation, muscle spasms and weakness, fatigue, blindness, and pain. The entire collection of symptoms that constitute multiple sclerosis can be explained by damage to the myelin sheath of specific axons in the brain and upper spinal cord. All the symptomology deriving from the interference of the normal communication between the brain and the rest of the body is due to what is tantamount to short circuits in axons that transmit life-sustaining information in both directions.

Specifically, damage is found around the axons that transmit signals to and from the muscles and sensor cells. Even though the impulse that runs down the axon is not identical to the flow of electrons that runs through an analogous electric wire, nevertheless the myelin must be insulated to provide for the security of the messages traveling through it and to prevent the bare axons from touching and allowing signal cross over between nerve cells or, even worse, the breaking of the unprotected axon itself. The one major difference in the appearance of the myelin sheath when compared to the insulation on an electrical wire is that the nerve cell's insulation is applied in numerous evenly spaced lumps, called nodules, that run down the length of the axon, giving a healthy axon the appearance of a strand of beads. Each nodule consists of many layers of myelin wrapped in one continuous band around the axon it protects.

The disease is called multiple sclerosis because usually the myelin sheath can be damaged at multiple sites in the brain. These sites are not haphazard; they have a pattern which is characteristic of the disease and consistent with the usual symptoms. Interestingly, these sites are identical to the sites affected during methanol poisoning.

MS damage to the brain always begins in areas adjacent to blood vessels. Dr. James Dawson at the University of Edinburgh in 1916 performed detailed examinations of the brains of patients who died from MS. His meticulous descriptions of the inflammation and swelling of blood vessels and the damage to the adjacent myelin sheath is valid to this day[620] and again is startlingly reminiscent of the damage caused by methanol toxicity.[15] This presentation, consisting of the damaged vessel and many adjacent axons which exhibit complete demyelination, is plaque. These plaques radiate out from the vessels around which they are centered. Plaques enlarge three-dimensionally over time from the central vein or small artery outward until they give the appearance of the growing limb of a tree. The analogy stretches to the bark representing the "active" area of the plaque, where we can find macrophages busy consuming the myelin sheaths of previously healthy axons as the plaque slowly grows with the progression of the disease by what appears so obviously to be diffusion of a deadly poison.

Each human nerve cell has only one axon, some of which can reach over a foot in length. These axons have to be insulated, padded, protected, and fed – functions that are not provided directly by the neuron (nerve cell) itself, because the distances are so great between the body of the cell and the end of the axon. Rather, the axon is cared for by other cells of the nervous system to be found along its path in the brain and spinal cord. It is the Schwann cell which takes it upon itself to maintain one short segment of axon. To do this it must stretch out a thin layer of its cell membrane and grow that layer around and around the axon many times. These windings are what become the myelin sheath. Thousands of these Schwann cells are spaced at remarkably consistent intervals along the path of the average nerve cell axon, giving the axon the look of a garden hose strung with evenly spaced rolls of paper towels. The Schwann cells remain attached and are physically very close to the axon, providing life support to the living myelin sheath. They can also act to regrow the sheath when it is in need of repair or replacement. The regrowth is slow, but it is precisely what accounts for the periods of remittance which follow the relapses that often occur in MS sufferers.

It is this symbiotic relationship that helps explain the major difference between Alzheimer's disease, which is caused by damage deep inside the axon and is irreversible, and multiple sclerosis, which is a disease of the myelin sheath and is repairable, causing multiple cycles of exacerbation and remission. The modus operandi of formaldehyde during the evolution of MS is identical to that of Alzheimer's – even to the attack on the axons of the nerve cells in close proximity to the small veins and arteries of the circulatory system of the brain. The difference is that during Alzheimer's, the formaldehyde penetrates into the axon of the nerve cell itself, attacking the basic tau protein within. This process eventually kills the entire nerve cell, which cannot be replaced. In multiple sclerosis, it is the protein of the myelin sheath, which is actually part and parcel of the Schwann cell, that is being attacked and consumed by the activated macrophage. The axon of the nerve cell is spared at first, just as what happens in acute methanol poisoning. To put this simply, Alzheimer's is a disease of the nerve cell (neuron), while MS really begins as a disease of the Schwann cell. Eventually, as MS progresses, the loss of the protective sheath will result in breakage of the axon and repair then becomes impossible.

Figure 9.1

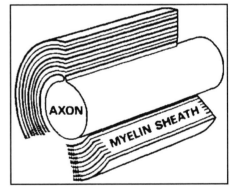

Figure 9.1 shows a close up diagram of what the layers of myelin look like wrapped around the axon. It reveals what happens as the myelin is devoured by hungry macrophages layer by layer, thus exposing once protected MBP to marauding bands of Crazy Hawks, leading to its modification by formaldehyde and its eventual consumption, and finally exposing the unprotected living axon of the neuron. Some considerable time is required to finally erode away the many layers of myelin. The fascinating thing is that many

Figure 9.2

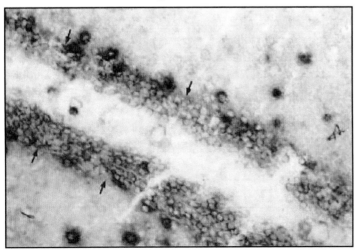

Schwann cells survive these attacks and can and do regrow their myelin sheath. Although once considered controversial, complete remyelination of demyelinated axons within even large plaques has recently been shown to be commonplace.[230] This explains the often complete disappearance of MS symptoms during remission in many MS sufferers. In most patients with MS the disease takes an up-and-down course with long periods of remission between attacks. This implies a valiant attempt of the Schwann cells to rebuild missing myelin sheaths consumed by the macrophages.[151] If we can stop the poisoning early enough by removing from the

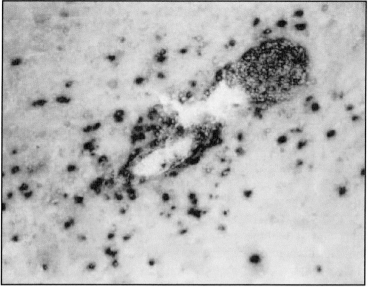

Figure 9.1

environment and food supply the poison that causes it – methanol, before too many axons break and Schwann cells are killed and the hope for complete recovery is lost, then perhaps MS can actually be cured.

The microphotograph of a section of a small vein in Figure 9.2[517] shows clearly the plaque formation surrounding the blood vessels in a patient with early MS. The dark spots are macrophages eating away at myelin. Figure 9.3[517] shows cross sectional views of the same tissue that can be more easily compared to the figures in the previous chapter of perivascular Alzheimer's plaque. As time progresses and plaques age and become larger, the unprotected thin axons may eventually break from lack of physical protection, cutting completely all communications and leading to the atrophy of muscles and organs and eventually death from lack of functioning of vital tissue.

Location, Location, Location

As you now know, human blood vessels are the location of much of the Alcohol Dehydrogenase Class I outside of the liver (extra-hepatic ADH). The intima and media of both the veins and arteries of the brain contain ADH,[220] which is capable of formaldehyde production from methanol. Once produced, formaldehyde will tirelessly search for a basic molecule with which it can react. The travel distance of formaldehyde within the human body is limited by its extreme reactivity. The formaldehyde hawks find much to keep them busy close to their point of origin and will not wander further than their nearest molecular prey. Yet it must always be remembered that formaldehyde is the smallest of molecules and is capable of going anywhere very quickly if not distracted. Much like a real hawk, formaldehyde that isn't reacting with something is constantly on the move. Once formaldehyde is produced from methanol it diffuses out, mostly in the acid form (Crazy Hawk), into the watery world of human tissue, hunting for prey.

What this all means is that much of the damage from methanol poisoning will be found close to home within tissue surrounding the blood vessels and in close proximity to the ADH sources. Only a handful of diseases are well-known to conform to this "perivascular" modus operandi with most, if not all damage clustered in sites surrounding blood vessels and, in particular, small veins. This anatomical behavior has always been lacking explanation. The two most important of these perivascular diseases are multiple sclerosis[517] and Alzheimer's. The reason that the vascular sites of ADH formaldehyde production are so critical to the elucidation of both these diseases of the brain is that, other than these sites within the lining of the cerebral veins and arteries, the brain is completely free of Alcohol Dehydrogenase Class I.[218] In other words, the plaques of MS and the damage of Alzheimer's *only* occur in the *precise areas* where the ADH that converts methanol to formaldehyde is found.

The good news for many, but obviously not all, is that the brain also has very significant,[327] but genetically serendipitous, distributions[216] of the good enzyme ADH III, which can destroy formaldehyde, turning it into the safe formic acid before it gets a chance to attack a basic proteins. Formaldehyde is, therefore, produced only by the ADH I found in the lining of the blood vessels of the brain and not in brain tissue itself.[528] It is a short journey from the blood vessel, where the formaldehyde is produced within the lining of the vessels, to the locations where MS plaque originates on the myelin sheaths of the numerous axons crisscrossing these vessels. It is noteworthy that some of the very first damage shown in the natural progression of MS is a swelling (edema) and thickening of the lining of these very vessels where the formaldehyde is produced, even before the nearby myelin appears to be affected.[517] It is again fascinating that this damage is identical to that found in unfortunate individuals who die slowly from acute methanol poisoning.[15] We can take this as an indication that formaldehyde does some damage to other proteins on its way to finding a more desirable nesting site like myelin basic protein (MBP). In Figures 9.2 and 9.3 MS can be seen slowly progressing along the length of these small arteries and veins throughout the brain and spinal cord.[517]

Please try to imagine flocks of formaldehyde hawk fledglings emerging from these blood vessels into the circuitry of the brain. Imagine wave after wave of hungry hawks looking for protein to attack, having to go further and further as protein landing sites are lost to competitors and then eventually consumed by macrophages, slowly but surely expanding the plaque as the years go by (Figure 9.4). It is worth noting that a single drop of diet cola sweetened with aspartame contains sufficient methanol to produce well over a hundred trillion of these damaging Crazy Hawks. What exactly are the Crazy Hawks attacking?

Details of Plaque Formation

Figure 9.4 shows us some older MS plaque with almost all of the myelin sheaths having been eaten away by those cute little big-eyed macrophages. This forces the Crazy Hawks (which, if you look closely, are emerging from the blood vessel in the foreground) to fly great distances to find more protein to attack at the war zone at the very edges of the plaque. What are the Crazy Hawks trying to find, and how do we prove

Figure 9.4

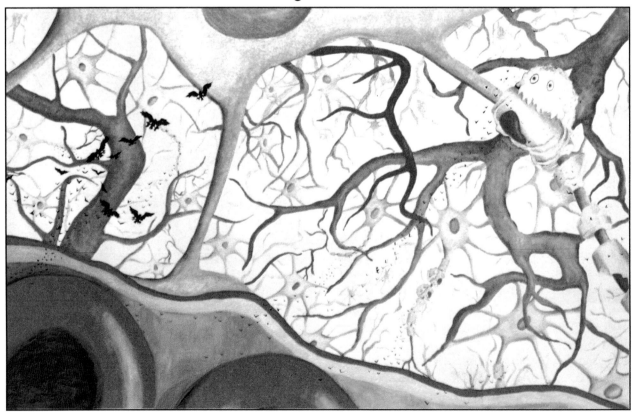

that they are indeed attacking that particular protein? In order for my explanation to go further you need to learn a little something about one additional molecule that will prove to be an extremely important part of our chain of evidence that will establish convincingly that MS is a disease of methanol poisoning. But first a little background.

The Look, Touch, Taste and Smell of Multiple Sclerosis

I lived what seemed a lifetime in Wellington, Colorado in the years I spent earning my master's and doctorate degrees in Food Science and then Nutrition at Colorado State University. It was there that I tasted multiple sclerosis for the first time.

I met her in my Urban Renewal office, where I moonlighted from my research assistantship at the university to earn enough extra money to lead a decent lifestyle in that rough-hewn western town on the Wyoming border. She was a striking tall blond woman with the deepest blue eyes and a blistering temper, and we became lovers in very short order. During the length of our relationship I lived with her multiple sclerosis in a more intimate manner than any specialist in the disease usually does. There was always a change in her that I could detect long before her suffering began, not in her mood or her movement, but in her taste and smell. I cannot say it was formaldehyde, but if formaldehyde had a sister it would have been that.

There is much more to multiple sclerosis then we may ever know, and we must be open to accepting evidence from every quarter. I doubt that Nature is an adherent to the scientific method and its null hypothesis.

The Kitchen Autopsy

One can never forget the vision of a scientist wearing a top hat and scullery apron bent over an oversized kitchen sink with his bare fingers thrust deep into the freshly removed brain of one of his MS patients. Jean-Martin Charcot, the discoverer of the disease, was notorious around the saltpeter institute, where he was chief neurologist, to have had subjected the freshly dissected brain of a patient who died from MS to a careful screening by running his fingers through the soft custard like tissue of her untreated brain, finding the long perivascular strands of leathery plaque that gave him the idea for the name Sclerosis (French for leather-like). The image of him doing this is reproduced in a book on the history of MS.[306] One can only imagine how he first encountered this extremely important telltale feature of the disease.

As the MS plaque grows larger, the formaldehyde hydrate produced in the lining of the blood vessels has to travel further and further to find new basic protein to bind to. The lingering of the Crazy Hawk as it wends its way to the outer reaches of the older plaque provides enough dwell time for some of the formaldehyde to react with deeper tissue within the plaque itself. This reaction of the formaldehyde with the already demyelinated plaque gives it a strikingly hard texture that is different from any other tissue to be found in the brain. This is what formaldehyde hydrate does to tissue and is one of the reasons that it is used for the tanning of leather and to plasticize other substances.[446] The original physical description of these areas by Charcot in 1846 might have led to a quick resolution of the cause of MS, if only formaldehyde would have been known to science at the time.

Charcot would have no idea what formaldehyde did to tissue, for unfortunately, it was not until 1868, more than twenty years later, that Hoffman was to discover and name the highly reactive substance so easily produced by passing methanol fumes over a platinum wire, (just as in my hand warmer). It wasn't until Ferdinand Blum was hired by the discoverer of formaldehyde to find uses for the extremely dangerous compound that its plasticizing effect on tissue was elucidated and exploited. But at that time it was considered to be a laboratory oddity and not discovered as a natural substance until years later. Much valuable time was lost to ignorance. The trail of the small molecule as the cause of MS grew cold and to this day is rarely revisited.

The fact that brain tissue is never touched with bare hands in the modern histology laboratory, not even after it is soaked in a solution of formaldehyde for days, makes this type of observation unlikely and esthetically barbaric to the contemporary histologist, who rarely removes the latex gloves from his hands. It is a sad reminder of the physical removal of modern medical practitioners from the real world of patients.

The Cause of MS is within the Thickening Blood Vessels

We owe a great deal to Dr. James W. Dawson, the Scottish pathologist who dedicated his professional career to the microscopic study of multiple sclerosis. Prior to his death in 1927 from a lifelong tubercular infection he published a detailed 230 page histological examination of tissue from nine cases of the disease. Dawson's Histology of Disseminated Sclerosis,[620] published in 1915, applied modern staining techniques that brought color and greater definition to the pathology of the disease. His work reinforced the perivascular nature of MS, along with revealing the details of the considerable thickening and damage to the walls of the blood vessels within the plaque. This well regarded work supplemented the microscopic analysis published by Charcot himself and numerous other scientists over the previous fifty years. Dawson's outstanding critical review of the scientific literature and his own summations give us a clear understanding and insight into the thinking of the medical community as to the progression and causation of MS during the critical early days after the first cases of MS were being reported. The noteworthy scientists of the early Twentieth Century were convinced that MS was caused by a toxic substance that, to their great disappointment, was invisible to them. James sums this up nicely as follows:

> The supposition of a selective poison acting through the blood-vessels, which has received the support of most recent investigators, is justified as an hypothesis but remains undemonstrated as a fact. ...This hypothetical toxin has not been isolated, but it is suggested that it forms in the body. ...It is admitted by all, except the supporters of the developmental nature of the process, that the distribution of the plaque areas points to the blood-vessels as the route of conveyance of this agent, and the assumption of an intoxication harmonizes with this relation to the blood-vessels."[620]

Though no animal model is reliable for studying either MS or methanol poisoning, when rabbits (one of the few animals used successfully to study some aspects of atherosclerosis in man) were forced to breathe methanol fumes for 8 hours a day for several months, all developed a marked increase in the thickness of their blood vessels similar to what is consistently noted in MS pathology. Dr. Eisenberg's microscopic examination of the rabbits' circulatory tissues attributed the changes to "the actual proliferation of the fixed tissue cells, as seen by the very marked thickening of the adventitia and media of the blood-vessels."[15] The most telling evidence of all can be found in one of Oluf Roe's ground-breaking articles, published in the early 1940s investigating a massive outbreak of methanol poisoning that killed and blinded numerous of his countrymen. Roe made a profound observation while investigating the optic discs of several of his poisoned patients. These men, one of whose age was only 32 years, had survived between 6 and 12 weeks after their acute methanol poisoning. Dr. Roe, the father of the use of ethanol to treat methanol poisoning, states:

> There was at the same time marked irregularity of the caliber of the large blood vessels with thickening of their walls. These changes resemble those seen in the blood vessels of the retina in arteriosclerosis."[49]

As is often the case it is the earliest of scientific investigators that make the real breakthroughs in discovering the cause of diseases. It is unfortunate that these great minds of the late 19th and early 20th Centuries did not have a way to visualize or detect formaldehyde. Although it was Charcot himself who first noted the thickening and obstruction of the small blood vessels of the MS plaque, it was Rindfleisch in Germany in 1863 who first identified the constant changes of the blood vessels in MS and presented what is today called the "vascular theory of MS." He noted the "enormous thickening" of the vessel lining within the plaque of the MS brain and proposed that whatever was being produced within these vessel walls was the cause of the disease.[230] What was being produced was formaldehyde.

Symptoms Mean Little Unless They Are Identical in All Ways…Then They Mean Everything!

We have spent time on the symptoms of MS in Chapter 6, showing how methanol kills. In summary, the symptoms of multiple sclerosis,[44, 83, 85,169] chronic and acute methanol poisoning,[13,144,189] and Aspartame toxicity[54, 58, 93,181] are in all ways identical. Nothing that happens to the human body from the toxic effect of methanol that has not also been expressed during the course of MS – *nothing*.[143,144] This generalization extends even to the remarkable ophthalmological conditions common to both: transitory optic neuritis and Retrolaminar demyelinating optic neuropathy with scotoma of the central visual field (which occasionally manifests as unilateral temporary blindness).[85,138,163] In fact, these ophthalmological symptoms have been thought for years in their respective literatures to be "tell tale" indications for the differential diagnosis for each of these maladies independently.[85,138,148,163,169] The common symptoms of headache,[13,83,181,189] nervousness,[13,83,181] depression,[58,83,189,181] memory loss,[18,147,85,169,181] tingling sensations,[13,85,168,138,169] pain in the extremities,[13,85,169] optic neuritis,[85,138,148,163,169] bright lights in the visual field,[139,83] seizures,[21,83,160] and inability to urinate or to keep from urinating[139,146,167] are all shared by each of these conditions and shared yet again by complaints from aspartame poisoning.[54,58,93,181]

I take these strikingly similar symptom patterns as evidence that these disorders act on identical components of the central nervous system and in the same way. In the early stages of MS, or when a non-lethal dose of methanol has been administered, blindness can occur often in just one eye. Complete recovery is a possibility. The only two afflictions for which such dramatic "remissions" are reported from identical neuromuscular and ophthalmological damage, including "blindness," are relapsing-remitting multiple sclerosis [85] and methyl alcohol poisoning.[138,163] The pathology of the two maladies is in all ways identical, particularly when it comes to destruction of the myelin sheath with no harm to the axon itself.[18,148,176]

It is not unusual for the modern medical practitioner to put little credence in the similarity of symptoms between disorders, and it is indeed true that certain very common symptoms, such as headache and depression, can be caused by all manner of bodily changes. However, the breadth of symptomatological overlap that we are putting forth here between methanol poisoning and MS is far too robust to put to neurological coincidence. In total, they reflect a link that cannot be refuted with any degree of scientific vigor.

Learn a Little About Arginine

Several important questions need to be answered when a poison is proposed as the cause of a disease. The first is what is the exact chemical interaction between the suspected etiologic agent and the biological molecule or molecules that initiate the disease process, and how can it be detected? For years the stumbling block of DOC elucidation was the inability to detect formaldehyde. An important new tool of scientific research, however, has recently made detection possible. To understand how this works we need to understand something about protein.

Our bodies are made of cells that are works of moveable art composed primarily of water and protein molecules. These protein molecules are the major constituents of all earthly life. The original recipe for each of these fascinating structures is protected deep within the nucleus of the cells, never to leave its safe haven in our lifetime. When a new protein is needed for repair or growth, that information can be copied directly out of the recipe book – or chromosome, as it is called – as long as the DNA that makes up the chromosome has not been previously turned off or methylated by formaldehyde (a methyl molecule). Just as your mom would copy a recipe from her tired old cook book onto a slip of paper and hand it to you to for reproduction in your own kitchen, so Nature scribes and passes out of the nucleus such individual recipes to be made into protein to build and repair your body. It is a fascinating structure called a ribosome that has the job of making each protein from the instructions on the recipe slip, putting together the required ingredients.

The ingredients are primarily amino acids. Floating around in the liquid of the cell (cytoplasm) are about 20 of these different amino acids, from which the ribosome can choose. These amino acids constitute the chemical alphabet that Nature links together for performing all of the purposes of living.

One of these amino acids is called arginine. This is the most important amino acid for those of us who have an interest in methanol diseases, and it will be the only one that we will take the time to study here. If you are a chemist you know about the structure of the arginine molecule, but what interests us is its behavior. Arginine is one of only three amino acids that are basic in nature and it is the only one that can provide three different nesting sites for our acidic Crazy Hawk. This means that formaldehyde can react with arginine and methylate it one, two, or occasionally even up to three times. Arginine is considered a formaldehyde capturer.[225] In fact, it is more than that – it is a trap for formaldehyde, and because of this it can be a tremendously valuable formaldehyde detector, telling us if brain tissue has made contact with formaldehyde. Thus, a molecule invisible for a hundred and fifty years now casts a shadow that can bear witness to its unwanted presence.

But before we can see formaldehyde's shadow, we must have a way to detect arginine as part of a protein. For then we could take protein from the myelin sheaths of MS sufferers and see if the arginine it contains has been modified by formaldehyde (or "methylated"). The good news is that we now have such a technique. The bad news is the evidence has been lost on those sleepy scientists who did not understand its significance. The story is a sad, yet hopeful one.

Myelin Basic Protein (MBP)

Myelin basic protein (MBP) is a major component of the healthy myelin sheath and, in fact, makes up over 35% of its total composition.[311] For many years this particular protein has been suspected as being the one protein most negatively affected during multiple sclerosis. Because of this it has been extensively studied. We know the exact structure of MBP; it is made up of 170 amino acids, 19 of which are arginine molecules. MBP contains a higher percentage of arginine than any other human protein. This extremely high percentage of arginine is what gives MBP its very basic nature[41] and from whence its name is derived. The Crazy Hawk, formaldehyde hydrate, is acidic and acids and bases will interact if given the opportunity. The Crazy Hawk would be naturally attracted to MBP, bonding to its arginine and eventually methylating it and leaving behind an excellent record of its presence as described above.

Even though changes in the MBP composition of the MS brain are considered the most important chemical milestones of the disease's progression, neurologists were surprised to discover that MBP often completely disappears from the center of the MS plaque itself.[707] Of greater significance was the discovery of an incredible selective loss of this basic protein in otherwise normal appearing tissue up to about a millimeter and a half beyond the edge of these plaques.[311] If you use your imagination to visualize the flight of the Crazy Hawks outward from their source in the vessels at the center of the plaque, if the formaldehyde modification of MBP would activate macrophages, then its phagocytosis (consumption) could account elegantly for the selective disappearance of MBP from surrounding tissue.

Looking for the Shadow of Formaldehyde

A few years ago while living in a small oceanfront New Zealand village with a population of less than 100 souls, I met a young German couple, both PhD chemists, who rented a home down the street from my cottage. We were quick to be friends and got together from time to time to discuss the chemistry of methanol and formaldehyde. The young woman was kind enough to translate some of the early German work done on methanol toxicity that I had in my almost complete collection of scientific literature on the subject. New Zealand happens to be one of those countries of the world with an extremely high rate of Multiple Sclerosis (the reason for which we will explain later), and so inevitably one day the topic of our discussion turned to MS.

I explained how I believed that the disease could be caused by methanol's transformation within the lining of the veins into formaldehyde, which then modified the basic protein of the myelin sheath, marking it for destruction by activated macrophages. I ended the monologue with my usual complaint that the reason this had not been discovered was the absence of a reliable way to determine that a protein had been modified by the little formaldehyde molecule. Without any hesitation my translator's husband informed me that in fact a new analytical method had been developed that could take large protein molecules, break them up into smaller bits and determine accurately if a change had been made by even a single formaldehyde molecule (one carbon atom) in any of the pieces.[706] The equipment (an ion trap storage/reflection time-of-flight mass spectrometer) was expensive, and it would not be easy to get time on it, but he had a friend at a German university who had access to one and for such a purpose he was sure he could schedule us the use of it. We immediately began putting together an experimental design that could prove or disprove once and for all if methanol was the cause of MS.

The brain tissue of MS sufferers could be compared to brain tissue from normal individuals. If we could show that the MBP from the normal brains contained arginine with little or no nesting Crazy Hawks (methylation) and, therefore, prove they had not been attacked by formaldehyde, this would be the first step. The second and most important step would be to test MBP from the areas close to and in the direct path of plaque formation in the MS brain to see if indeed more methylation of the arginine would be found there, giving us conclusive proof of formaldehyde modification. With that kind of evidence, surely the methanol hypothesis would be impossible to ignore.

We would have to apply to tissue banks around the world that stored frozen brain tissue from the cadavers of deceased MS patients and describe to their scientific committees our need for samples of their valuable tissue to perform our experiment. We would then use this fascinating new analysis method to determine if formaldehyde was setting the stage for the damage that became MS. Nothing else would be as effective in determining whether formaldehyde was altering the brains of MS patients as evaluating their brains for methylated arginine. Finally, we had found a way to prove methanol's formaldehyde as the cause of an important disease of civilization.

We parted in a state of great excitement. The real work started the very next day, with both of us hitting the computer and launching an intense review of the literature so that we would be able to write out proposals to the laboratories whose cooperation would be vital for us to carry out our research.

"Woody… They Have Done Our Experiment for Us…. But They Just Don't Get It!"

I will never forget the call I received the very next day. My friend was so excited that he spoke in German, and at first I couldn't understand what he was trying to get across. I only knew it had to do with what we had discussed the previous evening. The good news was that my German friend had found a reference that led him to believe that our experiment had been performed eight years before, in 2002, just as we had designed it. I asked him to email me the reference to the article so that I could read it for myself. The title was indeed titillating: *An Important Role for…Modifications of MBP in the Pathogenesis of MS*.[224] The bad news turned out to be that those doing the study had not a clue of the scientific significance or impact of what they had discovered. They had found gold and reported the glitter, but they had no use for it. But the results will not be lost on your prepared minds, I promise!

Finding the Shadow of Formaldehyde in the MS Brain:
The Smoking Gun (a Triple Blind Study)

Although it is tragic when lives are lost to ignorance, Nature is, by definition, uncompromising and has no inclination to follow the simplistic paradigms of man's seriously flawed scientific didacticisms. The natural world cannot be expected to be completely understood by even the most competent individual investigator if that investigator is only trained in science, but not nature. Thus the results of any scientific study can have many interpretations, the least reliable of which is very often the conclusion of the extremely prejudiced corresponding author of the manuscript in which it is reported. Scientists often only report what they were actually expecting to find, leaving any troublesome "outlying" data and conclusions that may offend their peers in the editorial trash bin. This is why the more removed the scientist is from the interpretation of his own data the better.

A single blind study is a scientific study performed on human subjects that are purposely kept in the dark as to whether or not they are part of the experimental group (usually a group being given a study medication or treatment, or suffering from the disease being studied) or the control group (usually a group being given a placebo or a group that is reflective of the general population). In other words, only the subjects are "blind" and, therefore, unable to purposefully or subconsciously act to skew the results. When the researchers are also kept from knowing this information until after the interpretation of the data, we have what is called a "double blind" study because both the researchers and the subjects are "blind," preventing either party from acting to affect the results. When researchers stumble on a result that they were not expecting and that they cannot explain, I call that a "triple blind" study because all pre-conception, prejudicial design, and ability to skew results has been removed, and the data is pure. Just as a double blind study is better than a single blind study, I consider a triple blind study to bear the most important fruit of all.

The original discoveries of the U-shaped curve that proved the protective effect of low levels of alcohol consumption against various diseases of civilization were all reported reluctantly by researchers who had discovered this association with no prior intent or expectation. These and other such discoveries have been invaluable in the development of my own view of Nature. The collaborative work done on MS brain tissue at the Department of Chemistry at the University of Michigan and the Hospital for Sick Children in Toronto will probably be the most important of all such studies, and it appears that their reporting was complete and flawless.[224] They were merely looking for changes – any changes – in the chemical composition of MBP between the brains of normal individuals and those with MS. Of the hundreds of changes they could have found, the only ones worth reporting were the ones that happened to show conclusively that formaldehyde was present in higher concentrations in the brains of those who had died with the disease than in the brains of the control group.

The researchers gathered the MS tissue for their study from brain tissue banks in Canada and Colorado. They carefully matched control cadaver samples by age and sex to normal brain samples obtained from violent or sudden cardiac deaths not involving brain injury. The samples gathered from the brain tissue of MS sufferers had well over twice the number of "Crazy Hawks" attached to the arginine that made up its MBP as the control samples. The results were astounding and went beyond our wildest dreams, for not only was the presence of formaldehyde verified by the large increase in arginine methylation,[200] but also another completely unsuspected outcome was reported. The phosphorylation of the MBP was "dramatically reduced" by over 90%, going from 60 sites in the normal brain MBP to only 4 in the MS samples. It is well known that formaldehyde inhibits phosphorylation at extremely low concentrations.[113, 404]

Do you remember the young black girl whose tragic death gave us the critical number for the minimum lethal dose of methanol in humans? Her dreadful last gasp for breath, which froze in vigor for all eternity, was caused by the ability of formaldehyde to destroy the enzymes in her mitochondria that cause the phosphorylation of ADP. By so doing, it robbed her of her ability to distribute life giving energy from her metabolism. No other phenomenon can explain both of these astounding changes to MBP in the MS brain; it can *only* be explained by the direct intervention of formaldehyde. It is well known that the mitochondria in the axons of multiple sclerosis plaque show significant signs of damage and oxidative stress[481] similar to that presented during methanol poisoning.[482]

Let me close this with a paraphrased quote from the authors of this revealing article that will help you tie together the last two chapters.

> *Although we do not have an explanation for the state of hypophosphorylation (reduced phosphorylation) at this time, studies in Alzheimer's disease demonstrated that uncoupling of mitochondrial oxidative phosphorylation resulting in decreased amounts of ATP-activation… and other forms of phosphorylation in the Alzheimer's brain.[224]*

Tragically the good scientists who performed our experiment for us knew nothing of the ways of the Crazy Hawk. Perhaps if they had, their good work would have led to the end of the mystery of the cause of MS and the beginning of the implementation of a real cure. Maybe now it can.

Evidence That Methanol Causes MS

MS Researchers Can Only Agree on One Cause for Multiple Sclerosis: Smoking

Science has been seeking the cause of multiple sclerosis for 150 years. In the early days of the disease it was repeatedly suggested that significant evidence implicated a small toxic molecule[153, 185] – perhaps a solvent.[74,140] Methanol is the smallest of solvents and one whose poisoning symptoms are identical to those of MS.

I will not take the time to go over all of the culprits that have been evaluated as a possible cause for multiple sclerosis. Bacteria, viruses, and most disease-causing agents known to man have at one time or another come under fruitless scrutiny. To this day, some still believe that MS is caused by a disorder of the immune system itself or by a sexually transmitted entity.[184] It is important to understand that for very good reasons the original researchers in the field, well into the early 20th Century, all held to the belief that MS was caused by a circulating toxin which they could not detect or identify.[153] Presently, however, the most regarded theory of causation puts full blame on the darling little macrophage.

The good scientists who held that the cause was a circulating toxin were at great disadvantage. Not only was methanol considered safer than ethanol at the time they were doing their laboratory work, but also formaldehyde had not yet been discovered. Even after the discovery of formaldehyde, researchers remained without any animal test subject for studying methanol poisoning and no way to detect the chemical changes made by formaldehyde to protein. Thus, even if it had occurred to them to do so, it was impossible to test the link between MS and methanol in the laboratory environment. In the article that I mentioned in the previous chapter by the neurologist Dr. Fredrick Wolfgram, he asks his collogues to reevaluate looking for a toxic cause for MS. The very last sentence of his conclusion is noteworthy, valid and insightful to this day: "Do we have any evidence as to whether there is or isn't a low-molecular-weight compound in the brains of MS patients that disrupts myelin? The answer is: 'No,' because no one has ever bothered to look." [153]

It is of the utmost importance that you understand the significance of the fact that during the last hundred and fifty years the search for a cause of MS has found only one culprit. The screening of literally thousands of viruses, bacteria and toxic chemical substances has to this day elucidated only one universally accepted causative agent for MS: cigarette smoking. Most significant of all, this one etiologic agent also just happens to be an important source of methanol. Tobacco smoke has been shown both to cause new cases of MS[67-70,337,338,339,340,71] and to induce the relapse of MS in patients who suffered from the disease but were in remission, transforming a relapsing-remitting clinical course into a much more serious and deadly secondary progressive course.[69]

Understanding the origin of methanol in cigarettes requires some knowledge of how tobacco leaves are processed into cigarettes. The leaves of the tobacco plant contain large amounts of pectin; and although most scientists are unaware of this, tobacco leaves are left in barns to ferment for weeks.[61,62,66] This fermentation releases some of the available methanol from the pectin into the leaf. Wood is then burned to flue-cure the tobacco. The smoke makes direct contact with the tobacco, its methanol-laden smoke soaking into the leaf, as the heat turns the tobacco a brilliant golden color before it is sold to be made into cigarettes.[65] Additional methanol is generated in the smoldering cigarette itself as the leaf is burned. Consequently, methanol is one of the most abundant poisons found in cigarette smoke.[63] Methanol has been detected in human breath following smoking,[64] indicating its absorption by the lungs and presence in the blood.

Looking back to the first discovery of MS it would certainly be difficult to link the disease to cigarette smoke, since the manufactured cigarette was not available in Europe until some time after 1860, when they were first being sold commercially in the United States. More important than this is the reality that many of those who develop MS, even today, do not smoke and in many cases never have. It is clear, therefore, that methanol has more sources than this one, but smoking should be considered a reliable source of methanol.

The Etiology of Multiple Sclerosis – Follow the Methanol

Every Disease has a Beginning, a First Performance – Just How Old is MS?

When an individual is suffering from the early stages of MS, it could easily be mistaken for many other diseases; however, the ultimate symptoms and unusual gate of the full-blown disease are unique, unmistakable, and so tragic as to still bring a tear even to my trained eye. Nevertheless, medical texts from the Middle Ages contain no descriptions of any disease which would be recognizable as MS.[230] The fact that this obvious severe symptomology is completely absent from any historical or even biblical literature is telling. Wolfgram even noted during his plea for the search of a small solvent as the cause of MS that "there is a curious lack of reference to the obvious symptoms of MS in the medical literature prior to the middle of the nineteenth century."[151] This is all proof that MS is indeed a disease of modern civilized man.

It was the discovery of the controlled use of fire that brought man and methanol into potentially dangerous proximity. In chapter two you learned that the smoke produced from the burning of plant material contains methanol. The impact of this methanol was probably minimal, depending on the relationship between various cultures and how they chose to use fire – and more importantly, its smoke. The smokeless flame of a clean burning wood fire contains no detectable methanol, as the blue flame represents the burning off of methanol. Charcoal is wood that has been heat treated in such a way as to remove all methanol and is safely used by many cultures for indoor cooking with no methanol risk. The cultures that developed a taste for food smoked for preservation purposes were probably the first to feel the sting of methanol disease, in the same way that today individuals who smoke cigarettes laden with methanol notoriously suffer from a higher incidence of all DOC.

It was not until the development of the canning of fruits and vegetables in the early eighteen hundreds that methanol was to begin its slow progression toward becoming a daily component of the diet of the civilized world. The daily consumption of methanol would be an important prerequisite for the continuous, unrelenting demylination that consistently exceeds the ability of the Schwann cell to rebuild itself, eventually leading to the complete removal of axon protection that presents as MS.

The History of Man's Methanol Consumption Corresponds to the History of MS

It is the Frenchman Nicolas Appert, the inventor of canning in 1807, who must take responsibility for beginning a process that was to eventually bring methanol into every civilized household throughout the mechanized world. By following the ebb and flow of the canning industry and the consumption trends of canned fruits and vegetables since those early years we can learn a great deal about the evolution of MS.

The first canning factory was fully operational in England by 1813.[46] Due to the expense involved in the production of the cans themselves, early canning was undertaken primarily with high value meats, which have no pectin content and, therefore, would not have caused methanol accumulation. Canning of fruits and vegetables, however, quickly followed as the wealthy acquired a taste for these products out of season. Over time canning became more prevalent and less expensive,[46] and the per capita consumption of canned plant material skyrocketed – as did the incidence of multiple sclerosis. As the canning industry flourished so did the practice of incorporating into recipes the "natural," methanol-laden juices from canned fruits and vegetables rather than discarding them.

Canned fruits and vegetables were, for many years, the major food source of methanol in the human diet. In the years that have passed since caning's humble beginnings, MS has transformed from a medical curiosity to one of the most important and common of the DOC. For 150 of the last 200 years the very best indicator of incidence of the disease in a population would have been the weight of canned fruits and vegetables consumed by the average citizen of the country being surveyed.

The incidence of MS increased slowly after its symptoms were first put to pen in the diary of the grandson of King George III in 1822. We see no official mention of the disease again until ten years later, when its anatomical details are depicted in a book of medical illustrations published in England by Robert Carswell in 1832. This was a time when canned fruits and vegetables were quite expensive and available particularly to the rich. The first officially documented case of multiple sclerosis was reported nearly 35 years later by Jean-Martin Charcot in a lecture in 1868 (discussed below),[45] although it is generally agreed that the "first identifiable instance of MS" was that of Augustus d'Este, whose symptoms started between 1822 and 1843.[45] During the 19th Century, MS was considered "quite rare," with Charcot reporting fewer than 40 cases during his long career.[45] Increasing numbers of cases were reported in the late 19th Century.[45]

During this same period it was discovered that if wood was heated in a large metal container it would produce a smoke that could be condensed into a dark foul smelling liquid called wood alcohol, the original name for methanol. The use of wood alcohol as a solvent for many industrial uses as a replacement for the much more expensive ethanol began about that time and, in fact, Paris was the first large city that would take advantage of the convenience of this liquid fuel, which was easier to transport than wood and could be used as a cooking fuel. It wasn't long before the rich had methanol burning stoves which, under conditions of poor ventilation, were responsible for exposing kitchen help to methanol fumes. It may not have been a coincidence that the first time multiple sclerosis was to be described in detail in a scientific publication was by Charcot in 1865. His first case was his own kitchen servant, whom he had convinced to donate her body, after her death, to his research.

The Early Years of the Multiple Sclerosis Timeline

- No evidence exists to suggest that MS is an ancient malady.
- MS was unknown until some time after Nicolas Appert of France invented canning in 1807.
- The first identifiable instance of MS was not until around 1822 (Augustus d'Este, Grandson of George III).
- MS was first illustrated in drawings done by Carswell in 1831.
- MS was first described in detail, but as a "rare" disease, in 1865 by Jean Charcot of France.
- MS remained uncommon until the 1890s, when the combination of several factors that increased contact with methanol coincided with the disease becoming common, with variable frequency.
- The beginning of the epidemic of MS over "the last 30 years" coincides with the introduction of Aspartame.

An Explosion of Methanol and Disease: the Turn of the 19th Century

The year 1865 was a noteworthy year for methanol in that it marked the end of the Civil War in the United States. It was during this long war that Union troops were often fed canned fruits and vegetables as sustenance while they were in the field. This was their first introduction to such delicacies, and they were greatly impressed. When the war was finally over, the soldiers brought home with them a ready appetite and market for the fledgling canning industry.

The invention of automatic machines that could make canned fruits and vegetables faster and cheaper than ever before slowly brought canned methanol-contaminated plant products into every home of the United States. It was at this time that the Ball family developed heat resistant jars that could be used by any homemaker to put away fruits and vegetables from their own gardens. Add to this the discovery in 1895 of a method for making the bad-smelling and -tasting wood alcohol look and taste just like ethanol. Subsequently, this new methanol began to be used as a substitute for ethanol in many industrial applications, such as in solvents used to make fast drying glues for the leather and shoe industry, and as an additive in many cough syrups and foods extracts, such as vanilla. It is easy to see a correlation between the steady acceptance of MS as a "common" disease during the first twenty years of the 20th Century and the steady increase in the methanol in the environment and the diet during the very same period of time. Meanwhile, some of the most intensive testing of the safety of methanol was being conducted in laboratories throughout the world, on every animal except man, and they all proved that methanol was safer than any other alcohol.

Up until the early 1880s the cigarette was a specialty item made by hand, sold for a penny apiece, and very much the stepchild of other tobacco products, such as snuff. But in 1883, an automated cigarette rolling machine, developed by James Bonsack, was put into use, revolutionizing cigarette production. The retail price was cut in half, and volume, which in pre-machine days had never exceeded 500 million, leapt to 10 billion by 1910 in the United States alone. There is no doubt that these few years between the nineteenth and twentieth centuries saw a sudden explosion in the incidence of all of the diseases of civilization, of which MS is a prominent member. This was also a time when the consumption of methanol, not merely from cigarette smoking, but from many different sources, increased dramatically in both the diet and the environment.

Innovations at the Turn of the 19th-20th Century that Increased Contact with Methanol

- Use of methanol for heating in Paris kitchens replaced dangerous wood burning stoves.
- Machine-rolled cigarettes increased smoking by a factor of 20 in less than thirty years.

- Use of methanol as a solvent for fast drying glues in the leather and shoe industries rose dramatically in shoe making centers such as Italy and New York.
- Home canning of fruits and vegetables was becoming extremely popular after the American Civil War; the returning troops loved the idea of eating fruits and vegetables in winter.
- Machines made cans extremely inexpensive and plentiful, and canned fruits and vegetables cheaper than fresh and available all year long.
- Tests on all animals proved methanol was safer to drink than ethanol.
- Methods for purifying and removing bad odor and taste of wood alcohol were developed.
- Methanol was allowed and frequently used in place of ethanol in food extracts, many medicines, and body salves, including witch hazel and other body ointments.

A Food Scientist's Nightmare Called Aspartame

The symptoms of multiple sclerosis, chronic and acute methanol toxicity, and aspartame poisoning are in all ways identical because they all reflect slight variations on the same theme. Nothing happens to the human body from the toxic effect of methanol that is not also expressed during the course of MS – not one thing.

Thirty years ago as Professor and Director of the Food Science and Nutrition Laboratory of Arizona State University I was unwittingly thrust into the aspartame debate with a great deal of publicity that accomplished only two good things. First, it brought to the public's attention the fact that a problem of some kind was associated with the new artificial sweetener. Second, it established me as a contact person with whom the public could share their experiences and information.

The calls from consumers started coming to my office at such a rate that for over six months I had to enlist student volunteers to man my telephone when I was in class or working in my laboratory. By far the preponderance of complaints were from women, and these reports consisted mostly of the classic symptoms of early MS.[58] Some even sent me MRIs depicting images one would expect of MS. I would talk directly to as many as my schedule would allow and encourage all who complained to stop their consumption of aspartame, suggesting that if they felt brave enough, they should wait a month and then resume consumption and share with me the results. Nearly every time, the symptoms disappeared within a week after aspartame consumption was stopped. Those who had the courage to retest all reported a return of symptoms in varying degrees of severity.

On one very notable occasion I was sent a clean MRI from a girl who had stopped diet soda for a year and whose prior MRI showed massive signs of MS. By the way, MRIs taken in the early stages of MS do not show demylination; they show edema in places where the high-fat brain tissue is being displaced by the microglia (the brain's macrophage) and the liquid of inflammation. That was what this girl's initial MRI had shown. At that time, MS was not within my scope of research, so when I had heard enough I made contact with the headquarters of the National Multiple Sclerosis Society in New York City and got the ear of their director of research. I shared with him, with the enthusiasm of a young scholar, why I thought that methanol might be the cause of MS. He asked me to send him what evidence I had, which I did with dispatch. To make a long story short, I never received even the courtesy of a reply to my extensive report and was never allowed to talk to him directly again. Medical researchers hate anecdotal information. The reasons for this are clouded in the evolution of a scientific mindset that specifies data must be generated in the perfect laboratory environment. Unfortunately, this approach does not work well in the absence of suitable animal test subjects in the laboratory.

In 1984, I published my first scientific article about the sweetener: *Aspartame; Methanol and the Public Health.*[1] In the article, I voiced my concern about the new sweetener and the fact that it was increasing the methanol content of the food supply – but made no mention of multiple sclerosis. Publication of the article, along with more publicity over my lawsuit against the Food and Drug Administration (FDA) (which eventually made its way to the US Supreme Court), brought a flood of additional calls and letters to my office from individuals who thought that they had been poisoned by the product. Many of these individuals also had symptoms of multiple sclerosis and some, in fact, were being tested for the disease. A local doctor also visited me to ask whether I thought his patients' consumption of large quantities of diet sodas in the intolerably hot Phoenix summers might be connected to their complaints about symptoms of MS.

Looking into the scientific literature I discovered several articles suggesting that I was not the first to identify methanol as the possible cause of multiple sclerosis. Dr. Hugo Henzi, a Swiss physician who, during his long career, cared for many MS patients, had been struck by the similarities of the symptoms of methanol poisoning and MS. Henzi's work consisted of a book published in 1980[5] and three scientific articles[6,8,10] that have never been referenced in any MS publication, save my own. I realized that aspartame had provided us with a way to track the public health to the quantitative change of methanol in the food supply. For all intents and purposes, aspartame was methanol, and I had consumption numbers for it. Ending the circumstantial nature of the etiological basis of methanol as the cause of MS would serve as good news for the future of world health, though it would provide little comfort for the innocent populations that had submitted to the Mengele-like enterprise that was the aspartame industry.

Unfortunately, it would take many years for the MS disease statistics from increasing aspartame consumption to build. When the data became available I was ready. I procured from the Centers for Disease Control its multiple sclerosis incidence data for the United States during the period that consumption of aspartame was building. This was data that could have quickly been made available to the Multiple Sclerosis Society.

Figure 9.5

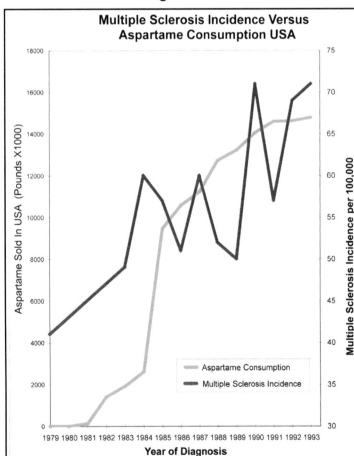

Multiple Sclerosis Incidence Versus Aspartame Consumption USA

Figure 9.5 plots the data in a linear manner just as we did for Alzheimer's disease in the last chapter. The data certainly appears to indicate a marked upward trend in the incidence rate of MS beginning early in the 1980s. In order to get some indication of the strength of this trend I have created another graph of the same data. In Figure 9.6 I have had the computer draw a trend line, sometimes called a linear regression line, in heavy black that shows more clearly the direction of the trend of the incidence of multiple scleroses during that important period of time. Just as I had feared, the incidence had gone up 60% during the first decade following the introduction of aspartame.

MS usually takes about ten years from first onset of symptoms to reportable diagnosis of the disease.[86,167] This early reporting was evidence, to me, of much worse to follow. How long did it take before the deaths from

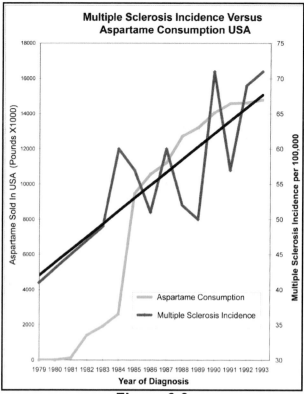

Figure 9.6

Figure 9.7

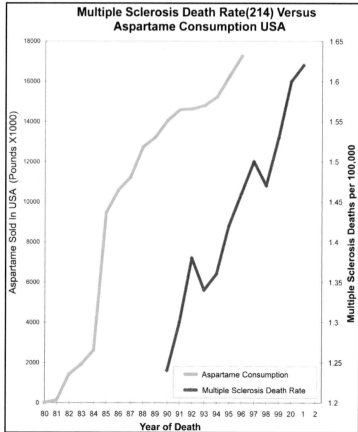

MS caught up to the consumption of methanol from aspartame? The issue of the death rate from MS has been a very important topic in neurology, particularly with the report of the steady decrease in MS deaths that was observed in the United States during the entire 1970s.[710] This decline would reflect a continuing decrease in smoking among young adults, as well as a clear change in preference of US consumers for cleverly marketed and delicious frozen fruits and vegetables, which began attracting consumers' attention away from the high methanol canned alternatives, beginning in earnest in the 1960s.

The neurological community was taken aback by the clear and apparent reversal of this trend during ten-year study period beginning in 1990, with a dramatic and steady increase in the death rate of MS throughout the period. Their concerns were justified, considering, as the investigators themselves noted, that the treatment of the disease had actually improved since the earlier study.[214] What they do not mention is that their study was performed just ten years after the introduction of what would be the most important source of methanol in the human diet. This allowed for plenty of time for the added methanol to take its toll on those already suffering from the disease.

I have plotted in Figure 9.7 the data from this study on our usual graph so we can compare the death rate from MS, as we did from Alzheimer's, with the consumption of aspartame. The results are again breathtaking. The mirroring of the two curves is obvious, although expressing a gap of ten years as compared to the 14 years it took Alzheimer's deaths to catch up with increased methanol consumption from aspartame.

You will notice that the MS death curve is not quite as smooth as the Alzheimer's curve, but this comes from the much lower number of people who die each year from MS as compared to Alzheimer's, which has a death rate over ten times higher than that of MS. One can, however, have absolutely no doubt as to the strong upward trend throughout the entire study period.

MS: a Disease of Colder Climates and Flush Toilets – before Aspartame

A number of unusual theories about the origin of Multiple Sclerosis have come directly from the scientific literature. To my mind the silliest of all is the present speculation being acted upon by some of the most influential of the world's pharmaceutical companies: that the innate immune system is its cause. Let me volunteer here, in the spirit of full disclosure, that some of my very closest friends are macrophages, a fact which I admit may cloud my thinking. But in all seriousness when a scientific thesis known as the sanitation hypothesis[85] comes right out and faults proper sanitation as the royal road to multiple sclerosis and correlates the number of flush toilets in a community to the long term disease incidence, it should give one pause. This is particularly the case when the assumptions on which it is based appear to be, etiologically, the most reliable proposed to date by the sum total of the neurological research establishment. If this scares you, then you may not have the stomach to be an MS scholar. No matter how misguided, the present medical establishment will consistently reference the most challenged of theories of MS origin – so long as those theories have nothing, whatsoever, to do with a food origin for the disorder. This prejudice against the dietary origin of this disease (or any disease) has always been a serious handicap of the medical community.

By now, if you have read the supporting literature referenced here, the most skeptical among you would have to find at least some merit in the possibility that methanol just might be the cause of MS. I will not waste time reiterating the massive amount of literature on this disease. Other fascinating facts about its distribution across geographical locations, occupations and gender need explaining, along with the changes in all of these categories that have accompanied the revolutionary introduction of the sweetener aspartame. This evidence is circumstantial, but still has considerable merit and is worthy of both your time and consideration.

One thing that you can take away from the latter part of this chapter is important: MS was once considered to be a "rich man's disease" in that its prevalence was positively correlated with the trappings of civilization, including modern sanitation practices.[85] It is a universal truth that the economically poorest among us – those who cannot afford toilet paper, let alone toilets themselves, those who farm only or forage for all of their sustenance and cannot afford canned fruits or vegetables or cigarettes or diet soda or any other methanol-containing mark of civilization, those poorest of the poor who still make up an alarmingly large percentage of the world's population – are free from autoimmune diseases such as MS.[168]

A World Awash in MS after Aspartame

Aspartame and cigarettes have two ignoble distinctions that they share: the first is the inordinate amount of money spent by their manufacturers for seriously compromised science,[249] political influence and extravagant advertising campaigns to assure the public of their safety; the other is that both are substantial sources of methanol, without any significant redeeming ethanol protection. They stand out in this latter regard, as no other such naked methanol sources could be listed as common consumables.

The epidemic of multiple sclerosis and other autoimmune disease throughout the world over the last 30 years cannot be denied.[79,337-346, 80, 347-349, 81,350, 82] Multiple sclerosis, once almost unknown in Japan,[44, 85,168] has now risen to menace a large portion of the population.[81,350] The lower latitudes and warmer climates, which once "mysteriously" protected people from the full brunt of this tragically debilitating disease,[83,85,168] have seen incidence and prevalence of MS climb to as much as four times what they were in the days before summer drinks were sweetened with aspartame.[79,338,340,342,343,344,345,80,347,348,349] The United States, which has long had a relatively high MS incidence, has seen at least a 50% increase.[77] Medical journals in Australia[82] and New Zealand[90] both report unexplainable increases in their inordinately high[168] "infection" rates.

I believe that just telling you this information is not going to convince you. My experience has shown that for most people, that is just so many words. In order for you to be convinced of something as important as the methanol theory of MS causation you need to take a little walk in my shoes. What I have done is put together a short slide show that is available on my website (www.whilesciencesleeps.com - "Chapter 9 Slideshow 1"), in which I present the literature that I just described above, in an annotated fashion, right out of their respective scientific journals. Excerpts from this can be found in Appendix 2, page 231. You will find their reference numbers in parentheses on the lower left corner of each slide. Please take the time right now to read through this personal slide show made just for you, and I will be waiting right here for you when you return.

As you can see, all the available data does show that the incidence of MS in the United States, and eventually the rest of the developed world, has clearly increased, and that increase appears to have begun with the introduction of the methanol-containing sweetener aspartame in July of 1981.[194586] Spend some time reviewing the maps done by Dr. John F. Kurtzke on slides 10, 11 and 12. John is a physician whose life work has been the epidemiology of MS. He drew these maps at different times during his career. When dealing with such depictions of data, it is a very important consideration that they are all produced by the same competent individual and to the same standard. We will talk more about John's work on the Faroe Islands later. Pay particular attention to the increase in MS incidence in the warmer climates. The growth of the disease into Mexico and South America is easier to see, but have a close look at Europe, where the entire northern Mediterranean basin is now an area of high frequency, and where all of Italy and both Portugal and Greece are now also subject to a high frequency in the disease.[195] John calls this "diffusion," and that is very descriptive, but to my mind it is all linked directly to the success of the marketing of carbonated diet beverages containing aspartame throughout all of Europe and, interestingly enough, the Netherlands. The second largest aspartame production plant in the world (Japan has the largest) had to be built in Italy in 1985 to supply the tremendous demand for the methanol-containing products by the burgeoning European market.

One last word about the marketing of diet soda – the advertising blitz throughout the South American countries of Brazil and Argentina was noteworthy and appealed quickly to the narcissistic tendencies of those countries' weight-conscious populations, a fact which probably accounts for the increase in their MS statistics. The enhanced importance of this unexpected increased incidence[77] is that it reversed a clear trend that had been going on for ten years during the entire 1970s[214] which, looking back, appeared as an apparent consequence of the reduction of smoking with the increased awareness of the health implications of tobacco smoke (which, as mentioned in Chapter 2, is the only known cause of MS). It took about eight years of exposure to aspartame before the death rate from MS began to dramatically reflect the increase in incidence.[214] The increase in death rate is an eerie mirror image of the graph of the increase in the consumption rate of aspartame and, therefore, of methanol (see Figure 6).

The only logical explanation for an increase in multiple sclerosis in the warmer climates would be an increase in the exposure to the causative agent. If that cause was methanol, then that implies that something consumed in warm climates would have to have had its methanol content increased dramatically. Before the summer of 1981 no diet drinks contained any methanol. Beginning that summer, only powdered drinks had aspartame and, therefore, methanol added to them. These drinks had to be mixed with water and were marketed mostly to women who had a kitchen available to them most of the day. In the fall of 1983, after I lost my bid to prevent aspartame from being approved for uses as an artificial sweetener in carbonated beverages,[56] the methanol content of diet drinks began an upward trend which was eventually to lead to their exposing consumers to more methanol than canned fruits and vegetables[1] – or any other food, for that matter. This trend definitely increased the general consumption of methanol in warm climates.

Change in Frequency of MS by Sex: Methanol's Source (Food or Smoke) Makes All the Difference

Modern women bear the brunt of the multiple sclerosis epidemic.[351,352,353] Presently three or four women get the disease for every man who does. We have become used to the reality that MS is a women's disease and, as you saw in the slide show, it is becoming more and more of a women's disease as time passes. It appears that each survey that is done and each study that is repeated finds ever greater numbers of women over men who suffer from the malady.[91] It has not always been this way, and the ratios appear to have changed considerably over time with no apparent reason; however, an explanation is indeed easy if methanol is what causes MS.

Well into the turn of the 20th Century, with the concomitant introduction of methanol into the environment and food supply, the incidence of MS had already grown from that of a rare disease and medical oddity to one of greater prevalence. Before long, it became the subject of much organized medical research and discussion. The group of nine neurologists who made up the New York Neurological Society met to discuss MS in 1902. Recorded in the minutes of that meeting was a general agreement that MS was a rare disease in New York.[153] MS increased dramatically (over 140%) in Germany and Switzerland between 1906 and 1940.[153] In 1921 this sea change prompted the American Association for Research in Nervous and Mental Diseases (ARNMD) to theme its annual meeting in New York City *Current Knowledge and Research on Multiple Sclerosis*.[306] The two day meeting featured presentations on the pathology, epidemiology, etiology and clinical features of the disease and were published the following year. The organization also captured a consensus of the understanding and state of medical research on MS presented by the gathered researchers and clinicians. The conclusions emphasized that MS was among the most common organic disease of the nervous system and that its cause was some "unknown toxin." Most important of all the organization concluded that "males are attacked more often, with a male: female ratio of 3:2" and that the disease occurs more in "skilled manual workers than laborers." It was at this meeting that it was also first noticed that MS is more frequent in the colder climates of both the United States and Europe.[306]

How methanol gets to the brain makes all the difference. If you were a skilled leather worker employed in one of the many shoe or leather factories in New York City or other major industrial centers of the Unites States during the early 1900s, methanol would be an ingredient in the glue and treatments you used and you would be breathing in these fumes during the work day. This would also be the case if you were a painter or one of any number of other occupations which used cheap methanol as a solvent or to clean surfaces before finishing. If you smoked cigarettes, as many men did during this time period when cigarette smoking was increasing tremendously with the advent of cheap addictive automatically-rolled cigarettes, then you would also be exposed to steady amounts of methanol. These occupational and recreational sources of environmental methanol would supplement the methanol to which both you and your wife were exposed at the evening meal when she opened up a few cans of vegetables and heated them up with their juices for your supper.

The details of how methanol reaches your brain differ, depending on whether you are getting your methanol via your lungs or in your diet. It is this difference that accounts for all of this tweaking of the sexual ratios of MS and some of the other DOC. All is sexually equal when methanol comes from cigarettes or exposure in the workplace air supply or via environmental fumes. Methanol entering the lungs goes directly into the bloodstream equally in both sexes. It is when methanol enters the body via the food supply that things get really interesting, and is what accounts for the difference across sexes in incidence of MS.

A modern study published in the *New England Journal of Medicine*[94] reports the result of biopsies of the gastric lining of men and women. The astonishing result proved that the concentration of ADH in the gastric lining of men was much higher than that in women. Men, therefore, have the advantage of having large supplies of ADH busily removing methanol from their food at a rate that is four times faster on an equal-body-size basis than women's bodies can remove dietary methanol.[94] The methanol that men consume, both in the food they eat and the diet soda they drink, is four times more likely to be removed from the blood before it ever reaches their brains. The male brain is spared the onslaught by the Crazy Hawks because the methanol is metabolized to formaldehyde in the gut where it can reap its havoc on a more forgiving organ that has a considerably greater regenerative capacity. Finally, we have an explanation for the disparity between men's and women's reactions to methanol poisoning and the diseases it causes. This may also help to explain why men have more gastrointestinal complaints from both methanol and Aspartame consumption.[93, 99]

The importance of this cannot be overstated. Those presenting their patient reports at the ARNMD meeting were reporting on a preponderance of victims from the occupational exposure to methanol in the workplace and smoking. Certainly, women were suffering from their dietary exposure, but their disadvantage to methanol toxicity was overshadowed by the industrial exposure and smoking to which their male counterparts were much more likely to make contact. During this time the use of methanol in the workplace was being investigated and was receiving considerable negative press, with the result that laws were eventually passed restricting its use and requiring warning labels be placed in plain site wherever it was stored.[17] As time passed methanol was reduced in the workplace but, unfortunately, not banned completely. The consumption of canned fruits and vegetables literally skyrocketed as canned foods became less expensive and more acceptable. Additionally, home canning of all manner of plant produce increased between and during the two World Wars.

In the 1940s, just two decades after the ARNMD meeting, the National Multiple Sclerosis Society found the incidence of the disease to be virtually equally distributed between the sexes. In the 1960s, Professor Schumacher found that slightly more women than men were contracting MS.[306] The '70s reversed completely the ARNMD ratios, with every series reporting women being more frequently affected than men, with the usual ratio being three woman to two men.[169] By the early 1980s the number of women with the disease rose just a little higher with 1.7 women to each man who had the disease.[166]

But the real sea change in the incidence of MS in women did not come until after the introduction of a brand new methanol source never before known on our planet or found in our food supply. A can of diet soda sweetened with aspartame has up to four times the amount of methanol as a can of green beans. Worse than that and of much greater significant is that while one would have difficulty consistently consuming six cans of green beans or tomato sauce a day for any length of time, in places like Arizona, Australia or Mexico such consumption of thirst quenching, good-tasting calorie free liquid would be commonplace and has now become customary. The great human health experiment that was begun in 1981 took a great leap forward with the sweetener's allowance as an ingredient in carbonated beverages in 1984, and is going strong right now with aspartame costing much less than sugar to sweeten. The result of all of this was presented at the 59th annual meeting of the American Academy of Neurology in Boston on April 26, 2007.[351] Dr. Gary Cutter, professor of Biostatistics at the University of Alabama, said women are now four times as likely as men to get multiple sclerosis: "It started at two-to-one and is now four-to-one."

The increase is more pronounced in younger people, with young women especially contracting it at an accelerating rate. "This rapid change suggests that it's not just the disease behaving as usual," Cutter said. "It is unfortunate, but it is an opportunity and we can use this information to learn what directions we ought to pursue." Nicholas LaRocca, a VP at the National MS Society, said, "This is an interesting phenomenon, and I'm not sure anyone knows why it's happening."

MS is going through the roof and nobody knows why! As a statistician, Professor Cutter deals with numbers. We thank him for his fine research. But to the victims of this dread plague it's more than "unfortunate," and more than "an opportunity" or "an interesting phenomenon."[91]

It is interesting to note here that 3:1 is the sexual ratio represented by adverse reactors to aspartame reported by the US Center for Disease Control in its study of serious aspartame health related reactions in 1984.[58] The Center found three women to every man whose aspartame consumption complaints were serious enough to warrant investigation.[93] Women's complaints also more frequently involve serious neurological complications that are identical to those of MS. The Centers for Disease Control could not put 2 and 2 together and claimed they could not see a "constellation" of symptoms that would cause them any concern about the new additive. This was after a very unusual two month delay in the release of the report to accommodate an emergency "executive review" of the original document. The executive review has never been released.

Can Methanol Really Cause MS?

The evidence that the formaldehyde produced from methanol causes multiple sclerosis is overwhelming and would be very difficult to refute, particularly if you are debating me, but unfortunately it can be ignored – and has been.

Back in 1990, after the Federation of American Societies for Experimental Biology refused to allow me to give an oral presentation at its annual meeting, I agreed to present a poster session showing a rat model of MS using methanol to damage axons.[2] I decided I would personally give the presentation, not wanting to put any of my graduate students in a position to take the heat for something that was not merely controversial, but perhaps more importantly, something which could impact the financial stability of many junk food and pharmaceutical goliaths. I had prepared myself to face the toughest questions and was, in fact, anxious to debate the issue as to whether methanol was indeed the cause of multiple sclerosis. To my surprise, however, I was relegated to what turned out to be a very remote corner of a satellite presentation hall with a few dozen foreign graduate students, none of which could converse easily in English – and no one came. It was as if my presentation had a little note attached that warned of the possibility that serious bodily harm would come to any who attended. Our data was submitted to various research publications, in one case several times, but was always refused without consistently remediable comment.

The fact is, sufficient information already exists in the scientific literature to show convincingly that long term exposure to methanol will invariably increase the incidence of MS in human populations, and conversely, to show that the absence of methanol is an important precursor to an MS-free population. Let's take a look at that fascinating data and you can decide for yourself.

MS Can Be Found in Some Places, but Cannot be Found in Others

Places Where MS Isn't on the Menu

You can find locations on this planet where MS simply does not exist. This alone should give hope to those who have the disease. The people who occupy these special places are, for all intents and purposes, made of the same stuff as those who are prone to contracting MS. It has been shown that when they immigrate, at an early enough age, to environments that do foster the disease and they eat the food and drink the water and breath the air of their new environment, they acquire the same risk of the disease as everyone else.[44] The good news from this is that it isn't you. It is something in what you eat, drink and breathe that is the cause of this disease.

The places where MS is nonexistent or extremely rare can change rather quickly, as we have seen happen over "the last thirty years." This is even more evidence that the disease is not part and parcel of the sunlight or the geography of these sanctuaries, but is strictly part of the changeable environment of food and air. We know that MS is absent from places where the majority of the population lives directly from nature with little or no access to – or need for – canned fruits and vegetables or diet products containing aspartame. Though the scientific literature points to tropical areas or areas of extreme poverty (where the laughable but statistically valid sanitation theory was born), these MS-free zones have never been strictly limited to the warmer, poorer countries of the world. The exceptions are glaring and can teach us something about MS.

Although central Africa,[184] Mexico, South and Central America, and good part of India did fit into the MS-free category in 1979 when Dr. Kurtzke produced his excellent MS distribution map, important exceptions to the warm climate rule could still be found. The Inuit or Eskimo people of extreme northern Canada have rarely known MS, and those who still maintain their customary diet remain free of the disease.[169] Japan is an example of a country which once enjoyed the lowest MS rate of any civilized country in the entire world, and yet it is extremely affluent, without a tropical climate, and has extremely high standards of sanitation.

All we need do is take a look at the diet of the Japanese people and we can lay to rest this whole muddled issue of the epidemiology of MS. The Japanese are sticklers for eating fruits and vegetables fresh and in season. They would not even consider opening a can of green beans or any other such canned plant product. Even though they do have a thriving canned food industry, it is primarily the canned fish and marine mammals that are canned for domestic consumption. The canned fruit and vegetable products make up a small part of the industry and are essentially all produced for export. Furthermore, the Japanese consume a consistent quantity of fermented foods which are abundant in ethanol, another great advantage that protects the population from methanol. In 1960 the prevalence of MS in Japan was a little over 2 per 100,000 population. Compare that to an island at the same latitude, England, at about the same time, where the MS rate was over 50 per 100,000.[169]

In January of 1985 I received a call from a colleague at MIT asking if I had time for a meeting with an important Japanese scientist and his translators. He was consulting for a major food cooperative in Tokyo, one of the biggest in the country. In Japan, if you have a product that you want the Japanese to consume it must be carried by one of these cooperatives, and they are very strict about what they allow into their stores. Aspartame was at the gate and the Japanese were concerned about what my friend was saying about the possibility that it was causing seizures.[368] When he showed them my article warning of the dangers of methanol consumption and exposure, they immediately wanted to see me. To make a long story short, we did meet and I did what I could to supply him with numerous articles and evidence that I had uncovered up to that time, but my efforts were fruitless. The fix was in. Ajinomoto, the Japanese chemical giant, had made a deal with Donald Rumsfeld's company and agreed to participate in the mass production of aspartame to supply a market that was expanding faster than anyone's wildest dreams. No one could have stopped the approval of aspartame in Japan with Ajinimoto behind it. To this day the company bears a heavy burden for using extreme political pressure and far worse to protect aspartame from proper scrutiny. Aspartame entered the almost perfect Japanese food supply shortly thereafter, and as the article that constitutes slide number 14 in the slide show indicates, the prevalence rate of MS in Japan has remarkably quadrupled "in the past 30 years."[81]

A Group of Islands called Faroe where a Lack of Trees Prevented MS

A group of 17 islands in the North Atlantic has played an inordinately important role in the history and study of multiple sclerosis. A number of medical professionals have made a name for themselves fruitlessly pursuing the cause of MS in those islands – to the point that the island government no longer appears to be interested in proffering its citizenry as guinea pigs for a failed cause.[195]

The Faroese are a semi-independent part of the Kingdom of Denmark. They are located as far away from Japan as one can get without heading back closer. This small group of islands is situated in the stormiest part of the North Atlantic, midway between Scotland and Iceland. The weather is cloudy and windy throughout the year and the summers are cool and sunless. Daily sunshine in the summer months averages only about four hours a day. If ever a place could be found that would be perfect for disproving the vitamin D deficiency theory of the cause MS, this would be it. The meticulously kept medical history of the native-born residents of this land of over 44,000 in population has been searched back to before the 19th Century began, without finding one single case of MS – until July of 1943. What makes this truly amazing is that this location could be considered to be the geographical heart of MS country. The nearest land masses have MS prevalence rates that are the highest on the planet. Scotland has 62 per 100,000, Iceland has 72, Orkney Island has 108, Shetland Island approaches 300, and so on.[169] All these countries and islands were originally settled during the same Nordic migrations, thus ensuring populations of similar genetic descent, making the conundrum even more interesting.

The event that occurred that apparently triggered the first case of MS on the Faroe Islands was the occupation of the islands by British military forces for five years during World War II, beginning in April of 1940 and ending in September of 1945. This event is believed to have triggered the "epidemic" of MS on the Faroes. The epidemic began in 1943, after two years of contact with the troops or something they brought with them, and consisted of 21 patients. It is generally believed that the troops brought either an infection or a toxin that was to cause the disease.[195]

A careful study has revealed that those individuals most affected were those who had been in direct contact with the troops and who lived in close proximity to their numerous bases.[168] It is at this point where the silliness begins, culminating in a scientific piece accusing MS of being a "sexually transmitted infection."[184] The toxin idea was put to rest early on when it was clear that the disease didn't go away after the troops left and subsequent "epidemics" occurred.

In a review written in 2003 by a man who had spent years on the island looking for the cause of MS, Dr. John Kurtzke explains the phenomenon in an important paragraph which I will quote here exactly.

> *The troops therefore brought something to the Faroes which later resulted in an epidemic of clinical MS. This had to be either an infection or toxin, with either one geographically widespread on the islands from 1941. Now a toxin could not be responsible for later epidemics. Therefore, if there are such (and there are), then there must have been an infection carried by a large proportion of British troops (because of its wide distribution) in asymptomatic fashion (because they were healthy troops). This must be a persistent infection which takes time (here two years) to be transmitted to a naïve populace, the Faroese. As noted, we call this agent the primary multiple sclerosis affection, which have defined as a specific, but unknown, widespread, persistent infection that will only rarely lead to clinical neurologic MS years after its acquisition.[195]*

I can't emphasize enough the importance of this paragraph, which exemplifies the extent to which physicians will go to try and show that all disease is caused by bacteria, virus or some other living thing, no matter how far they have to reach. This is the medical mindset and it has cost literally millions of lives to poisonings and nutrient deficiencies throughout the ages. This is not John's fault; this is the fault of his medical training.

The most egregious misstatement in John's paragraph is, "Now a toxin could not be responsible for later epidemics." The troops brought with them items such as canned foods, fruit preserves, marmalades and other rations, along with the ubiquitous cigarette, all of which would be very desirable to the island people, especially during time of war. It is very possible that any of these methanol-containing treats were traded or gifted to the locals, who acquired a taste for, or, in the case of cigarettes, an addiction to them and subsequently became a staple after the troops departed. If this was the case, then of course the "toxin" would have lingered.

To me, the methanol explanation makes much more sense than the strange-new-alien-disease-causing factor, of which the good doctor and all of his many colleagues have never actually been able to find even a trace. Because of the preponderance of physician investigators with preconceived expectations, the diet of the islanders was essentially ignored during the early years when good data could have been gathered from the population while the occupation was still fresh in their memories.

In the more than 60 years since MS mysteriously found the Faroes, only one scientist has put any effort into looking at the diet of the islands and has studied seriously the food consumption of the Faroes and its relationship to MS. His work was not published until 1989 and is actually a review of cook books and importation records of foods to the islands before the occupation and shortly afterward. He stresses that until the war, the traditional diet was indigenous and based primarily on fish, as well as mutton, whale, wild birds, and potatoes. This very limited diet is still maintained to some extent, particularly in the smaller villages, which are still free from MS.[82] This scientist does confirm that after the war, a "rapid" evolution introduced many new food products into the diet, though unfortunately he is not specific about which foods were introduced.[82]

The truly fascinating angle that the author, Klaus Lauer, takes on the Faroe diet may, in fact, explain exactly why they had been completely exempt from MS all throughout its dramatic increase in the rest of the civilized world and, in particular, their close neighbors during the early 1900s: the complete absence of smoking. By that, I do not mean cigarette smoking, but rather the smoking of fish and other meat products. Unlike the traditions of the islands' neighbors, smoking of meats is not practiced as a traditional method of food preservation in the Faroes.[82] They preserve fish and other meats by air drying, as is done with cod in many cultures. Their cook books describe in detail salting and wind drying, but do not mention smoking.

Outside the Faroes, that area of the world is famous for its smoked foods. The Scots and Icelanders, for instance, have perfected the art of preservation by smoking and it is not unusual for them to offer smoked fish along with their jams and preserves with every meal.[487] The Shetland Islands have a special process called "reesting" in which they smoke their food slowly over a peat fire.[82] Unfortunately, the smoke from burning peat contains three times the methanol level of wood smoke.[180] This could help explain why the Shetland Islands have the dubious honor of having the highest incidence of MS in the world, approaching 300 per 100,000 and climbing.[169] But what these other cultures have that Faroes do not is trees and/or peat bogs to provide the heat, smoke and methanol to make the food smoking process work. The North Atlantic archipelago is known for its treelessness. Climatic and geographic conditions and centuries of sheep-breeding have left the Faroe islands all but treeless.

After publishing the Faroe diet article, Lauer published an article attempting to link the disparate incidence of MS in various provinces of France and Switzerland to the use of wood smoke to preserve meat.[69] He made a convincing story of the high incidence of MS in populations that would customararily smoke meats as compared to to those who air dried their meats. Though he was not aware of the possible impact of methanol at the time, it is interesting and important that he put to pen a clear association between MS and diet that needed exposure. His writings have been largely ignored by the medical community.

Methanol consumption was overlooked as a factor in all the studies done on the Faroes. The fact is that even after the work of Henzi, methanol has never been seriously explored as the possible cause of MS. The Scandinavian countries and portions of the Slavic nations have some of the highest incidence of MS of any population in the world.[354,168] In these countries consumption of both commercial- and home-canned fruits and vegetables is high, as is consumption of smoked food as describe above.

Moreover, methanol can be found in traditional liquors made from rotted fruit culled off the ground during harvest and rotted in barrels for months. Some of these liquors have a high enough methanol content to exclude them from international commerce. It may not be a coincidence that the highest incidence of MS is found in cultures which had the potential for very high methanol consumption even before the advent of aspartame.

The Little Village of Wellington: the World's Highest MS Incidence Rate

It seems like many significant things in my life happen in towns called Wellington. I met MS in Wellington, Colorado. I discovered the very rare dark side of the little country of New Zealand in its capital of Wellington. And as you soon will probably agree, the most interesting Wellington of all was one where I have never been and have no desire to ever visit, the Village of Wellington, Ohio. It isn't that I have anything against Wellington, Ohio. It's just that it appears that an old enemy of mine, multiple sclerosis, chose to take up residency there for a time.

The real mystery of this story is how I discovered this little burg in the first place. With a population of 4600 people – one tenth that of the Faroes, and with absolutely nothing of great importance ever having happened within 100 miles of the place since the last Ice Age, we have the Internet to thank for bringing us together. The juxtaposition of the word's methanol and multiple sclerosis plugged into the Environmental Protection Agency's website brought up something I had never seen before: a Health Consultation. It seems that it is type of investigation done by a group that serves under the US Centers for Disease Control called the Agency for Toxic Substances and Disease Registry. The study was conducted in 2005, during the George Bush administration.

I knew the chances of the work being slanted toward industry and away from the public health were strong. I went to the report's conclusions first, just as one would look ahead to see whether a cheap novel had a good ending before deciding whether to waste much time reading it. As I suspected, it was clear that the anonymous researchers who had conducted the study (none of their names were attached to the document) were themselves unwilling to make a difference.

The conclusion began with "no significant contaminants of concern were identified in human exposure pathways." Reading further, however, there appeared a bit of a surprise that made my heart skip a beat or two: "The causes of MS, the primary health concern in this community, are unknown; the disease is believed to be caused by a combination of genetic and environmental factors." Then this highly unusual statement: "This evaluation did not suggest any additional hypotheses for the cause of MS."[578] Obviously, this little town had suffered a serious outbreak of MS, but the population was very small and it was located in the middle of farm country, surrounded by rolling hills of grass. The researchers could only point to a mysterious environmental factor, but could not identify the cause of the outbreak.

The other promised word I had entered into my search criteria, methanol, was nowhere to be found in the conclusion. This often happens with modern search engines finding every use of the word. I am often disappointed to find "methanol" being something less than important in the documents found by such searches, with the only use of the word in some minor subscript. Throwing my concern for the forests aside I quickly printed out the entire document and devoured and annotated it in what seemed like no time at all. The document, hidden in the archives of a government agency under siege during the worst of years for public safety issues, contained information that was enlightening and extremely helpful and confirmed my fears of what could/would happen to a population that was consistently dosed with small amounts of methanol over a long period of time. Unlike aspartame, this methanol came from the air.

The report was oddly written as if by someone who was new at such things. It did not disclose exactly why the federal government was called in to investigate this outbreak of MS until halfway through the report itself.

Chapter 9

Under the topic of "Community Health Concerns" I found that the Ohio Department of Health had, in 1998, identified enough cases of MS in this little community to give Wellington an MS prevalence rate of 600 cases per 100,000. To put this into perspective, this gave Wellington the dubious honor of having the highest MS rate ever recorded in the entire world, worse even than that of the Shetland Islands, which had not yet reached 300. For twenty five people in this little community to have been diagnosed in a period of less than ten years with multiple sclerosis was bad enough, but it did not end there. The incidence of other suspected autoimmune diseases and cancer had also risen to the point of great concern to local authorities. The other disease that most interested me was lupus, another methanol disease which we will discuss in the next chapter.

By the time I got to this earth-shattering bit of information, which was treated with the greatest of nonchalance, I had already learned that the EPA did not arrive at Wellington until September 4-5, 2003 – a year after what it turns out was the offending foundry had fired its workers and closed its doors for the last time, thereby limiting the chances of gleaning any valuable information from the fresh memories of its disgruntled former employees. It seemed, in fact, that this group of Washington bureaucrats came to this village to allay fears and participate in a cover-up of a major cluster of MS that could have done for them precisely what their conclusion said it did not do: "suggest an additional hypothesis for the cause of MS" – methanol. For you see, the *only* chemical that this group's investigation found that was being flagrantly dumped into the environment and that could have caused this tremendous increase in the MS rate of this little community was methanol.

The report contains a review of the literature in which the researchers admit knowing "a weak association between solvent exposure and the development of MS may exist," but the statement is couched in such a way as to make it appear that the anonymous authors are essentially attempting to cover their own rear ends, since at the same time they also recognize the fact that methanol can cause "damage to the central nervous system" without any reflection whatsoever on the situation at hand.

In this age of computerized searches, the literature review by all rights should have mentioned the works by Henzi that clearly and specifically implicated methanol as a causative agent for MS. Obviously, they chose not to mention this, for any competent researcher would have stumbled across Henzi's work and included it – but then they would have been required to explain away the possible association between the methanol exposure in the little town and the resulting MS epidemic.

It would be far too easy to get carried away with politics at this point; suffice it to say, it is clear to me that if this Health Consultation is anything it is a political piece. The long and short of it is that methanol is at the very heart of the health problems that confront the people of this little Ohio community. This methanol came from Sterling Foundry, which was located on the very southwest edge of the city limits of Wellington, just a few hundred feet from the drinking water plant and reservoir for the town. In 1990, new owners bought the foundry out of bankruptcy and it appears that the trouble began at around that time. The prevailing wind in this area of Ohio blows out of the southwest and it wasn't long before townspeople began complaining of "odors" emanating from the plant.

The State of Ohio Environmental Protection Agency investigated the facility in 1995 and discovered the plant was operating without any effective air pollution control equipment, all of which had stopped working during the time the plant was in bankruptcy and out of commission. The plant had "unregulated on-site storage facilities" for large amounts of methanol, with between 20 and 40 tons of it stored on site, outside the plant proper. Nothing anywhere in the report indicates exactly what the intended use of the methanol was, although usually in such facilities it is used to clean freshly cast metal work as it comes out of hot molds. This process usually takes place in outdoor areas to prevent the buildup of dangerous vapors. We can only guess at this point why the foundry workers were never asked by researchers how the methanol was used or why such enormous amounts of methanol were kept on the property at any one time.

After the first Ohio EPA investigation in 1995 the plant was required to keep records of the amount of methanol it kept in storage and to "estimate" the evaporative losses from these storage facilities. The self-reported Toxic Release Inventory from the Sterling Foundry facility in the last three years before it closed (the only inventory available) indicated an annual leakage from storage to the air on-site as 5000 pounds a year. The Ohio EPA admitted that this was evidently not regulated or monitored and never itself did any testing of the atmosphere or verification of any kind. The researchers mentioned this methanol leakage and restated that "methanol can be toxic to humans, targeting the central nervous system." The same paragraph, without scientific reference, states that methanol released into the atmosphere is "rapidly oxidized to carbon dioxide," thus justifying the next statement that the data does not necessarily mean that off-site residents were exposed to methanol at concentrations that would amount to any health concern. The first statement is a lie and the second is silly.

Methanol is very stable in the air and its oxidation to carbon dioxide requires either that it be burned or that it be exposed to the presence of a very special bacterium not found in the atmosphere.[723] I believe the smells from the foundry that for years had instigated complaints from the townspeople located downwind from it were in part methanol that was leaking from those storage facilities and being used for some unknown purpose outside the facility. The very sad thing is that we could have had a very good idea of just how much methanol was going into the air of Wellington. The foundry was buying its methanol from somewhere and the companies that sell such dangerous substances keep good records of those sales. Why didn't the CDC "investigators" track down Starling's methanol source and ask the right questions? The only possible answer is that they just didn't want to know. Sadly, the only thing we do know is that it was enough methanol to raise the rate of MS of the citizens of Wellington to a level higher than anywhere else in the world.

Industrial Exposure to Methanol – Jobs that Can Last for an Eternity

Organic Solvents and the Risk of MS: Only One Solvent at Cause

According to a review article published in 1996, the theory that prolonged contact with organic solvents can cause MS was first proposed in 1982.[74] This theory is correct and this book backs it up fully. Only one problem remains, and it brings us to a very important issue. Only one organic solvent, methanol, is the cause of MS; the other few thousand organic solvents have nothing to do with MS. Most important of all, only one other organic solvent, ethanol, can, if properly applied, stop or even cure MS, by preventing methanol from transforming into formaldehyde and, therefore, preventing symptoms. This means if you wanted to prove the theory, disprove the theory or reverse the theory you know how that can be done by carefully picking your organic solvent.

It was clear in the early 1900s that workers in the leather and the shoe-making industries developed multiple sclerosis more often than workers in other industries.[59] The major reason that MS was considered a disease of men in the early 1900s was because methanol was used freely in industry, particularly in the manufacture of glues and many other sorts of liquids used by businesses that hired only men. Methanol was common in industry for two important reasons. First of all, methanol is an outstanding solvent, better than ethanol for use in all manner of glues, paints and varnishes. Second, it has a lower boiling point than ethanol and evaporates off much more quickly, drying paint or hardening the glue faster and reducing labor costs. Methanol is also an outstanding and very inexpensive solvent for cleaning and removing stains and oily contaminants.

I mentioned the association between exposure to solvents in general and incidents of multiple sclerosis in the previous section. The scientific literature is peppered with articles on the pro and con side of this issue, and now that you know more about methanol than the average scientist you can see that the premise is correct, but only for methanol and no other solvent. Knowing that all solvents are not equal when it comes to causing MS, you can wade through the industrial solvent MS literature and cull the useless articles from the others.

The removal of methanol from industrial glues has been a very slow process since the advantages are so great. The shoe industry was the last to convert to other solvents, although records are difficult to obtain on such industrial secrets as the exact makeup of this type of product. Unfortunately, the MS rate of a particular factory is the most reliable indication as to whether methanol is being used as a solvent or not. The first published study addressing the question of MS and solvent exposure found that in the late 1970s, the incidence of MS among workers in the shoe and leather industry in Florence, Italy was five times higher than that of the general population.[245] Another Italian prevalence study done in the mid 1980s reported a prevalence of MS among shoe workers of over three times above the general Italian population, a number that was still extremely high but probably reflecting a reduction in methanol use by the leather industry around the world.

The fact of the matter is that in modern times the danger associated with methanol contact with industrial personnel and the large number of deaths from industrial accidents caused by improper use of methanol has limited the number of occupations and industries where workers make contact with this dangerous organic solvent. Painters were often exposed to methanol in the old days, but again methanol has slowly been removed from most paints due to the danger of both its manufacture and its ultimate use. Its presence in paint is bound to account for the twofold increase in risk of MS in painters over construction and food processing workers found during a study of 50,000 workers followed over a 16 year period in Norway beginning in 1970.[480]

Industrial Contact with Methanol

These days warning signs abound and the use of methanol in all industries and even science laboratories is accompanied with stern visible and documented warnings of blindness, irreversible neurological damage and birth defects associated with methanol. In fact, a definite disconnect seems to prevail. The only individuals who seem not to be take methanol seriously are the bureaucrats working at the Food Safety Authority of New Zealand or the Food and Drug Administration of the United States or even the European Food Safety Authority, where I am consistently and repeatedly told that "there is nothing to worry about because methanol is a food."

At any rate, the workplaces of the modern world treat methanol with great respect and it is difficult today to find any profession in which individuals daily and consistently make contact with methanol. Two exceptions, however, help prove my point.

Those Who Work with Hot Wood

The paper and wood industry have a great deal to fear if methanol is banned completely from the workplace,[553] as it must eventually be, because it can actually be produced as a byproduct of these industries' general operations. Methanol is, after all, just another name for wood alcohol. The heat required to release methanol from wood as a gas into the environment is not as great as one would suspect. No flame is required, and the temperatures at which paper is made from scrap wood fall well within the methanol production range. Even the heat produced from the friction of the blade of a chainsaw can produce methanol when trees are felled. The paper industry does not like to talk publically about methanol, although we know that all 300 paper mills throughout the world produce what they call internally a "methanol-water waste stream," and each must find a way to dispose of it. Some do much better than others. This stream, which comes off the processing wood pulp, is often exposed to the atmosphere, where it releases both methanol and a group of sulfur-containing compounds called mercaptans that smell very bad (like some paper mills). Chances are very good if you smell a paper mill, you are also smelling some methanol.

Some mills incinerate the methanol streams to destroy the methanol, while others turn the methanol into formaldehyde for sale to other industries.[70] Methanol produced by paper mills and wood processing plants is not carefully regulated by most governmental agencies, due most likely to the political power of organizations such as the American Forest & Paper Association, which collects and uses large sums of money from its members for the purpose of lobbying, much like the methanol and formaldehyde lobbying groups we discussed earlier. Keep in mind that any process that heats wood to high temperatures can and does produce methanol. With the proper precautions, plants can be and have been designed to keep this methanol from causing harm to their employees or the nearby community. Sweden sets a good example of how paper can be made safely.

In a fascinating epidemiological study a number of industrial activities in four European countries were randomly screened to determine if any of them had higher risk than any other for their workers developing multiple sclerosis. Paper manufacturing was by far statistically the most closely associated with MS in all countries tested except for Sweden. Paper manufacturing was followed by wood processing in Norway and Switzerland and leather processing in those same two countries. The author points out that the "association between MS and paper manufacturing is all the more surprising, since this industry played only a minor role in the respective countries."[13] This study is in agreement with the high correlation of MS with the felling of coniferous trees in Norway and earlier observations of a high MS rate associated with wood processing occupations in Europe.[334] This data would mean little if other industries showed a high correlation to MS. The fact is that multiple sclerosis is found more frequently in industries where methanol is used or made as a byproduct that can contaminate the working environment.

It would be ideal to find an occupation that would not be considered one in which practitioners would normally make contact with any toxic chemicals except for methanol. Then we could look at health records and see just what happens to these people in the course of their working lives. It sounds like a scientists daydream - and yet we have done just that in the next section.

Teachers' Paradigm

Methanol is a powerful killer of humans. Our tolerance to acute dosages is low, much lower than the toxicology literature reflects. This discrepancy is due primarily to the accompanying ethanol that is almost always co-administered with the methanol, either as a portion of the lethal concoction or as an attempt at life saving that goes hand-in-hand with dialysis.

A patient who survives the first week of an acute bout of methanol poisoning may not always enjoy a complete recovery, but the patient usually lives. We don't know experimentally what chronic administration of methanol over a long period does because it can only be tested on humans. To my mind the perfect human testing has already been done by the double blind introduction of aspartame to the world's food supply. I have shown you where that testing has gone, but due to the magnitude of my claims I felt it important to find another human study group with another approach to the administration of methanol – one that allows for consistent administration of methanol on as regular a basis as would be feasible with a human test population while at the same time limiting the contact these individuals might have with other dangerous industrial chemicals.

Where was I to find such an idyllic study group who would stand still and expose themselves willingly for their entire careers to this dangerous poison? Little did I imagine that this perfect experimental study group would turn out to be one of which I was a member for a number of years.

A Cold Awakening in Riverton

I woke up with a start in the middle of a wintry New Zealand night late one July with something on my mind. I ran to my office without properly protecting myself from the cold, turned on my computer, which seemed to take forever to find the Internet, and, teeth chattering, I inputted the key word, "Ditto."

I had started teaching right after graduating from the New Mexico Institute of Mining and Technology. My high school chemistry and physics teacher and mentor, Oscar Weisberg, was not about to allow his protégé to get killed in Viet Nam. Oscar had heard that I was back in New Jersey staying at my parents' summer home at the Shore. He called, and after we had a good catch-up he summoned me to his laboratory. Although Oscar was essentially a high school teacher, he was also a brilliant scientist who was exempted from service during the Second World War to work on the atomic bomb. The short story is that he would be taking a sabbatical and I was the only one he was willing to trust to teach his flock while he was gone. I told him I was a scientist and had no intention of teaching, having taken not one class that would count toward a teaching certificate. All he had to say was, "Well, you are going to let me down then."

Somehow he managed to obtain an emergency certification for me that would allow me to teach in my old high school while he was gone. After a little initial awkwardness teaching a summer school class in chemistry for practice, I found that I loved the experience enough to begin taking night school classes that would allow me to continue teaching for a few years. Eventually, I was lucky enough to get a fantastic job at one of the best teaching establishments in the world, a private school called Colorado Academy just outside of Denver. In all, I taught young kids in secondary schools for five years before I went on to earn my Doctorate and return to University.

So why am I telling you this? Part and parcel of learning to teach, particularly in secondary schools with large classes, was learning and gaining proficiency in the care and use of a device called a Ditto machine. The dream I had many years later on that chilly Riverton morning was one of me back in New Jersey working in the faculty lounge at my high school. I was retrieving a rectangular one gallon metal can of liquid from a closet stacked high with such cans. In my dream I was looking at the label and, sure enough, it was Ditto fluid. I turned it over to view the contents declaration. What woke me up was the horror of seeing only a brightly colored cautionary skull and crossbones and noticing that one of the eyes in the skull was looking back at me with a slow, menacing wink. Fear quickly turned into curiosity and my search began.

A Ditto machine (also referred to as a spirit duplicator) is a low-volume, very inexpensive printing method used by primarily by schools. The term "spirit duplicator" comes from the alternative term for alcohol, which is "spirits." Methyl alcohol was the only component of the liquid in that can. It is used as a solvent to transfer inks from a template typed by the teacher onto the blank paper that would become the handout for the students in class that day. The spirit duplicator was invented in 1923 by Wilhelm Ritzerfeld. The best-known manufacturer in the United States was Ditto Corporation of Illinois, hence that name. My search turned up some amazing information about this ubiquitous secondary teaching tool. By ubiquitous I mean that the duplicators were everywhere, but particularly in the teachers' lounges of every school where I ever taught or visited. Our school had four of them, and they were always kept in tip top shape. While other teachers were having a coffee or chatting or preparing for their next classes, someone was usually busy in the background inserting their templates and running off purple copies.

I taught secondary science classes that required numerous handouts, as do most secondary school classes. I remember doing some presentations in the primary school on occasion and having to wait in line at their one and only machine. It sounds silly, I know, but this bit of information will turn out to be important very soon. Even the advent of the Xerox machine didn't change this; because of the inexpensiveness of the Ditto machine copies and of the machines themselves, teachers even today are encouraged to use the Ditto to make the copies for their classes. The copies that come from the Ditto machine have a distinctive light blue print and a strong methyl alcohol smell that some find appealing. I can't tell you how many times I would watch as my colleagues would pick up a ream of Ditto copies and fan them in front of their face and smell to see if they were dry enough not to smear as they handed them to their class that day. Often the pages coming off the machine would be saturated with methanol and would have to sit on a desk in the faculty lounge to "dry." The reason that ethanol would not work as a substitution for methanol in these machines was that it would take too long to evaporate and was not a satisfactory solvent for the ink that was impregnated into the original template.

All this methanol – but what was it doing to these poor teachers? I would like you to see what I saw as I progressed through my literature review. You can find a slide show on my website (www.whilesciencesleeps. com, "Chapter 9 Slideshow 2") that is an abbreviation of what I found and which may mean more to many of you than my discussion. Please take the time right now to read through it.

Safety Studies – but Nothing Changes!

My computer search of Ditto machines brought up some fascinating information and good evidence that over the years concerns have been raised about the methanol from these machines and just how dangerous exposure to it might be. These machines have been used in schools since the 1930s. The first investigation was by the Connecticut State Department of Health, which found that the average Ditto machine, without a great deal of use, could easily evaporate up to a gallon of methanol a day, all of which was subsequently vaporized and went into the atmosphere of the room in which the machine was located. Researchers measured methanol concentrations of well over 200 parts per million in the air of the rooms that contained heavily used Ditto machines.

Researchers warned of this in the 1948 issue of the *Industrial Hygiene Newsletter* and again in 1954 in an article entitled, "Exposure To Methanol from Spirit Duplicating Machines," which was published in *The Industrial Hygienist*.[411] This article was specific and stated that "this type of duplicating machine is in common use in schools and business offices." The article further stressed that all of the duplicating fluids contain methanol, with some being made up of 100% of this solvent and rarely any containing less than 40%. One gallon of the fluid can produce between 8,000 to 12,000 copies with wide variability. The paper came out of the machine wet with methanol and, as the copies were handled or riffled, large volumes of methanol vapor rapidly evaporated into the room air and the lungs of the operator, who was often exposed to concentrations of over 1000 parts per million of the poisonous substance. They warned that they tested the air in one very large 5000 square foot office with a 10 foot high ceiling, even leaving the door in the room open during the run. This decreased the methanol concentrations, but even so, they remained above the allowable limit. In the end, researchers recommended that all such machines be hooded and vented out of the building.[411] I taught in several schools between 1967- 71 (twenty years later) and visited many others, and I can attest to the fact that I never saw a single vented Ditto machine until in 1997, when ASU began a program to put vents above all spirit duplicator machines in the University, including the one in our department.

This was not the end of the warnings. Again in 1980 and 1981the US National Institute for Occupational Safety and Health (NIOSH) was called in to investigate two major cases involving numerous complaints. The first was in the Everett School District in Everett, Washington, where operators of spirit duplicators throughout the very large public school district were reporting MS-like symptoms and blaming it on the duplicators. Then they were called in to do another extensive Health Hazard Evaluation Report for very similar complaints, this time to the main campus of the University of Washington.[208] These cases were the most extensive studies done to date on the exposure risks of individuals operating Ditto machines, researchers verified that within just 15 minutes of operation, 75% of the duplicators they tested produced concentrations of methanol that were well over 1100 parts per million. They also noted that 45% of the operators experienced symptoms such as blurred vision, headache, nausea, dizziness and eye irritation, all of which are consistent with the toxic effect of methyl alcohol. The conclusion was that "a health hazard due to excessive exposure to methyl existed in the operation of spirit duplicators."

Teachers, it seems, had been exposed to methanol for their entire careers. This has been going on certifiably since at least 1948. But when did it stop? On March 21, 1995 the nationwide newspaper, *USA Today* published an article entitled "Ditto Sheets in Schools Hazardous."[209] The piece was written as a result of the release of a study done by the American Federation of Teachers at the request of numerous member teachers complaining of health problems that they had linked to their use of Ditto machines. The article starts, "Those smelly, purple-ink sheets that teachers regularly crank out on low-tech Ditto machines may be hazardous to everyone's health." The study revealed that a spot check of schools from all over the country, including the most populous states of California, Pennsylvania and Michigan, found that the Ditto machines are still in frequent use. Most important, the study showed that exposure to methanol in schools can be much higher than levels allowed in workplaces by the Occupational Safety and Health Administration. The article goes on to reveal that methanol has a "high odor threshold," and by the time you smell it, "you've already been overexposed."

Teachers Become the Perfect Test Animal for Methanol Poisoning

We can document that at least in the United States, most teachers have been exposed to methanol on a workday basis for their entire careers. We can't say that they received equal doses as we could if we were experimenting with rats in a controlled laboratory environment, but we can make up for that by having a large population of exposed teachers over a very long period of time. We know a little more about our subjects as well; we know that those who teach on the secondary level have been consistently exposed to more methanol than the average primary school teacher, who has need for fewer handouts. We know that some equanimity may be found among these two classes of teachers because even though some teachers have used more handouts than others, the machines have usually traditionally been located in the teachers' lounges, thus exposing even those teachers who didn't do many handouts.

The Diseases of Teaching

While still in secure self exile in New Zealand I continued my literature review, looking to see if teachers' health was any different from that of the general public. The results of my search shook me seriously to my very core. It was while still in lovely Riverton among my many Kiwi friends that I really did begin to wonder whether some sort of conspiracy could have been involved in the fact that science seemed to have entirely missed the connection between methanol exposure and MS. The title of this book, "While Science Sleeps," was thus born, as was my determination to circumvent the establishment and bring all of my findings directly to the public – the people who needed it most.

The first article I remember reading was a review that described a French survey which had the perfect title: *Do teachers have more health problems?*[215] Sure enough, the author admitted that the literature comparing diseases between teachers and the general public was rare, but he pointed me in the right direction to other articles that have shown an increased incidence in breast and thyroid cancers in the teaching population, two methanol-sensitive organs that we will talk about in the cancer chapter. The "Eureka!" moment, however, came when I read this phrase: "and surprising enough, there is an association between school teaching and mortality from autoimmune diseases." I just wanted to stop right there, go no further, and avoid the risk that the reference was a weak one or poorly done, or worse, that it had a strange sample selection. I think that I floated on the little bit of good news for at least an hour before I built up the courage to look up the reference number in the bibliography.

When I did finally look it up I was both relieved and pleasantly surprised. The article had been published in one of the few journals in the area that I regarded as both untouchable and prestigious; I would trust the results of any article its editors selected to publish. *The Journal of Rheumatology* published only the best work, and now I couldn't wait to get the article into my shaking hands. When I did, I was blown away by it, and I think you will be, as well.

Excess Autoimmune Disease Mortality among School Teachers

The name of the article was "Excess Autoimmune Disease Mortality among School Teachers."[210] The work was faultless and the data was conservatively compiled from the death certificates of all deaths in the US for the ten year period between 1985-95. School teacher deaths were compared to those of persons in other professional occupations. The conclusion: "Our results substantiate excess mortality from autoimmune diseases among teachers and suggest that, relatively early in their careers, teachers experience an occupational exposure that increases the risk of autoimmune diseases." They found that "excess mortality was significantly greater in secondary teachers than elementary teachers." Most astonishing of all, "the greatest relative excess in autoimmune disease mortality among teachers occurred for multiple sclerosis."

In fact, the rate of multiple sclerosis among secondary school teachers was almost twice that of their professional counterparts. "The autoimmunity disease mortality was most strongly elevated among secondary school teachers. In particular, significant excess mortality from multiple sclerosis and lupus occurred in the 35-44 age interval of secondary school teachers." We will discuss lupus and the other autoimmune diseases that this study found associated with secondary school teaching in the next chapter and the cancers of methanol in the chapters after that. The one other statistically significant statement that can be taken directly from this study was that "among white males teaching was associated with excess mortality from multiple sclerosis."

In explaining the rationale behind doing this study the investigators said that the National Institute for Occupational Safety and Health had produced a survey of occupational mortality that unexpectedly pointed to elevated autoimmune disease mortality among school teachers during the 1984-88 period. "Our results show that significant elevated mortality also occurred in the subsequent 1989-95 period."

MS Treatment – Pharmaceutical Placeboes or Perhaps Worse

All modern treatments for MS and all treatments that are in "the pipeline" are dangerous and should be avoided at all cost. MS has no known cure, and after reading about all of the many modern treatments,[615] I can only conclude from the evidence provided that over the last 50 years the only one that showed statistically valid improvement in double-blind studies, albeit for a relatively short period of time, is plasmapheresis.[186] Plasmapheresis involves removing the liquid portion (plasma) of a patient's blood, then returning the red and white blood cells to the patient without the plasma. The reason this procedure has a positive effect may very well be something other than the official reason it is performed; you see, the process could be expected to remove much of the methanol from the bloodstream, reducing its concentration substantially in the tissues. Transfusions seem also to have similar effect.[43] I cannot recommend these two treatments because it would be far easier to just avoid methanol.

Conclusion and Review

You can see for yourself now that the daily administration of methanol to the human organism does not go unnoticed by the immune system. The evidence is simply far too overwhelming for the pharmaceutical industries to credibly justify ignoring it any longer. As a scientist I can do little more than present a coherent molecular theory, and then prove the hypothesis using three paradigms with two distinct methods of methanol administration. Viewing methanol toxicity as the etiologic cause of MS answers all of the nagging questions and unexplained anomalies that have stalled the search for the cause of this disease. I realize that absolutely nothing can convince the pharmaceutical giants, who are now heavily invested in developing their own useless palliatives for MS, to give them up and rally around the methanol hypothesis. In the end, however, I believe that the truth will win out. Henry Miller prophesied over 50 years ago:

> *It is possible that the cause of multiple sclerosis lies buried somewhere in these lengthy protocols waiting to be found by someone ingenious enough to unearth it.*[306]

Review

1. MS is a disease that begins around brain blood vessels, adjacent to the exact locations where methanol converts to formaldehyde, very much like Alzheimer's disease.
2. MS was first discovered long before formaldehyde, making the determination of its cause impossible.
3. The vast majority of early researchers believed that the cause of MS was a "toxic substance" that forms in and is distributed via the blood vessels of the brain. "Whatever is being produced within the vessel walls is the cause of the disease."
4. All symptoms of MS can be found during the course of methanol poisoning if the patient lives long enough.
5. Myelin Basic Protein (MBP) is the protein of the myelin sheath that is removed during MS plaque development. MBP contains a high percentage of arginine, which acts as a trap for formaldehyde. The MBP of MS patients has been shown to have reacted with formaldehyde and cause a marked increase of the methylation of its arginine.
6. The MBP of MS brain tissue has been shown to be severely deficient in phosphorylation, which we know can be caused by formaldehyde.
7. The Smoking Paradigm: Cigarette smoke is high in methanol and is the only etiological cause of MS that is generally accepted by the scientific community.
8. Consistent circumstantial evidence links increases in methanol-containing food consumption and in industrial use of methanol to corresponding increases in MS incidence during the transition from the 19th Century into the 20th Century.
9. The advent of aspartame, a methanol carrier, has introduced an opportunity to quantify additional methanol in the food supply since 1981.
10. The Aspartame Paradigm: statistics show convincingly that as more and more aspartame is consumed by the US population the incidence of – and perhaps more importantly the death rate from – MS has also increased dramatically.
11. The higher incidence of MS in colder climates was due to the higher consumption levels of canned fruits and vegetables in temperate climates. This began reversing shortly after methanol-containing diet sodas and other thirst quenching products became popular and inexpensive in the tropics.
12. MS was at one time a disease of men when it was caused by industrial contact. It is increasingly more of a women's disease. When methanol is inhaled as a gas during cigarette smoking or industrial contamination the distribution tends to be equal between the sexes. The stomach of the man, however, has 4 or 5 times more ADH in its lining than that of a woman. When methanol is consumed via diet soda, the ADH removes methanol before it can get to the brain, so less of it reaches men's brains than women's brains. As more and more methanol has become a dietary poison, the shift from male to female disease has followed.
13. The Faroe Islands are surrounded by countries with very high incidence of MS, yet the country traditionally did not have the disease represented in its population until after the occupation of large

numbers of British Troops during the Second World War. Faroes have no trees or peat deposits and, therefore, developed methods to salt and air dry fish and other meats for preservation, unlike its neighbors, who dine on smoked foods at each meal. The indigenous diet of the Faroans contains no methanol.

14. The Village of Wellington, Ohio experienced an epidemic of MS that should have been traced to the escape of methanol fumes from a foundry, affecting the populace located downwind of it.

15. Professions such as shoe making and papermaking that have been shown to have high incidence of MS can also be shown to have exposes their workers to levels of methanol.

16. The Teaching Paradigm: The US teaching profession might just be the best profession by which researchers could link methanol exposure to increased incidence of MS. Secondary school teachers suffer an incidence of MS almost twice as high as their professional counterparts. They also can be shown to have had consistent workday exposure to methanol fumes by the ubiquitous use of Ditto machines that use high concentrations of methanol as a print transfer agent.

It has been over 30 years since I heard my first unsolicited plea for help from an aspartame consumer who had linked consumption of the product to her suffering. My first thought after an hour's listening was that this courageous young woman would soon be diagnosed with Multiple Sclerosis. It is in her honor and in the memory of my friend from Wellington, Colorado that I seek to explain the compelling link between methanol and MS.

Post Script: A Word about Depression, a Common Complaint
of Methanol Poisoning and All the DOC

We have charted two methanol diseases that have long gestation periods. However, methanol poisoning, MS and aspartame consumption have one symptom that is a quick responder (24-48 hours) that permeates the literature of both methanol poisoning and MS and is a constant anecdotal complaint from aspartame consumers. Depression was the second most reported complaint from aspartame consumers, next to headaches, in the study done by the CDC when it finally took a cursory and shallow look at the health impact of aspartame in a very conflicted and highly unusual report published by them in 1984.[58]

A comprehensive double-blind crossover study designed to ascertain whether individuals with mood disorders were vulnerable to developing depression after consumption of moderate amounts of aspartame concluded that "individuals with mood disorders are particularly sensitive to this artificial sweetener and its use in this population should be discouraged."[54] The results of this experiment were statistically significant even though the experiment was halted prematurely by Ohio University's College of Medicine Institutional Review Board, due to the severity of reactions within the group of patients with a history of depression. Such major reactions are uncommon in the aspartame toxicity literature. The reason for this may have to do with the difficulty in procuring the chemical for testing purposes without having to rely on the honesty of the manufacturer. Dr. Ralph G. Walton, Chairman of the Department of Psychiatry and the first author of the article explains in his own words what he went through.

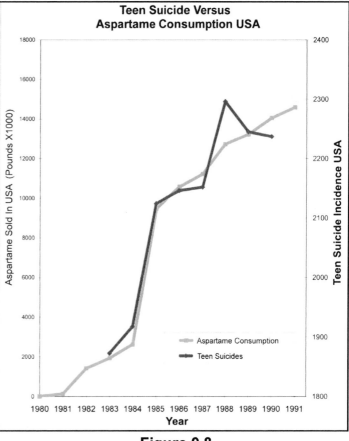

Figure 9.8

"Nutrasweet Company did try very hard to prevent me from getting aspartame for our double blind study. The company had stated that they would supply aspartame and placebo capsules free of charge to any 'legitimate researcher.' As a full professor and chairman of a department at a major medical school I think I qualified as 'legitimate' but they refused to provide it to me. When I pressed they said it was 'unnecessary' research. At that point I said I was willing to buy it from them rather than have it provided free. They still refused. I then turned to bottlers of diet soda and was told that they had been instructed by the company not to sell it to me. We did eventually obtain aspartame, but only after a world-wide search. In retrospect I am glad that I did not get the aspartame or placebos from the company – who knows what they would have sent me?"

As a teacher, I immediately noticed that college students and teenagers, in particular, were quick to pick up on the great-tasting aspartame sweetened diet sodas as a way to keep their weight down. I asked the CDC for the data it had collected on successful suicides of teenagers during the years after aspartame was added to carbonated beverages and its consumption exploded. The response was startling. Figure 9.8 represents this data in the usual fashion. Unlike Alzheimer's, with a 14-year delay until death, the teen suicide rate of this important period spirals around the aspartame consumption curve like the two snakes slithering up the caduceus.* This quick response would be expected since the mood alterations generated by both methanol and aspartame take hours, not years. There is also some evidence that the anhedonia (inability to experience pleasure) produced by methanol may be identical to that induced by alcohol withdrawal and may linger for some time.[38] This striking yet tragic illustration required the deaths of 1600 teenagers above the normal rate in the US to generate. Their parents would not consider their loss anecdotal.

* The caduceus is the magic wand of the Greek god Hermes (Mercury) and is used by the medical pharmaceutical establishment as its symbol. Hermes is considered the protector of merchants and thieves.

Chapter 10
Classic Autoimmune Diseases Lupus and Rheumatoid Arthritis

The *Excess Autoimmune Disease Mortality Among School Teachers*[210] article we reviewed in the last chapter was a revelation to me and I am sure it will help you appreciate classic toxicology and the importance of keeping track of disease expression in various populations. The statistics associated with the teaching profession, smoking, and aspartame consumption all present powerful evidence of the long term deleterious consequences of methanol exposure. School teachers are particularly important test subjects because, unlike smokers, their exposure is to pure methanol. When teachers were compared to other professionals on a disease-by-disease basis they suffered from a higher proportional death rate as a result of 11 out of the 13 autoimmune diseases investigated.[210]

Methanol poisoning and autoimmunity make direct contact in two places. These points of impact between a toxic substance and a requisite disease process are invaluable in linking the suspicions of epidemiology to the reality of causation. It is the modification of protein by formaldehyde at the molecular level that activates the macrophage and causes the slow consumption and self-damage of this class of diseases. The macrophage then, due again to formaldehyde modification, can initiate the production of antibodies to self protein that increases the magnitude and the scope of the destructive process. This chapter will cover how this occurs.

We have already discussed multiple sclerosis (MS), which was found to be the most statistically significant autoimmune killer of teachers, who suffer it at twice the rate of a comparable population. Now we will go into greater detail with two of the other autoimmune diseases – systemic lupus erythematosus S.L.E. (lupus) and rheumatoid arthritis, both of which significantly contributed to increased death rates for teaching professionals in the years from 1985-95.

Before we discuss these diseases, let's take a closer look at the immune process and see how formaldehyde has been used during the development of immunity to disease through vaccine production and the impact that formaldehyde from methanol may have on the evolution of the diseases of autoimmunity and their auto-antibodies.

The Scene of the Crime: the Antibody

Autoimmune diseases, as we have already seen, appear to be caused primarily by phagocytosis (eating of self) by macrophages.[514,519] This is probably caused directly by formaldehyde modification of self or indirectly by the marking of self protein by "autoantibodies." If you read the present scientific literature that discusses macrophage disease interactions you will often come across the technical term "apoptosis," a Greek derivative coined to poetically imply the falling of petals from a flower or leaves from a tree. The implication is that healthy cells are "selflessly" committing suicide in order for life to proceed over their devoured bodies. Indeed, true apoptosis is alive, well and required for the massive physical changes that the human embryo experiences as it morphs through a billion years of phylogeny into an infant and then the massive resculpting of that baby into a physically very different adult.

I do not agree, however, with this term being used to describe the macrophage-induced decimation associated with autoimmune disease, which appears to be more of a rout than an orderly mass suicide. What is being implied by the use of the term "apoptosis" is that the genetically scripted, vitally important process of apoptosis has gone awry in autoimmunity and that indeed must explain the cause of these tragic diseases, pointing the blame, again, toward an error of Nature and away from a manmade poison. Nature, however, never makes mistakes; it is man who creates them. By now you know what causes these diseases: methanol's conversion to formaldehyde, a process caused by a very human error in food processing and industrial environmental husbandry. We will now present more proof by discussing another outcome of these so-called "autoimmune" diseases.

The production of antibodies to self (auto-antibodies) is an important indication that macrophages are primarily and not secondarily involved in the disease process. Antibodies are Y shaped proteins that are very uniform in shape and structure except that the two tips of the Y are custom made specifically to bind to things that the macrophage determines the body does not want. The unwanted substances are called antigens and can be anything from a viral protein to a substance on the cell wall of a bacterium. In the case of autoimmune disease, the antigen is one of the molecules coded on our own DNA.

The production of antibodies to an antigen is a very significant step in the removal of that substance from the body; however, as we have seen, it is not a necessary step. The macrophage is capable of destroying anything it deems harmful or damaged without any antibody involvement. Antibody production simply reduces the time required for antigen removal and can act as a memory for those antigens previously discovered by individual macrophages, which live for mere months, while antibodies have been known to persist in the blood for years.

When our macrophages are working the way Nature intended, it is a very good thing. The process can save our lives by quickly, protecting us from disease-causing life forms before they can reproduce in our bodies. Conversely, it can be a very bad thing when, during the course of an autoimmune disease, we produce antibodies against something near and dear to us that we would rather not lose.

Just how much damage can an antibody do? Remember our girl Venus and her brain cell the size of Manhattan Island? You probably recall that an ADH enzyme was about as big as one of the brownstone houses that surround Central Park. Well, antibodies are also proteins, but are not that big; they are the size and shape of one of those modern football goal posts at your local high school, the ones with just one post in the ground to cut in half the chance of anyone crashing into it during a game. To that same scale an average virus would be about the size of a New York City bus. You can see that it wouldn't take too many attached goal posts to incapacitate a city bus. But what about a bacterium? Well, that is another story. A medium sized bacterium would be about as big as a 7 to 10 story apartment or office building. A few antibodies attached to something that size are not going to do much to interfere with its functioning.

Although antibodies can, by themselves, isolate and keep us protected from some small antigens, the real purpose of an antibody is to mark the enemy for destruction by the big guns of the immune system. They work like a laser tag for a rocket attack. Once an antigen has been marked with an antibody it is much easier for the population of macrophages to find it and eventually devour it.

All of this works well in the normal course of living where the macrophages that roam the body are looking for foreign materials like bacteria and such. The macrophage and other similar cells in the body also do a tremendous amount of housekeeping by removing our older or damaged cells or tissue that is no longer useful or has died for one reason or another, including apoptosis. Even cancer cells are routinely dispatched and eaten by macrophages. The cells that are being routinely devoured and recycled into their original amino acid building blocks still contain our "self" protein, even though they are old or defective. The macrophage knows this and would not think of calling for antibodies to be made to them. Such an error would harm the organism they are programmed to protect – us! So why does it happen?

I don't want to lose you in the minutia here because we are dealing with some important issues where a basic understanding will be much more valuable than if only a few of you became experts on the trivia of the immune system. So let's back off a bit and look at what the macrophage really is. This gentle giant has two jobs. First and primarily, it is a janitor – or more respectfully, a custodian of your body. It travels around looking for our dead or damaged tissue to clean up and recycle. Its other function is keeping a sixty kilo chunk of delicious warm meat from being devoured by a planet chock full of hungry microscopic predators. This function often brings our macrophage into direct contact with armed intruders from the outside world. This is the point at which our gentle janitor has the ability to transform into the equivalent of a member of the Seal Team 6, armed to the teeth and ready to kill and eat anything in its path.

Autoantibody Production Enhanced Dramatically by Formaldehyde Treatment

While wearing its custodial hat, the macrophage, for reasons mentioned above, has no occasion to begin the process of producing antibodies. It is when it is activated into the commando mode that antibody production becomes a priority. We know then that it is vital to the life of the host of the macrophage that not every protein it devours be turned into a template for the production of an antibody, because some of what it might need to remove would be damaged "self" protein. We have no idea how the macrophage makes that extremely important decision about what is "self" and what is not, but it is clear that most of the time it makes the correct decision. We can surmise that the decision process must be somewhat conservative because even when remnants of virus or dead bacteria are injected directly into the bloodstream they will not always elicit antibody production, even though it is within the job description of the macrophage custodians to routinely clean such material from the blood. We do know – and are very lucky to know – that one form of treatment for these foreign antigens, if performed before their injection into our bloodstream, helps guarantee high levels (titer) of antibody production. Subtle treatment with formaldehyde hydrate (the Crazy Hawk) almost always acts to guarantee antibody production to an antigen.

During the evolution of vaccines, not long after the pioneering work of Jennings and Pasture, the pharmaceutical industry noticed and took good advantage of the "trick" of toxoid production.[75,114,179] A toxoid is a bacterial or viral protein that has been treated in the laboratory with formaldehyde.[26] The full scope and depth of the ingenious use of formaldehyde for such vaccine production will never be fully revealed, as it remains a proprietary secret of the pharmaceutical industry. We do know that they began treating bacteria and viruses with formaldehyde in order to kill them so they would not cause infection when injected into humans. In doing so, they discovered three things. The first was if they used too high a concentration of the formaldehyde Crazy Hawk for too long a period of time, the antigens were so changed that the antibodies produced became nonsense antibodies, and when the treated antigen was injected it did not work against the disease they were trying to prevent. The second was if they let the formaldehyde reaction go on for too short a period of time, the virus or bacteria would not be killed. The third, and most important to us, was they found that by using very low levels of formaldehyde over a period of days at human body temperature they would often produce a "toxoid" which, when injected, would cause a much better antibody production and, therefore, a much greater immunity than even the injection of pure antigen painstakingly extracted from the original organism.

Let me give you some examples here because knowledge of this industrial use of the Crazy Hawk will reveal the power of formaldehyde as an indispensable adjunct for the production of both antibodies and, perhaps, autoantibodies as well. Few realize that in order to guarantee that antibodies are produced to target certain antigens injected into the human body during vaccination, that antigen must first undergo prolonged treatment for a week or more with very low levels of formaldehyde. For instance, venoms from dangerous snakes are first treated at human body temperature with low concentrations of formaldehyde hydrate in water solution for several days before they can be injected as "antivenoms" to encourage the macrophage to call for antibody production to the venom.[114] For vaccine production the use of low concentrations of formaldehyde is extremely important, as high concentrations render the material ineffective for immunization.[114] The perfect reactions with formaldehyde at body temperature often take weeks in the case of influenza vaccine production.

What we learn from all of this is that the modification of protein by formaldehyde is a key component that can guarantee the production of antibodies against antigens. The formaldehyde that is produced within the body from methanol cannot be overlooked as a possible adjunct for antibody production to self molecules that have been modified by it. Each of the autoimmune diseases originate in locations within the human body where ADH sites are known to occur. The possibility that this formaldehyde binds to our basic protein in such a way as to not only cause their macrophage phagocytosis but to also occasionally induce the macrophage to call for antibody production to this self protein cannot be overlooked. This may, in fact, be the trigger that encourages the macrophage to class certain self molecules as antigens.

Systemic Lupus (SLE) and Rheumatoid Arthritis (RA): Two Sisters of Atherosclerosis

Lupus (SLE) is more of a disaster than a disease. It is accompanied by an "explosion of autoantibodies" to over a hundred self molecules, including DNA.[520] The damage done by lupus is massive and all-encompassing. It is as if the body was at war with itself. It would take a hundred pages to describe the entirety of the symptoms and tissue damage caused by SLE. Much like that forest fire that I imagined being

Table 5.2: Target Organs of Methanol Toxicity

Methanol Target Organ	ADH 1 Site (reference)	Formaldehyde's Potential Target
Brain	Vascular tissue (218, 220)	Tau Protein
	Vascular tissue (218, 220)	Myelin Basic Protein
	Vascular tissue (218, 220)	Vascular Lining
Eye	Found with retinol dehydrogenase	Retina
Blood Vessels	Intima, media (220) Aorta	LDL
Skin	Fibroblast (221, 638)	Fibroblast
	Fibroblast (221, 638)	Fibroblast
	Skin and Perivascular	All ADH Organs
Breast	Epithelial (357)	Epithelial
Kidney	Epithelial Tubule (637, 640, 503)	Epithelial
		Epithelial
Bone	Synovial Fibroblast (563, 514)	Synovial Fibroblast
Pancreas	Langerhans Islets (637, 503)	Insulin Production
Lung	Fibroblast (221, 503)	Fibroblast
	Fibroblast (221, 503)	Fibroblast
Fetus	None in placenta (503)	DNA Methylation
	(503, 640)	Liver, Lung, Kidney
Liver	Highest in Body (503)	Various

investigated by a race of aliens that knew nothing of the phenomenon of fire, the minutia would take a lifetime to describe in proper scientific detail – and to what avail? I am not going there with these classic autoimmune diseases because the cause of lupus is far more interesting than the tally of the aftermath. This is a methanol disease and I will give you evidence of that.

All the organs and tissue that ultimately come under attack during the course of SLE and its sister, RA, are hiding places for the enzyme ADH Class I that you can review in Table 1-*Target Organs of Methanol Toxicity*. These include the joints, kidneys, heart, lungs, brain, blood, and skin. The symptoms of lupus include achy joints, fever, arthritis, kidney damage, chest pain and skin rash.

Rheumatoid Arthritis is considered an "overlap" disease of SLE, due to the frequency of the two diseases occurring together in the same individual. If indeed these are both methanol diseases, then we would expect that they should also coexist with atherosclerosis, the most common of the methanol diseases. The evidence for this is overwhelming in both diseases considered together ("It is well established that patients with rheumatoid arthritis and SLE die prematurely and that cardiovascular disease is an important driver of the increased mortality in these populations."[516]).

It is also overwhelming in each of these diseases individually ("Atherosclerosis occurs prematurely in

(Bad ADH Sites)

Disease Manifestation	Incidence ↑ Last 35 Years	Reference Incidence	U-Shaped Curve	Smoking Methanol	Aspartame Causation
Alzheimer's	↑10,000% (100X)	540, 533	531, 534	643	
Multiple Sclerosis	↑100% Women higher	77, 214		332	586
Headache, Seizures	↑	471, 181		376	471, 328
Cancer Glioblastoma	↑200%	329			
Macular Degeneration	↑30-40%	668		667,3,37	
Atherosclerosis	↑	532	485	345	
Skin Cancer	↑400% Young women	95		645	229
Dermatitis	↑			227, 437	328,545, 630
Lupus (SLE)	↑300% Women higher	536	73	73	228
Adenocarcinoma	↑50% Adenocarcinoma	250, 193		242, 574	50,48,197
Kidney Cancer	↑200%	577, 646		652	50
Kidney Function ↑	↑100% (Aspartame link)	577, 646		651	588, 659
Rheumatoid Artritis	↑After decades of decline	635	295, 642	332	
Type II Diabetes	↑1000% Adolescent Females	629	650	648, 647	647
COPD	↑100%	523, 641		345	
Adenocarcinoma	↑With decreased smoking	655		655, 656	657
Autism other Terata	↑2500% (25X)	525		644	159, 659
Preterm Delivery	↑	653	654	654	617
Hepatic Cancer	↑300%	577		332, 345	657

patients with systemic lupus erythematosus and is independent of traditional risk factors of cardiovascular disease."[515] "That people with rheumatoid arthritis would have a high rate of cardiovascular disease morbidity and mortality seems surprising… due to the predilection of the disease to occur in women and its frequent treatment with aspirin and other nonsteroidal anti-inflammatory drugs which would be expected to protect these patients from cardiovascular disease."[634]).

Even though we are approaching these diseases as a continuum of chronic methanol poisoning, the magnitude of the association of these diseases with cardiovascular disease is stunning and dramatically reinforces our original hypothesis. Please reread the quotes above until the magnitude of what the researchers are trying to say sinks into your consciousness.

Compared with the general population, patients with rheumatoid arthritis had a 4-fold higher risk of new cardiovascular events over a one year study,[516] while another study showed a 52-fold increase in cardiovascular events in 35-44 year old women with SLE even after controlling for heart disease risk factors. The researchers reviewing these studies state that their "data support the hypothesis that inflammation associated with RA and SLE contributes to accelerated atherosclerosis.[516] Of course, they make no mention of methanol poisoning, but by now you and I know better.

Cigarette Smoking Increases Risk of Both Lupus (SLE) and Rheumatoid Arthritis

Secondary school teaching is not the only exposure to methanol that is responsible for increasing one's risk of SLE and RA. To date, three case-controlled studies have reported significantly increased odds ratios for the development of SLE in smokers.[332] In 1987 the first study looking into the increased risk of rheumatoid arthritis among women smokers showed they had an unexpectedly high, 2.4-fold increased risk of RA. Since that time eleven case-controlled and four cohort studies have confirmed the increased risk of rheumatoid arthritis with cigarette smoking. "Cigarette smoking is now the most conclusively established environmental risk factor for rheumatoid arthritis."[332]

The U-Shaped Curve of Ethanol's Protection from Autoimmunity

What better way to protect from the deleterious conversion of methanol to formaldehyde than through constant low level consumption of the only cure for methanol poisoning: ethanol? Here again we have powerful evidence indicting methanol as the cause of these autoimmune diseases. What else can explain the "marked highly significant negative association between alcohol consumption and SLE… which becomes stronger with higher weekly intake of alcohol."[73] In other words, researchers found those who drank moderately suffered significantly less frequently from SLE. The negative side of the U-shaped curve of alcohol consumption by SLE subjects did not appear to effectuate until over 30 drinks of alcohol a week (over three drinks a day) were consumed, although too few subjects fell into this very high ethanol consumption group to "analyze statistically."[73]

The most startling evidence of all is found in a study published in 2010 in the journal *Rheumatology*. In this large study, non-drinkers had statistically over four times higher risk of acquiring rheumatoid arthritis as compared with subjects in the highest alcohol consumption category. The conclusion of the study was "our data suggests that alcohol consumption has an inverse and dose-related association with both risk and severity of rheumatoid arthritis."[642] As an aside, similar results also showed strong U-shaped curves of protection by ethanol consumption from Osteoporotic Fracture due to low bone density.[295]

How can we help but to be drawn directly to the ADH hiding in the synovial fibroblast of human joint tissue,[563] just waiting to convert dietary methanol into formaldehyde in the absence of ethanol? What better way to induce the cartilage and bone destruction which is mediated by synovial macrophages[563] doing their custodial duty of removing formaldehyde modified (damaged) protein? The evidence showing the direct involvement of activated macrophages in the development of full blown rheumatoid arthritis is far too overwhelming to ignore.[514] It is well known that no natural disease of animals mimics arthritis.[562] Interestingly, the only known procedure to produce experimental arthritis in laboratory animals is to inject in the vicinity of their joints a very dilute solution of formaldehyde at regular intervals, inducing macrophage invasion and a self-maintaining chronic granuloma resulting in a syndrome tellingly called "formalin-arthritis." [561]

Is Aspartame the Cause of the Epidemic of Autoimmunity over the "Last Thirty Years"?

The incidence of systemic lupus erythematosus (SLE) has tripled since the introduction of aspartame into the American diet.[536] The change started almost immediately after the introduction of the artificial sweetener into foods and increased along with its consumption rate. When we graph the lupus numbers provided by the Centers for Disease Control of both incidence (Figure 10.1) and death rate of the disease (Figure 10.2)[701] we see the same pattern we have seen with other of the methanol diseases. You now know what to look for in these charts. Please put some time into their perusal. You will not be disappointed. Remember also that lupus was cited as "possibly" having played a part in the outbreak of autoimmunity so ineptly investigated by the CDC in the little town of Wellington, Ohio.[578]

Rheumatoid arthritis is the slowest to develop of all the methanol diseases and because of this we will be waiting a long time for our data here. Even so, we do know that its incidence was declining dramatically in apparent conjunction with a decline in smoking incidence during the 30 year period from the early 1950s to the early 1980s. Investigators now believe, albeit with little hard evidence, that the "incidence and prevalence of rheumatoid arthritis in women appears to have increased during the period of time from 1995 to 2007" for reasons which are unknown, but which may be "environmental."[635]

Figure 10.1   Figure 10.2

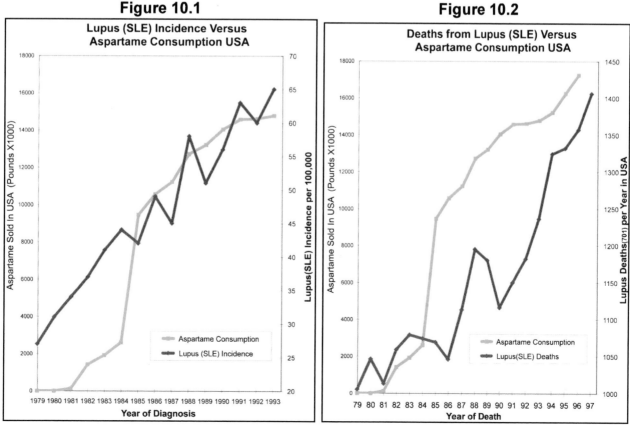

A Few Words about Diabetes

Two Very Different Diseases: Diabetes Type I and II

Diabetes I is a true autoimmune disease. It has been shown conclusively that it is caused by macrophages consuming an entire group of self tissue called beta cells that are normally located only in the pancreas. The pancreas is a complex organ composed of many types of cells that serve various functions. The beta cells are the sole tissue in the body capable of producing insulin. These cells are found only as a major constituent of little groups of gland-like cells dispersed throughout the pancreas. These cell groupings have the lovely name "islands of Langerhans." Under a microscope they do indeed look like isolated little "islands" dispersed throughout the pancreas. About a million such islands exist in the average pancreas.

Table I indicates the pancreas has sites of ADH I and is, therefore, a target organ for methanol poisoning. Interestingly enough, an unusually high concentration of ADH I is found within these same "islands of Langerhans."[637] This has little or no bearing on the development of juvenile onset diabetes type I, which is a disease most likely caused by immunity to a component of cow's milk found in all human infant formula;[715,714] however, it may prove to be pertinent to the origin of adult onset diabetes type II, in which the beta cells appear to be damaged or poisoned, but not destroyed completely as in diabetes type I.

Cigarette Smoke

It has recently been revealed that active cigarette smoking is associated with an increased risk of type II diabetes.[648] Of tremendous importance was the discovery of a "dose-response phenomenon" with diabetes type II increase found to be greater for heavy smokers, with almost a doubling of the rate of the disease for those who smoked over a pack of cigarettes a day.[648]

U-shaped Curve of Alcohol Consumption

Fully three independent studies have conclusively shown that a U-shaped association can be found between alcohol intake and diabetes type II. The risk of type II diabetes in one small study was 2.4-fold higher in nondrinkers than in those consuming moderate amounts of alcohol daily, while heavy drinkers assumed the same risk as nondrinkers.[283] The relationship between insulin resistance, considered a pre-diabetic symptom, and alcohol is "minimal in individuals with regular mild to moderate alcohol consumption and increases in both heavy drinkers and subjects without any alcohol consumption."[650] In 2004, a very large meta study of 15 original smaller studies comprising about twelve thousand cases of type II diabetes in a population of over three hundred and fifty thousand individuals showed a greater than 30% reduced risk of diabetes in moderate alcohol consumers, with no risk reduction in those who consumed over six alcoholic drinks a day.[289] Most startling and provocative of all was a report evaluating the long term symptomology of over three thousand patients with type I diabetes. The complications of long term type I diabetes are retinopathy (damage to the retina of the eye), neuropathy and vascular complications, all of which we have discussed as associated with methanol toxicity. This study showed that moderate alcohol consumption in these individuals protected against all of these complications by a protective factor of as much as three times compared to non-alcohol consumers in what the researchers concluded was a "U-shaped fashion."[297]

Diet Soda: the Incidence of Type II Diabetes among Adolescents in Greater Cincinnati Increased 1000% Just 12 Years after Aspartame

Recently, during a study of over six thousand individuals performed in six widely dispersed clinics in the United States, it was revealed that the consumption of at least one 12 ounce can of diet soda a day for four years was associated with a statistically significant sixty-seven percent increased risk of type II diabetes.[702]

The possible effect of increased type II diabetes as a result of consumption of diet products by our burgeoning population of obese children causes me great concern. I noticed early on that children and young people in general became true believers of the powerful, relentless marketing of aspartame. Television advertisements showing children pouring little blue packages of pure aspartame sweetener down their throats followed by big smile on their faces were a powerful call to childish mimicry and the eventual poisoning that ensued. It will take time to sort out the ultimate outcome of this mass illusion of safety, if indeed we can find anyone interested in its elucidation. I hope that the discussion of the potential link to diabetes will light a fire under some of you to dig deeper into the connection.

I will leave you with this one research article published in the prestigious *Journal of Pediatrics,* but lost on many who know nothing of the all important timing of the aspartame plague. The medical researchers discovered that in 1994, 33% of all the diagnoses of type II diabetes were among patients 10 to 19 years of age. After digging deeper they discovered that the incidence of **adolescent** type II diabetes in Greater Cincinnati increased over **1000%** from 1982 to 1995, going from 0.7/100,000 in 1982 to an unbelievable 7.2/100,000 in 1994.[649] Further, females were found to suffer about twice the incidence of males and were being diagnosed up to a full year earlier than their male counterparts.

Diabetics in Danger

Among the organizations that received millions of "marketing" dollars from the company who invented aspartame were the various diabetic associations and the American Dietetic Association (ADA) which counsels many diabetics. For over twenty years I was a registered dietitian and professional member of the ADA. The G.D. Searle company purchased full page ads in the journals of these organizations, sponsored gala events at their conventions and appear to have been given considerable status at administrative levels of their governing boards. The ADA had a toll free "aspartame hotline" installed at its Chicago main office that dieticians could call to be assured that aspartame was safe. This contributed to the fact that diabetics, as a group, consume considerably more aspartame per capita than the average American. Perhaps this is why recent studies have shown:

1. Diabetes doubles the risk of Alzheimer's.
   http://www.huffingtonpost.com/2011/09/19/diabetes-alzheimers-disease_n_970803.html
2. Diabetes and obesity are linked to autism (see Chapter 12 for more on this subject).
   http://www.webmd.com/baby/news/20110511/diabetes-hypertension-obesity-linked-to-autism
3. There is a link between diabetes and multiple sclerosis.
   http://www.medindia.net/news/view_news_main.asp?x=12360
4. Diabetics have a higher incidence of breast cancer.
   http://care.diabetesjournals.org/content/26/6/1752.full

Do you see what I see?

Chapter 10

Chapter 11
Cancers of Aspartame

Aspartame's proclivity to cause cancer in humans should be a surprise to no one. The unimpeachable biochemical pathway whereby its methanol transforms into formaldehyde at cancer prone ADH-containing tissue locations throughout the human body constitutes sufficient scientific basis for considerable concern. Animal feeding studies of aspartame show statistically significant, dose dependent increases of breast and kidney cancers in test animals even though these animals are known to be more resistant to the toxicity of methanol than humans. The Centers for Disease Control SEER program, which monitors the wellness of the US population, has published data showing an alarming increase in these and other important cancers that mirrors the popularity and consumption of aspartame over the last 30 years. The real question is, why hasn't this overwhelming commonality of logic and fact been sufficient evidence to remove aspartame from the marketplace?

Considerable evidence against the safety of aspartame comes directly from its regulatory file history, stored in the vaults of the US Food and Drug Administration. Aspartame's carcinogenity (ability to cause cancer) in laboratory animals is documented in studies done on the sweetener before its approval.[57] Cancerous brain tumors found in laboratory rats in a dose-dependent relationship to the content of aspartame in their diet were among the most compelling reasons it was consistently rejected for use in foods.[56] It took the hiring, by the G.D. Searle company that invented the sweetener, of a Washington insider, Donald Rumsfeld, as CEO in March of 1977 to force aspartame into the food supply.

The exquisite and pivotal laboratory work done by Professor Marie Alemany despite the strenuous, though unconvincing, objections of the opposition[40] is proof conclusive that aspartame and, therefore, methanol does turn into formaldehyde within the living organism. Dr. Alemany skillfully used radioactive tracing of the methanol component of aspartame and thus clearly and unequivocally demonstrated methanol's evolution into the formation of formaldehyde modified proteins and DNA.[7] How strange it seems now that anyone would ever doubt that formaldehyde is produced from methanol or be convinced to think otherwise! For his exquisite work, Dr. Alemany had his university funding revoked and, like so many other scientists that dared go against the corruption that abounds in the western bureaucracies, was made to endure indignities designed to discourage dissension.[222]

Laboratory animals that take our place in safety testing have catalase enzyme in sufficient quantity within their bodies to protect them from the lion's share of the carcinogenetic effect of methanol's formaldehyde. When an animal does show signs of cancer the ramifications for humans are ominous. Therefore, when it comes to making a fair determination of the carcinogenic potential of methanol or aspartame, we are dependent on careful epidemiological observation of exposure of human populations to either methanol or aspartame. Nothing is wrong with this approach; it brings us back to the roots of the health sciences where observation leads to the application of logic and, in more cases than modern practitioners of medicine would like to admit, to the development of methods to prevent disease.

For aspartame, we have excellent data of its consumption rate during the extremely important time its popularity was ramping up in the United States. The entire US population has been a study group, with no knowledge or forewarning of its participation in a ghastly experiment. Using this data may be the very best way that its cancer causing potential can be determined. Toxicologists could only dream of such a large blind research population, which normally would make the job of the epidemiologist quite simple. Unfortunately, many toxicologists owe their allegiances to various industrial and pharmaceutical groups who insist they waste their skills proving how safe new chemicals are rather than showing the havoc that they might cause. No worries; we will see for ourselves where the truth lies and make our own determinations by looking at the graphs of the aftermath of thirty years of aspartame consumption. We will put ourselves in the position of the ancient Aztec, Inuit or Judean intelligentsia whose insights guided their people away from foods that might do harm. The edge we have over the ancients is that our culture has uncovered knowledge of the chemistry of nature, and this can reinforce our observations with reasonable insights as to the molecular details that might lead to cancer production.

Formaldehyde's Cancer-Causing Prowess is Enhanced when it Comes from Methanol

What exactly is the link between cancer and aspartame's methanol component? Without a doubt, a poison such as methanol that produces formaldehyde within cancer-prone tissue throughout the human body will eventually cause cancer. On the very day this paragraph was begun, June 10, 2011, the government of the United States finally caught up with the rest of the world[451] and officially declared formaldehyde a "known human carcinogen."[11]

A full grown human can die from ingestion of just a "few drops" of formaldehyde with death from acute formaldehyde poisoning often taking only minutes.[448] Air contaminated with formaldehyde, even at very low concentrations, is now known to cause cancer in humans.[11] Again let me stress that formaldehyde is one of a handful of chemicals classed as a Group I carcinogen by the IARC, the International Agency for Research on Cancer, Lyon, France. No known safe level of formaldehyde exposure exists; it is in all amounts a dangerous carcinogen[11] and mutagen.[86]

Even so, were it not for one major obstacle, formaldehyde might reach the status of one of the most perfect and powerful of carcinogens. Its only weakness is that it is so highly reactive that its destructive power is usually used up before it can travel all the way to the nucleus of the cell, where cancers originate. Like an overanxious lover, it spills its energy long before it makes its mark, prematurely squandering itself prior to reaching the perfect site for its application. On the other hand, methanol as a source of formaldehyde acts as a partner to its carcinogenic potential, easing it into places much closer to where it can more successfully work its dark magic, potentially producing cancers in all the human sites of ADH activity, including the liver.

It only takes one cell succumbing perfectly to formaldehyde's attack to produce a full blown cancer. Other methanol diseases, such as multiple sclerosis, atherosclerosis and Alzheimer's, are all slowly developing diseases that require years of collective damage caused by countless formaldehyde interactions that eventually add up to a defect that manifests as a chronic disease. Not so with cancer. A single cell's bad encounter with a carcinogen can initiate cancer progression that is virtually unstoppable. The exact behavior of the cancer from then on depends on which type of cell is affected and how quickly it can multiply. In some cases, individuals have been exposed to known cancer-causing agents for years and never experienced cancer, but in others, after just one encounter with asbestos, plutonium or formaldehyde, a cellular change was induced, turning one cell into the seed of a fatal malignancy.

Does that mean that just one sip of diet coke could start a cancer? Regrettably, the answer is yes. Cancer, therefore, is a purely statistical phenomenon in a game of environmental roulette. We turn the wheel each time we take a sip of diet soda or a puff of cigarette smoke and the wheel does not stop spinning until all the resultant formaldehyde has found its final home. If science understood the exact details of what cancer "really" is, I would certainly spend time in its explanation. Here again, we have put our trust to find the cure for cancer into the hands of those who have the most to lose when a remedy is found. We know little more about the truth of cancer than we did when lone scholars worked long hours in underfunded university laboratories out of the reach of Big Pharma.

What we do know with certainty is that unwanted methylation[560] and inappropriate cross-linking of chromosomal tissue[449] play a major part in the production of cancers. Both these phenomena are the handywork of our Crazy Hawk.[596] Formaldehyde is actually just a reactive methyl group, a "methyl molecule" that is essentially a methylation machine. It is capable of the methylation of DNA as long as enzymes are available, as they are in the living cell, to finish the job.[564] Over 60 methylation defects of DNA from human cancer cells have been identified thus far.[567] This hyper-methylation of DNA causes the shutdown of the expression of genes involved in preventing the production of important proteins that have been coded into the methylated portion of DNA. These are the changes that also come into play during the evolution of Autism and other birth defects, which we will discuss in the next chapter.

As for cross-linking of DNA, few chemicals are more likely to form a bridge between a DNA molecule and protein or other DNA than formaldehyde hydrate. The indiscriminate attachment of formaldehyde to the chromosomes in the nucleus of a living cell has been shown time and time again to cause the inappropriate linking together (cross-linking) of these molecules in such a way as to induce cancer.[596, 633] This works much the same way as the linking together of the Tau proteins, resulting in Alzheimer's. In humans, the methanol placement of formaldehyde is the key to its ultimate perfection as a carcinogen. Methanol is a very small and nonreactive molecule. It can go anywhere in the body with no effort at all, as a Trojan horse delivering formaldehyde to where it can cause severe damage.

You should come away from this discussion with the knowledge that the ultimate cancer-causing agent in humans just might be a trinity of unfortunate circumstances allowing methanol to make contact with ADH, which converts it to formaldehyde. Show me a place where ADH can be found in the human body and I will more than likely be able to show you a cancer that has increased in incidence since that fateful day in 1981 when a new source of methanol was forced into the diet of the unsuspecting consumer.

Thousands of Carcinogens Exist

We have a number of new chemicals in our environment which, to my way of thinking, have not undergone proper screening for carcinogenity. This is the result of a lack of genuine governmental oversight and the extraordinarily unrestrained involvement of chemical and pharmaceutical interests into the bureaucratic decision-making process relative to the safety of chemical substances (along with the largely industrial leanings of the toxicological and epidemiological professions in general). It is still technically against the law of the United States to allow any chemicals known to cause cancers in man or animals to be an ingredient added to foods (pesticides have been exempted). Since we now know that aspartame turns into a cancer-causing agent, we need to look at what the effect of adding millions of pounds a year of that carcinogen to the food supply over the last thirty years has done to the cancer rates in the US. We will concentrate on those cancers that originate in the known centers of ADH I

Figure 11.1

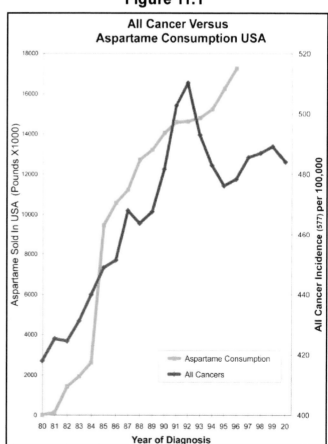

concentration in the human body where formaldehyde is the predictable outcome of aspartame consumption.

Cancer statistics for the United States are published by the Surveillance Research Program of the National Cancer Institute, which manages the Surveillance, Epidemiology, and End Results (SEER) Program. The SEER program is an authoritative source of information on cancer incidence in the United States. SEER collects and publishes these statistics from population-based registries covering 26% of the US population.[577] Looking first at an overview of the total cancer burden for the United States, I have plotted the CDC SEER data for incidence of "all cancer" occurrences in the United States for the period since the introduction of aspartame (Chart 1). This chart clearly shows the full impact of the sudden increase in aspartame consumption. But why does the cancer incidence appear to peak in 1993?

The Sensitive, Vulnerable, and Susceptible Will Be Lost First

To answer that question, I will need to relate a story. A few years back, upon landing in Christchurch on one of my many flights from the States to sanctuary in New Zealand, I was contacted by a good friend who asked if I wouldn't mind sitting for the filming of a TV interview that might never see the light of day. The interviewer, a Kiwi with a reputation as a hard-hitting investigative journalist, was said to have an interest in aspartame, but he didn't think he could talk his managers into what would be an outright challenge to the cola industry, a major source of advertizing dollars to his company. New Zealand media, once run by the government with no need to pander for its survival, had deteriorated quickly to the US model after deregulation. I accepted and we asked the airport hotel to let us use an unoccupied garden area as a temporary studio.

I will never forget one of his questions, obviously something that he had researched and which had been on his mind for some time. "Professor Monte, do you think that the unexplained increase in teen suicides in New Zealand has anything to do with allowing carbonated diet beverages into the tucker (school lunch) programs?" I explained that I did not realize that New Zealand had experienced a similar problem to ours in the US. My answer was in the affirmative, and followed the lines of logic that I used to explain the chart in Chapter 9 of the teen suicide experience in the US. He quickly countered with a question that I am sure he hoped would please his employers. "Well, how do you explain that the consumption of diet soda has been steady over the last few years and the teen suicide rate is now in decline?" Without hesitation, I countered with "It is obvious your advertiser has succeeded in killing off the most sensitive kids."

The show never aired, but I relate the incident to you because it points out a common outcome of toxicological experimentation done on large populations of test animals. The introduction of a poison into the diet of a colony of test animals is the very most important stage of the experiment. It is at some point after this that we expect to see the most susceptible individuals of the colony, never before stressed at these levels, killed off. I have done such experimentation myself and know what to expect. The horror of this, to me personally, is that the curve I would expect to see in a laboratory study of a deadly poison would be shaped very much like Chart 1, with a spiking of incidents followed by a slow down as the more resistant animals remain alive and in the study. The time it takes to achieve this peaking of the curve varies, depending on the characteristics of the poison administered. The most interesting indication of this phenomenon is the curve never drops all the way back down to the baseline (where it started before the experiment began) for as long as the poison is being administered to the colony. This indicates a definite cumulative effect on the population as a whole. The "depletion of the weaklings" is what we used to call it before we came to realize that in the case of aspartame each of these data points represented a person.

Brain Cancer: the Killing Begins

<u>Increasing Brain Tumor Rates: Is There a Link to Aspartame?</u>[329] is the title of an article published in

1996 by the American Association of Neuropathologists and written by the renowned research neuroscientist John W. Olney. John cites the results of the original aspartame animal studies I mention above "revealing an exceedingly high incidence of malignant brain tumors in aspartame-fed rats" and notes that "spontaneous brain tumors in laboratory rats are quite rare." He goes on to point to the relevancy of a Public Board of Inquiry that had been called together by the US Food and Drug Administration in 1980 to evaluate these studies, and had "included prominent neuroscientists Walle Nauta and Peter Lampert." This Board subsequently concluded that "aspartame may contribute to the development of brain tumors in the human population." They recommended that the Food and Drug Administration withhold approval of aspartame as a food additive. Within months of this decision, Donald Rumsfeld's team was in control of the White House, and within days aspartame was a "food."

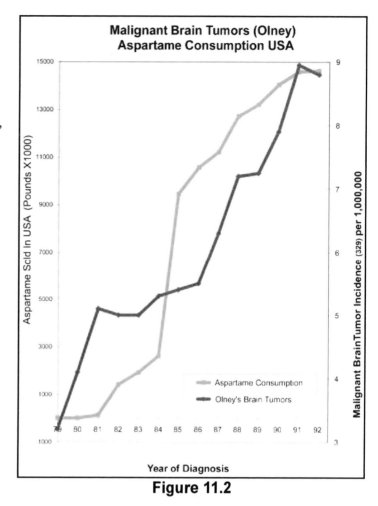

Figure 11.2

Nauta points out that a sharp upward trend in deaths from brain tumors was detected in the mid 1980s in countries that approved the use of the sweetener, including the United Kingdom, France, Germany and Italy. Nauta found during his study similar increases in brain cancers in the States, noting that "it was not a fleeting phenomenon. Rather, it was the initial phase of an upward swing in the brain tumor incidence which evolved into a sustained increase in both the per capita number and malignancy of brain tumors, a phenomenon that has endured for at least 8 years."

I have taken the liberty to chart the data from Figure 3 found on page 1119 of Dr. Olney's article on our standard graph of aspartame consumption (Chart 2). You can see from this chart that the brain cancer rate in the US population more than doubled after the introduction of aspartame. Olney goes on to warn that "Compared to other environmental factors, aspartame appears to be a promising candidate for explaining the surge in brain tumors in the mid-1980s." In his concluding sentence he pleads for a "reassessment of the carcinogenic potential of aspartame which is currently being ingested widely throughout many parts of the world."

John's fine article is a professional plea from a world renowned scientist and physician who is respected by not only his neurological peers, but by the scientific community in general. The plea is in the form of a scientific article that had been reviewed and published in the premier journal of a leading neurological association whose scope includes this exact type of research. Reading the article you will see the high standard that is used to evaluate the potential of aspartame to act as a human carcinogen. John asks three questions: 1) Does the agent have carcinogenic potential? (This is John's weakest argument since he cannot use the formaldehyde link); 2) Do experimental animals show an increased incidence of specific types of cancer when exposed to the agent?; and 3) Do humans show an increased incidence of the same types of cancer when exposed to the agent? John claims, rightly so, that "aspartame appears to meet all three criteria."

This man could not have done anything more. He is an expert in his field and he proceeded in the proper way, and yet absolutely nothing changed. He was ignored by the FDA and all the other such public organizations of the world that are charged to protect their respective populations from poisons. The argument used against John's premise was the so-called "ecological fallacy." The meaning of the fallacy goes something like this: "The temporal coincidence of two events observed at an ecological level without examination of individual data can lead to faulty conclusions regarding risk association." In other words, because two things happen at the same time, that doesn't mean they are related. This, of course, could be true in this case except for the ignored fact that John went beyond this and made a good case for the science behind the cause of the cancer and showed that the same cancer was demonstrated in laboratory animals. John did all this and his premise should have won the day. His argument should have swayed the FDA to immediate action against the use of aspartame in foods. He, in fact, went well beyond the standard used to remove Thalidomide from the marketplace.

Breast Cancer

Something quite remarkable happened during the aspartame feeding studies done by Dr. Morando Soffritti – something that prompted him to break with tradition, go beyond what John Olney had done and call publicly for an "urgent reevaluation" of the current guidelines for the use and consumption of aspartame. During a long term aspartame feeding study done by the industry-independent European Ramazzini Foundation headed by Dr. Soffritti it was shown conclusively that Sprague Dawley rats, which have the highest resistance to methanol toxicity of any laboratory animal, developed breast (mammary) and other cancers on a statistically significant and dose dependent basis when fed aspartame at low levels.[50] Morando reports the results eloquently in his own words: "Our study has shown that aspartame is a multipotential carcinogenic compound whose carcinogenic effects are also evident at a daily dose of 20 milligrams per kilogram of body weight (mg/kg), notably less than the current acceptable daily intake of aspartame for humans."[50] The horror that Morando witnessed happening to his test animals was a partial reflection of what the aspartame-consuming world has been going through for "the last thirty years."

The considerable evidence linking breast cancer to methanol is very convincing. There is good reason to believe that the epidemic of breast cancer over the last thirty years has more to do with the introduction of aspartame into the food supply than any other proposed cause. The production of breast cancer in laboratory animals fed aspartame, the increased rate of breast cancer in school teachers exposed to occupational methanol (see below), and the direct implication of high ADH tissue levels in those more prone to developing breast cancer over the course of their lifetimes goes a long way to prove methanol as an etiologic agent of breast cancer.

Why is the Human Breast Particularly Sensitive to Methanol?

Methanol travels easily to breast tissue and has been found in human milk.[219] The cells that produce milk within the breast, cells prone to develop the most common of breast cancers, adenocarcinoma,[358] contain high concentrations of ADH enzyme,[358] allowing methanol's conversion to formaldehyde. Mammary epithelial cells have no way to protect themselves from formaldehyde[216] – no means to render it harmless. They, unlike other breast tissue, contain no aldehyde dehydrogenase enzyme[216] (ADH III) that could transform formaldehyde into the non-carcinogenic formic acid.

Of particular interest are recent findings implicating ADH as playing a pivotal role in the formation of breast cancer, documenting a greater incidence of the disease in women with higher levels of ADH I activity in their breasts.[357] These articles go on to indict acetaldehyde as the potential culprit.[357] Remember acetaldehyde, as stressed in previous chapters, is essentially vinegar that results when ethanol is changed by ADH; it is a largely benign molecule with no link to cancer in humans. The role of acetaldehyde must be questioned when the same researchers report: "Very heavy drinking has <u>not</u> been associated with increased breast cancer risk relative to moderate drinking. We cannot explain why we have not observed an increase in risk from heavy lifetime consumption of alcohol."[501] What they are saying is that those who are constantly inebriated would have the cells in their breasts continuously producing acetaldehyde, thereby increasing the chances of breast cancer if acetaldehyde was indeed the culprit. This, of course, is not what actually occurs. Acetaldehyde is not the problem. Formaldehyde is the problem. The correct answer here is that the cause of breast cancer is not the ADH metabolite of ethanol, but rather the ADH metabolite of *methanol*. As you know it is ethanol in the blood that keeps the ADH busy and prevents it from producing formaldehyde from methanol.

School Teachers Have Higher Risk of Breast Cancers

In Chapter 9 we learned of the long term exposure of school teachers to methanol vapors from Ditto machines and the increase of autoimmunity that appears to be endemic in that group.[210] Statistically significant evidence, developed from several different sources during large cohort studies, shows that teachers in the United States and Canada also have been at much higher risk of developing and dying from breast cancer than professional women in any other occupation. In a comprehensive study done of school teachers in British Columbia from 1950 to 1984, long before aspartame was allowed into carbonated beverages, it was shown that school teachers had a 70% greater chance of dying from breast cancer than women in other occupations.[217] A study done at the Yale Cancer Center of breast cancer incidence in Connecticut women found only one occupational group of women with a statistically increased risk of breast cancer. That group – teachers – had twice the chance of developing breast cancer even after adjustment for other major breast cancer risk-factors.[241]

An article entitled <u>High breast cancer incidence rates among California teachers</u>,[213] published in 2002, found that "teachers have long been suspected to be at high risk of breast cancer." In a mortality study done between 1979-1981, the California Department of Health Services noted a substantial excess mortality from breast cancer in California teachers. A large cohort study of over 133,000 California female teachers showed these women were statistically more likely to develop invasive breast cancer, in-situ breast cancer, and localized invasive breast cancer than other female professionals with 51%, 67% and 65% respective greater risks.[213] The Yale study cited above points out that increased breast-cancer risk among teachers is "consistent with most earlier studies." It continues, "it is currently unknown, however, what factors may explain the observed increase," however, "considering teachers represent one of the largest single occupational groups among employed US women, further investigation of this association is warranted."[241]

Aspartame Causes Breast Cancer in Human Feeding Study Done by Searle

Remember from the introduction that in the summer of 1983 I spent time in a cramped conference room in Washington, DC that housed the docket file and application made by the G.D. Searle company to the US FDA to allow aspartame into carbonated beverages. A nameless FDA employee handed me one of the files he had been reading. Staring straight into my eyes he said in a whisper, "Did you see this?" I was taken aback, but before I could ask any questions he had disappeared, just as other such angels had into the endless corridors of that bleak federal building.

The study he handed me was damning evidence of the danger aspartame posed to the public. It was a long-term human study of diabetics who consumed 6 capsules daily containing a total of 1.8 grams of pure aspartame for 13 consecutive weeks.[48] This dosage of aspartame is tantamount to taking 200 milligrams of pure formaldehyde daily. This was the equivalent to the daily consumption of the amount of aspartame to be found in between three and 5 liters of diet cola. The subject base consisted of a total of 77 individuals, only 39 of which were aspartame consumers, while the others were controls. As a prerequisite to being accepted into the study, each participant had to pass a through physical examination that included considerable blood work. It was a double blind study, so neither the subjects nor the researchers had any idea who was taking the aspartame capsules or who was taking the placebo until the end of the experiment or until the subject was dropped from the study or died. Yes, one of the aspartame-consuming subjects died, while two others from the aspartame group developed cancer (one of these was breast cancer) during the study.[48]

Three subjects had to be dropped from the study before the 13 weeks ended. The culls had three things in common: they were female, they were dropped due to disease developed during the study, and they were all from the group that was consuming aspartame. None were dropped from the control group. The one death resulted from a stroke experienced after 8 weeks of aspartame consumption. The remaining two women survived 11 weeks on aspartame before developing epithelial cell cancers, one of the lining of her stomach, with hyperplasia reported in her lymph nodes during her pathology. The other woman's breast cancer resulted in a mastectomy and she was diagnosed with adenocarcinoma.[48] Both breast adenocarcinoma and hyperplasia had been found in laboratory rats fed aspartame during the testing of the product by Searle.[197]

This damning animal carcinoma information tragically was kept from the pathologist who reviewed the tissue samples from the two women who developed cancers during the study. In the final report of the results of the feeding study it states that the reason these human cancers were ignored was because there was no instance of carcinogenicity in animal feeding studies. To quote the report, the cancers were considered "coincidental … in view of information showing no evidence of such carcinogenesis in animals who received large amounts of Aspartame over a prolonged period.[48]"

The pathologist's report was sent directly to the G.D. Searle company. He refers to viewing slides of breast and stomach tissue from the long term rat studies done by Searle. It is obvious that the cancerous tissue slides were kept from him.[48] To my most profound horror, the executive summary of the human diabetic study concluded, "In summary, aspartame appears to be well tolerated by diabetic subjects as a safe sugar substitute." The rationale used to ignore the fact that fully 8% of the Aspartame consumption subjects, developed epithelial cancer during the study was that "no such cancers were seen in the numerous animal studies."[48] The Bressler Report, which resulted from an audit of all of Searle's aspartame experimentation by a group of FDA investigators, reports that this was a lie, and that breast cancer was indeed an outcome of the animal feeding studies. [197]

There are only 2 ways to get Formaldehyde into the Human Breast

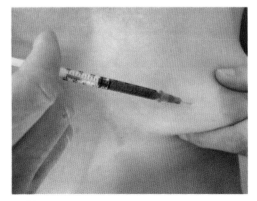

The cancers found in the diabetic women should never have been ignored. Such a high mortality and cancer rate in a human study should have raised red flags and prevented aspartame from being rushed into the market against the clear intent of the US food law, which prohibits cancer causing additives.

The Scene of the Crime

The only reliable way that formaldehyde can reach the mammary tissue, aside from purposely injecting formaldehyde solution into the breast,[122] is to administer the formaldehyde as methanol

Matching Epidemics of Breast Cancer and Multiple Sclerosis: the Legacy of Aspartame

I don't always remember to bring my reading glasses with me when I go to professional offices, but only once did I not regret the oversight. Since my only chore on this occasion was to pick up a good friend who had been deposing another attorney at the offices of that attorney I had no intention of spending much time in the waiting room. As fate would have it, the deposition was taking longer than expected and the receptionist said that I could make myself comfortable in the lounge. Without my spectacles I had to look through the pile of surprisingly up-to-date periodicals for something that might have lots of pictures – big pictures. I found a favorite, *Time Magazine*, that looked as if it would fill the bill and sat down to make myself as comfortable as I could in what was essentially enemy territory.

I quickly came to a two page fold-out map of the world, big enough to easily make out the countries. From the shading I was certain I was looking at a recent full color rendition of one of Dr. Kurtzke's Multiple Sclerosis disease distribution maps that can be found in the second of the slide shows in Chapter 9. It would be great news if *Time Magazine* was doing an article on the MS epidemic, I thought. I returned to the receptionist and told her my story and she not only found me a pair of magnifying glasses, but she also gave me the magazine. I was awestruck by what I could finally see clearly. Here was a feature article about the epidemic of breast cancer, not MS.[190] How could I have missed this epidemic? One look at the disease distribution throughout the World (Figure 11.3) and I knew I was looking at what would turn out to be the twin sister of MS. Breast cancer was a disease of well-to-do northern women, a disease of "affluence,"[250] that was now spreading quickly to their poorer sisters in the warmer climates – all coinciding with the timing of the popularity of aspartame. I shook with a strange mixture of rage and excitement as I vowed to learn all I could about this epidemic of breast cancer.

Figure 11.3

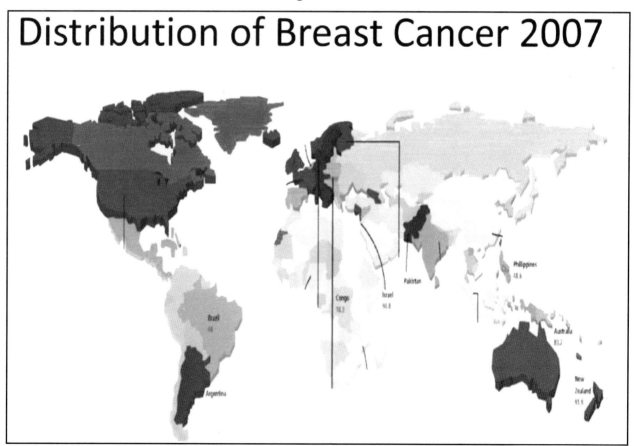

It turns out that breast cancer is no stranger to women suffering from multiple sclerosis. Those afflicted with MS have over a twenty percent greater chance than women in the general population of developing breast cancer. This increased risk is cannot be attributed to reduced parity or delayed first child birth, and is an increased risk that the authors of the study who found the association admit it is "consistent with previous observations and remains unexplained and warrants further attention."[658]

A quick look at Figure 11.3 will bring back memories of Chapter 9 on multiple sclerosis. The darker shades of grey in the map of Figure 11.3 indicate higher incidence of breast cancer. Note the abundance of countries that seem to have matching high or low incidence of both diseases, particularly in the most recent MS distribution chart. Take note particularly of Argentina and how that little country was so quick to become a nation committed to consuming aspartame.

Breast Cancer Increases as Does Popularity of Aspartame

Figure 11.4 illustrates the SEER numbers for the incidence of breast cancer in the United States during the ramp up of aspartame in the US diet.[577] The tight relationship of the two curves is indicative of a relatively short time period between methanol consumption and breast cancer development. However, it is important to note that methanol began increasing in the US diet with the growth in consumption of aseptic canned juice drinks some years before aspartame's official introduction. This was also a period with an increase in breast cancer screening, which may account for the meandering of the incidence curve between the years 1987 to 1994. Implementation of more accurate screening methods will only temporarily appear to increase incidence with a sudden rise for a period of time and then a snap back a few years later. A good example would be a haystack that contains only so many needles, and whether you count them by hand, which may take a long time, or use a magnet to gather them more quickly, the end results is always the same number of needles. This improved screening effect has been used to explain away the apparent incidence increase in breast cancer over "the last 30 years," but the truth is that it cannot fully account for the relentless rise in the cumulative breast cancer rate since the introduction of aspartame.

It can be shown that the incidence of breast cancer has increased over the last 30 years,[219] and particularly in populations exposed to aspartame.[194] The uneven distributions of both MS and breast cancer throughout the world show a disarming similarity,[193] including the unexplained increases to epidemic proportions in the same regions, such as Japan,[192] over that short period of time.[190] Chart 3 shows a disconcerting and abrupt rise in the incidence of breast cancer coinciding exactly with the ramp up of aspartame consumption after it was approved for sweetening carbonated beverages in the United States.[194] The breast cancer rate of the

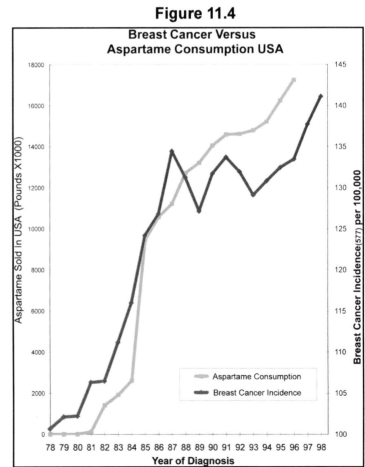

Figure 11.4

Breast Cancer Versus Aspartame Consumption USA

other countries throughout the world, even in countries with normally low breast cancer rates, also appears to have risen soon after aspartame was introduced into their diets.

Genetic Distribution of Slow ADH Verses Fast ADH Linked to Breast Cancer Risk

In Chapter 7 we discussed the discovery that three different genetically defined versions of ADH I exist. They vary based on the speed at which they metabolize ethanol. Our genetic makeup determines which one of these is distributed throughout our bodies. The fast-ADH is 2.5 times faster at removing ethanol from the bloodstream than the slow-ADH. When it comes to heart disease, individuals who are genetically endowed with the slow-ADH that metabolizes ethanol 2.5 fold slower than the fast-ADH have a 86% reduction in risk from developing myocardial infarction – but only if they consume ethanol on a daily basis.[483]

Interestingly, the role of ADH metabolism in the development of breast cancer mimics exactly its role in the development of heart disease. Women who are genetically endowed with the slow-ADH have less of a risk of contracting breast cancer during their lifetime than those that remove ethanol more quickly from their blood. This remains true even when both groups consumed the same amount of alcohol on a daily basis.[501] Fast metabolizers who drank 15-30 grams of alcohol a day had a 2.3 greater risk of breast cancer even than non-drinkers who were slower metabolizers.[501] The only explanation for the advantage to having an ADH that more slowly removes ethanol from the blood would be the ability of these individuals to maintain low levels of ethanol in the body fluids for longer periods of time, thus preventing the ADH in their breast tissue from converting methanol into the powerful carcinogen formaldehyde.

The U-shaped curve of ethanol's protective effect against breast cancer has not yet been elucidated, and the present mindset of the breast cancer community may never allow for such a study to be performed. Time will tell, but this information would be vital before we could make a recommendation as to safe levels of ethanol consumption. The literature clearly indicates that the beneficial effect of ethanol for women is limited to one standard alcoholic drink a day, and no more. One issue that must temper the enthusiasm of all of us who consider low dose ethanol beneficial is the results of one large study that claims to show an increase in breast cancer among women who drank.[279] Avoiding methanol consumption appears to be the best way to help prevent breast cancer (see Chapter 2).

Exposure to Organic Solvents and Breast Cancer

An article published in 1997 stresses that the incidence rates for breast cancer have increased steadily in both the US and Canada over "the last 25 years." The author points to the increasing number of women in the workforce and the possibility that the problem may be caused by occupational exposure to hazardous agents. No such increase was seen during the entire Second World War, when women, in mass, replaced their solider husbands in heavy industry. That aside, the author has some insight into the sensitivity of breast tissue to solvents such as methanol. He reminds us that solvent molecules quickly reach the breast epithelium cells, where they cannot be detoxified effectively because of the reduced activity of the "necessary enzymes" (aldehyde dehydrogenase) in breast cells. Second, because of the unique physiology of mammary glands, solvents or their "metabolites" accumulate in the milk ducts long enough to exert detrimental effects locally.[219]

Cigarette Smoking with a U-Shaped Twist

Women with a history of having smoked are more likely to develop breast cancer than those who never smoked.[574] It has been shown that a consistent dose-response enhances the plausibility of an increased breast cancer risk due to cigarette smoking.[191] Most intriguing of all is that women who start smoking as teenagers and continue to smoke for at least 20 years have a statistically significant (50% greater) chance of developing breast cancer compared with never smokers. This association, however, only applies if the women studied were nondrinkers of alcohol. Drinkers who smoke showed no significant increased in breast cancer incidence in the same study.[191] This appears to be an indication of the protective effect of ethanol against methanol's conversion to formaldehyde.

Cancer of the Kidney (Renal Cancers)

Kidney: a Target Organ of Methanol Poisoning

Early pathology of humans who die from methanol poisoning consistently shows considerable gross anatomical and histological damage to the kidneys and the lungs.[416] These organs both have extra hepatic stores of ADH I. The adult kidney contains ADH in measurable quantities.[640] The exact location of these ADH rich tissues coincides with the epithelial tissue of the kidney, which remarkably is where the cancers in question originate.[636]

Cigarette smoking has been the target of 24 investigations looking into its contribution directly as a cause of renal cell carcinoma. A Meta-analysis of all 24 of these studies published in 2005 shows a strong dose-dependent increase in risk associated with the numbers of cigarettes smoked per day and a substantial reduction in risk for long-term former smokers. For those who smoked over one pack of cigarettes a day the risk of developing renal cancer was about twice that of non smokers.[652]

Spontaneous carcinomas of the kidney are extremely rare in laboratory rats. During the Ramazzini Institute study described above, male and female rats that had been fed aspartame developed statistically significant and dose related increases in kidney cancers. Twenty one carcinomas of the renal pelvis developed in their study whereas the control rats had none.[50] The generation of cancers of the kidney, liver and lungs by aspartame was intrusive and unexplainable except by the unpopular formaldehyde theory. The results for all three cancers were not only highly significant but strongly dose related, showing that stronger doses were having a greater cancer-causing impact.[50] The real tragedy here is that similar cancers were generated in test animals by the company that invented aspartame 30 years before the Ramazzini study. The data was kept out of sight of the FDA until the Bressler investigation,[197] which came too late and fell on deaf ears.[39] This becomes remarkably important immediately upon the visualization of the human experience with identical cancers exploding in the US population in the years since aspartame

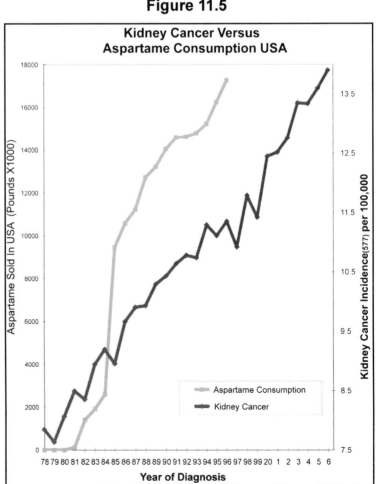

Figure 11.5

entered the food supply. Kidney cancer incidence rates, for instance, have inexplicably doubled "in the last thirty years."[646]

I have plotted the Centers for Disease Control SEER data for the US in the customary format in Figure 11.5. A *Journal of the American Medical Association* article entitled <u>Rising Incidence of Renal Cell Cancer in the United States</u>, published just months ago, unsuccessfully attempts to link the soaring rate of these adenocarcinomas (remember this term) to increased detection techniques. Its authors admit in their conclusion that increased detection alone "does not fully explain the upward incidence trends of renal cell carcinoma. Other factors must be contributing to the rapid increasing incidence of renal cell cancer in the United States, particularly among blacks."[646]

Kidney Damage beyond Cancer

The constant production of formaldehyde from methanol within the epithelial cells of the kidney as a result of consuming diet soda may be responsible for other damage beyond cancer. Aspartame has been shown to damage the kidneys of fetal rat pups whose mothers were fed it during pregnancy.[659] We can learn something from the autopsies and histological workups done to those who have died from acute methanol poisoning. The tubules of the kidneys of these individuals often reveal extensive degeneration.[416] Formaldehyde is a fierce deactivation agent for a number of enzymes, and even the mitochondria, which plays such an important role in kidney function, is itself extremely vulnerable to formaldehyde's presence.[582] It has been convincingly shown that heavy cigarette smoking more than doubles the risk of Chronic Renal Failure.[651] A recent study done at Harvard Medical School looking into the possible association between consumption of sweetened beverages with kidney function decline showed no such relationship, but the collected data inadvertently resulted in the conclusion of the report that more than two servings of diet soda a day is responsible for a statistically valid two fold increased risk for kidney function decline.[588] One liter of diet beverage, sweetened with aspartame, contains the same amount of methanol to be found in the average pack of unfiltered cigarettes.

Melanoma and Cancers of the Skin

"The Incidence of Skin Cancer Is Increasing at an Alarming Rate"

"The incidence of skin cancer has reached epidemic proportions. Only through heroic efforts by health care professionals and the general public to prevent the development of progression of skin cancer will this epidemic be abated."[718]

This quote from <u>The Epidemiology of Skin Cancer</u>, an article published in the *Journal of Dermatological Surgery*[718] in March of 1996, indicates that this increase in skin cancers had been going on for the previous 25 years. What makes this particularly confounding to dermatologists is that although nonmelanoma skin cancer is directly related to cigarette smoking,[645] the nonmelanoma skin cancer incidence has climbed steadily since the end of the of the late 1970s[95] during the same period of time in which cigarette smoking has steadily declined. The explanation tying this cancer increase to the thinning of the ozone layer can apply well only to sparsely populated segments of the Earth that lie close to the world's polar extremes. For all other areas the ozone layers have healed with no timely response from the skin cancer curves.

Skin Fibroblasts Are an ADH I Stronghold

Dr. Nelson Novick, whose patient developed macrophage-filled deep skin lesions (granulomatous panniculitis) over her lower body after consuming aspartame proved that it was indeed aspartame consumption that caused that serious skin reaction.[228] The skin contain numerous fibroblasts that contain ADH I.[221] This ADH will convert methanol to formaldehyde as easily as the ADH found in the other tissues we have discussed.[638] The reaction that Dr. Novick's patient had was an inflammatory response to something produced in her skin from the aspartame that caused the attraction and eventual activation of her body's macrophages.[555] We know that macrophages respond in such a way to formaldehyde modified protein.[25] The truth is that it would be very difficult to propose an alternative to the formaldehyde mechanism for such a skin reaction to occur from the consumption of aspartame, a substance made up only of two amino acids and methanol. Fibroblasts, when activated, are associated with cancer cells at all stages of cancer progression.[656] Their functional contributions to cancer production may emerge to have more to do with this unappreciated production of formaldehyde from environmental methanol than anything else. In the mean time, what better mechanism to increase the incidence of skin cancer than the production of formaldehyde directly within the skin?

Formaldehyde from Aspartame

The confirmation of aspartame's formaldehyde in human skin is important to our present discussion on aspartame skin issues.[7] Though methanol has been known for almost a hundred years to cause several forms of dermatitis,[227] the descriptions of which vary widely.[437] Individuals who are extremely sensitive to formaldehyde can develop contact dermatitis reactions to a minute amount of it, such as that found in newsprint.[438] Dermatologist have used this "exquisite sensitivity" of the human immune system to formaldehyde to show compellingly the connection of aspartame consumption to formaldehyde formation within skin tissue.

Two professors of Dermatology from the University of Kansas Medical Center, in a case report titled <u>Systemic Contact Dermatitis of the Eyelids Caused by Formaldehyde Derived from Aspartame,</u> published in the journal *Contact Dermatitis,* were the first to report eyelid dermatitis caused by aspartame consumption in one of their formaldehyde sensitive patients.[545] Since then, "severe systematized dermatitis" has been confirmed to be linked directly to aspartame consumption in patients who have tested positively for formaldehyde sensitivity.[630] It is interesting to note that positive reactions to formaldehyde on patch testing have now repeatedly been linked to both "systemic contact dermatitis" and a new syndrome called "aspartame-induced migraines," often presenting in the same patients.[328] In the most recent article confirming the positive link between formaldehyde sensitivity, systemic dermatitis and migraines[544] you may find the published rebuttal letter from the manufacturer of aspartame, Ajinomoto, both enlightening and entertaining.[543]

Young Women Take the Burden of the Epidemics of Two Skin Cancers

Dermatologists from the Mayo Clinic reported

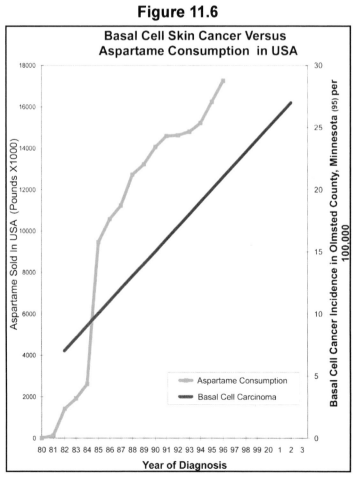

Figure 11.6

in the *Journal of the American Medical Association* (JAMA) in August of 2009[95] that they had been keeping track of the incidence of Basal Cell Carcinoma in their home county of Olmsted in Minnesota since 1976. They documented and histologically confirmed that since exactly 1980 the incidence of that non-melanoma cancer steadily increased by 400% (see Figure 11.6). This county, in which Rochester is a major city, is halfway between the North Pole and the Equator – far from any ozone hole and in an area with average daily sunshine saturation.

The most sobering aspect of the research reported in JAMA is that women younger than 40 years were at a significantly greater risk than their male counterparts. The exact quote is "This incidence of skin cancer is significantly higher for women than for men. A trend toward higher incidence of basal cell carcinoma in young women than in men has been reported by others."[95]

By far the most deadly form of skin cancer is melanoma, the origins of which are controversial. In fact, it appears to be much less related to UV light exposure than traditionally thought, and in fact is often found in areas of the body where scant exposure to the sun's rays would be expected. The year before the JAMA article was published another much more ambitious study performed by investigators from the National Cancer Institute's (NCI) Division of Cancer Epidemiology and Genetics studied the incidence patterns of invasive cutaneous melanoma throughout the United States. Figure 11.7 shows the change in incidence of melanoma for the population as a whole in the years since the introduction of aspartame. The study done by the NCI and published in the *Journal of Investigative Dermatology* broke down the original data to look for trends based on age and sex. I will let the National Cancer Institute's results speak for themselves. "Invasive cutaneous melanoma, the deadliest form of skin cancer, increased among Caucasian women in the United States aged 15 to 39 by 50 percent between 1980 and 2004." Further, they conclude, "Our analysis of SEER data suggests that melanoma incidence is increasing among young women."[557]

The outcome again goes to our premise that methanol in food will always have a more devastating effect on women due to their reduced ability to detoxify methanol in their guts. This is compounded considerably by the poorly kept secret that young women are the prime target of multimillion dollar diet soda advertisement campaigns, which we can presume have been very successful.

It is a hot summer day on a lovely Mexican Pacific coast beach. A beautiful young person is lying on the white sand renewing her tan before she hits the surf just one more time before lunch. She reaches into the cooler and pulls out an

Figure 11.7

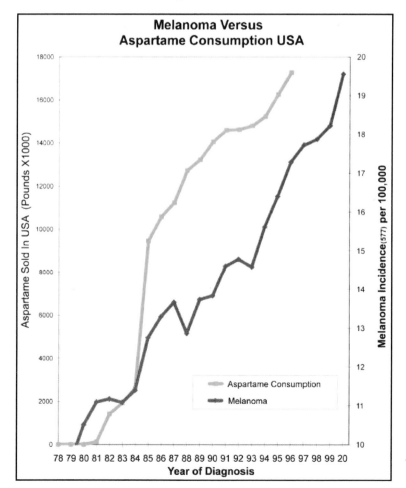

ice cold diet cola to quench her thirst. The soundtrack now switches to the unforgettable theme from Jaws. The aspartame in the carbonated beverage starts to turn to methanol before she can empty the bottle. By the time she hits the beach again after lunch, the methanol is already turning into formaldehyde in the fibroblasts of her skin. Fibroblasts are known to have a pivotal, yet little understood role in cancer formation. Her skin is already under attack from the very short UV radiation from the equatorial sun. Does this sound to you like the makings of a perfect surfer movie or a perfect storm?

Cancers of the Liver and Lungs

The Liver: The Ultimate Source of ADH

Alcohol Dehydrogenase Class I (ADH I) is also called Human Liver Alcohol Dehydrogenase because it was originally discovered in – and is still mistakenly thought by many to only be found in – the liver. In fact the highest concentration of ADH I in the body *is* in the liver[221] and this is what may account for the considerable carcinogenic stress on that organ from aspartame consumption. During the aspartame feeding studies of Swiss mice by the Ramazzini group, results showed a significant dose-related increase in both liver carcinomas and adenomas.[657]

We have said many times that the liver contains large quantities of protective enzymes such as aldehyde dehydrogenase that help protect it from formaldehyde. However, since cancer is a statistical disease that only requires one molecule of formaldehyde in the wrong place at the wrong time, it is probably the number of molecules of formaldehyde produced in the liver that will eventually work against a heavy aspartame consumer. When we look at the tripling of the incidence rate of human liver cancers in the US during the aspartame years (see Figure 11.8), nothing more needs to be said.

What about the Lungs?

One cannot come away from the study of methanol without having some very serious concern about the lungs. All the autopsies in the older literature of humans killed by methanol ingestion always point to oddly congested or hemorrhaging lung tissue. Often lungs at autopsy show marginal emphysema with petechial hemorrhages.[416] Again we have a significant dose-related increase of alveolar/bronchiolar lung cancers in the aspartame feeding studies done by Dr. Soffritti. Why? Lung tissue contains fibroblast tissue[221] with a heavy burden of ADH that is ready and able to turn methanol into formaldehyde.[503] During our experiments with pregnant rats fed methanol, we often autopsied pups with lung damage, as can be seen in the slide

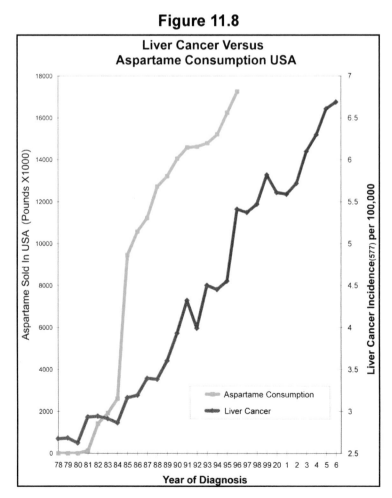

Figure 11.8

Liver Cancer Versus
Aspartame Consumption USA

Aspartame Sold In USA (Pounds X1000)

Liver Cancer Incidence(577) per 100,000

Aspartame Consumption
Liver Cancer

Year of Diagnosis

78 79 80 81 82 83 84 85 86 87 88 89 90 91 92 93 94 95 96 97 98 99 20 1 2 3 4 5 6

show from Chapter 12 (see www.whilesciencesleeps.com, Chapter 12 slideshow, "Birth Defects Caused by Aspartame").

Cigarette smoking has a direct and undeniable correlation and dose relationship to lung cancer. Most scientists would find it difficult to associate lung cancer or Chronic Obstructive Pulmonary Disease (COPD) with a food product. In the last thirty years, however, a considerable decrease in smoking in the United States has not been paralleled by a degree of decrease in lung cancer as was expected. Instead, the incidence of fibroblast centered lung adenocarcinoma has increased. The incidence of COPD has more than doubled, and in the last ten years the mortality from COPD has gone up over 20%.[641] Could this all be related to the methanol from aspartame? I just don't know; however, I can say with certainty that a lung bombarded daily by methanol-placed formaldehyde should be under suspicion for such developments. There would be good reason for serious consideration of methanol's role in these disorders.

The Strange Case of the Female Thyroid Gland

During the Bressler investigation of the hidden aspartame toxicity files, one of the tumors that were recovered from those "lost" from Searle's animal study of aspartame's safety was of the thyroid gland of one of the experimental animals.[197] Since that time a methanol vapor exposure study of Sprague Dawley rats of both sexes noted in particular that "The thyroid gland in females appeared to be a target organ for methanol."[593]

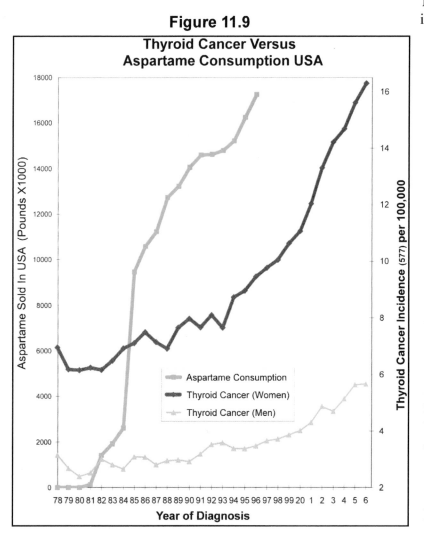

Figure 11.9

This all would have been of little import had it not been for a Swedish study that identified, in particular, school teachers who were in the workforce between 1971 and 1989 as having a significantly increased incidence of cancer of the thyroid.[405] The California teachers study that we used to point out the considerable increase risk of breast cancers gives the teachers they studied a 16 % greater chance of developing thyroid cancer.

We cannot do much more with this limited data. I was able to procure from the CDC SEER data thyroid incidence data that separated out the sexes. When graphed in the usual fashion, the data produced Figure 11.9, which does indeed seem to indicate that the thyroid gland may indeed be an organ sensitive to methanol that has been overlooked by those who have searched for sites of ADH activity.

Limitation of Animal Studies

I have mentioned a number of times

now that animals are not an acceptable venue for testing methanol safety. Only humans will suffice for testing methanol. We have been very fortunate to have good scientists, such as Morando Soffritti and his dedicated staff at the Ramazzini Institute in Italy, who are willing to spend the extraordinary time, effort and money to do long term animal studies. We must make the most out of it. To do that we have to understand the limitations of the species with which they are working. Rats and mice are not only between one and two hundred times less sensitive to the acute lethal effect of methanol, but also are blessed with a powerful enzyme, catalase, that protects them in ways that we don't understand from its many toxic and disease outcomes. To use the results of their testing we must take seriously any disease outcome that their experimental animals exhibit in excess of the controls and allow the experimenters to use, at the very minimum, a hundred fold greater dosage concentration of methanol than the equivalent dose to extrapolate to humans. Even at this level, some human diseases or cancers will never become apparent in these poor surrogates, no matter how long the study.

The only appropriate test animal for methanol's toxicity is the human. The innocents who have suffered and died to unknowingly test the safety of aspartame and, thus, methanol must not be allowed to have given their lives in vain.

Chapter 12
Autism and other Birth Defects

This is the last chapter. It comes now, not because it is the least important chapter – indeed it is probably the most important – but because the biology and chemistry from earlier sections are needed to understand the nature of what is really going on and why.

Methanol is required to be labeled as a poison with a skull and cross bones warning of extreme danger. Those of us who purchase it for our laboratories are cautioned, "fetal tissue will not tolerate methanol" and it will "probably cause birth defects."[93] Why then would the US Food and Drug Administration, or any other governmental agency, condone the purposeful addition of methanol into a food likely to be consumed by pregnant and lactating women? What would be the outcome of such a bad decision? How many would suffer? I report here what 30 years of experience has taught us about the folly of exposing unborn children, our most precious natural resource, to a poison whose true nature is yet to be completely understood. It is my most sincere hope that you can learn enough to become an irrefutable champion of the strong message this chapter teaches.

Methanol released from aspartame in diet soda passes through the placenta and into a pregnant woman's developing child as easily as water. Methanol saturates the brain of the fetus within an hour of consumption by the mother.[103] The human placenta, which protects the child from so many other poisons, has no alcohol dehydrogenase (ADH) and because its human catalase enzyme is unable to metabolize methanol it has no means by which to defend the fetus from transplacental methanol exposure.[503] Unfortunately, the developing human fetus does contain ADH and, therefore, has the means by which to convert methanol from the mother's diet into formaldehyde. Tragic proof of this is found in an incident in which a full-term infant suffered the classic methanol symptoms and subsequently died after having been delivered by Caesarian section from her mother, who was herself dying from accidental methanol poisoning.[267]

Previous chapters have taught you that the major target organ of methanol poisoning is the brain. All deaths caused by the acute administration of this poison result from the ultimate destruction of the central nervous system. The damage done to the brain by methanol poisoning has been likened to an intracranial catastrophe, the neurological details of which are still a mystery.[21] No wonder, then, that in the thirty years since aspartame was condoned as a food additive, all of the birth defects that have increased dramatically have had their greatest impact on the mind, the mood, and the memory of our children.

The developing fetal brain has been shown repeatedly in laboratory animals to be subject to damage from both methanol and aspartame. These injuries range from the grossly obvious neural tube birth defects[677] to a much more subtle but significant inability to interact normally with the environment,[492] with a general cognitive slowness[92] that might be as close as animal pups can bring us to autism.

Increase in Birth Defects in the U.S. as Aspartame Consumption Rises

A steady, yet unexplained increase in the incidence of three birth defects has been observed in the United States since the year aspartame became part of the American diet. Each of these diseases has its own reason for not having been immediately linked directly to its cause – the increase of methanol in the human diet. This now appears, in retrospect, to have been something that a small group of FDA and G. D. Searle insiders could have both foreseen and prevented. We will never recover from this; we can never reverse the great evil that was done, but we can and we must see to it that this will stop now and never happen again.

The increase in neural tube birth defects has been hidden from the press and the general public until this writing. A large number of prematurely terminated fetuses with neural tube defects were – and still are – disposed of without their numbers being tallied or included in any statistical tracking data related to the frequency of neural tube defects. As a result, the actual statistics have been obfuscated. Evidence of the existence of this "lapse" can only be gleaned by carefully reviewing insinuations scattered throughout the obscure literature of a neglected arm of the US Centers for Disease Control.

This deceit was compounded by the complacency of the US Food and Drug Administration personnel, who kept secret internal memos and corporate research data from as early as 1974 that would have revealed the discovery of multiple neural tube defects in the infants of animals fed aspartame.[677] The reality of an increase in this birth defect in the US population was to be hidden from public view and overlooked for years due to a peculiarity in basic data collection protocol by the Centers for Disease Control. This peculiarity still has not been corrected and thus keeps the statistical count of children succumbing to neural tube defects artificially and unrealistically low.[721]

Other birth defects were also to undergo large percentage increases since 1981, the year aspartame was approved for use in diet sodas.[525] Arguably the most tragic of all of these was the sudden explosion of the once rare organic personality defect first described in 1943[735] as autism. Autism was to see a twenty-fold increase from a rate which had remained remarkably unchanged for 40 years prior to aspartame's introduction into the diet of pregnant women. Fetal alcohol syndrome (FAS), a rare disorder, more than trebled (3.7 times) in frequency during this same time period.[356] We will discuss each of these birth defects and put their unprecedented increase into perspective relative to the increase in popularity of the methanol-containing aspartame.

Birth Defects Caused by Aspartame's Methanol

Neural Tube Birth Defects

Neural tube is often a grotesquely disfiguring malformation of the infant that encompasses a spectrum of disorders ranging from cleft palate, through spina bifida, to the always fatal presentations of horrifically deformed skulls with exposed or missing brains.[721] The proper medical term for the chemical transformation of the miracle of birth into an event of unforgettable horror for both mother and child is *teratogenesis* from the Greek, literally meaning *monster making*. Though this discourse concerns their origin and development, it is not my intention to belittle these unfortunate children; the fact is, the monsters of this chapter are those responsible for causing this plague of birth defects and those who harbor or protect them and keep their secrets.

I began writing Chapter 12 on the day of an encounter that broke my heart. It was a rare sunny afternoon on the Oregon coast with big white clouds and bright blue skies. Stopping for a traffic light I glanced to my right and caught sight of a very small person in a wheel chair holding a sign. His age was hard to guess; he was probably in his late twenties. Behind him was his adoring companion pushing his chair with practiced skill. The sign asked for help in a pleasant, neat hand, but one sees so much of this, the authenticity is always in question. I steeled myself to look straight ahead and pass, but something about the love in the expression of his companion, probably his mother, made me turn back to look again for a reassessment just after the light changed. The young man was clutching that beggar's sign tightly with both hands and close, as if to hide the shame of his need. The effect was to conceal his countenance – except for his unforgettably sad eyes. As my quick rear view glance caught his visage, the movement of the wheelchair over the curb brought the sign down enough to see that this poor soul was the survivor of a serious neural tube birth defect. Tears welled in my eyes and my soul drained from my chest. I couldn't breathe and a feeling of abject grief and helplessness came over me that I had only experienced at the death of someone I loved. I knew that nothing in my power to give could make those two ruined lives in any way whole. But in a sudden epiphany, I finally understood fully why the women in my laboratory would instinctively cry when yet another methanol rat pup was born a "monster." The ultimate horror of it all was the realization that the burden now was on me to finally put an end to something that I had been trying to stop since before the birth of this little man who now was long past being helped by anything that I am able to do.

Hidden Memo Revealed

In an article published in 1985 warning about potential health dangers posed by the methanol from aspartame,[1] I stated that the scientific literature contained no studies addressing the critical question as to whether aspartame or methanol would cause birth defects. I was incorrect in saying that, but only because I was purposefully prevented from seeing a key FDA memo dated September 11, 1978 describing the details of birth defects and serious developmental brain damage found in the offspring of laboratory rabbits whose mothers had been feed aspartame during pregnancy. This memo and the research data it describes were kept secret for over thirty years until January of 2011, when the memo was finally released as the result of a Freedom of Information request.

In that detailed US Food and Drug Administration memo, which was authored by Dr. Thomas Collins of the Animal Toxicology Branch to the Chief of the Food Additive Evaluation Branch, Collins reports the disturbing discovery of "significant" multiple neural tube (and other) birth defects in rabbit pups whose mothers were fed aspartame during the course of several different toxicity studies done by both G.D. Searle and Hazelton Laboratories between 1974 and 1975. It appeared to be Dr. Collins' assignment to evaluate the studies and his conclusions were stunning: "In both rabbit studies, aspartame appeared to cause birth defects."[677]

To my knowledge, this book is the first time this memo has been discussed publicly. Like most of the scientific community, I had no idea that aspartame had tested positive for producing neural tube birth defects. It was not until January 16, 2011 that this

Figure 12.1

ROUTING AND TRANSMITTAL SLIP — Date 7/22/83

TO: (Name, office symbol, room number, building, Agency/Post)

1.
2. *Ant—*
3.
4.
5.

Action	File	Note and Return
Approval	For Clearance	For Conversation
As Requested	For Correction	Prepare Reply
Circulate	For Your Information	See Me
Comment	Investigate	Signature
Coordination	Justify	

REMARKS

Dr. Woodrow Monte of Arizona State has an appointment to see this plus. 9:30 August 2nd

memos have been removed

DO NOT use this form as a RECORD of approvals, concurrences, disposals, clearances, and similar actions

FROM: (Name, org. symbol, Agency/Post)

A. P. Brunetti

Room No.—Bldg.

Phone No.

5041-102

☆ GPO : 1982 O – 381-529 (223)

OPTIONAL FORM 41 (Rev. 7–76)
Prescribed by GSA
FPMR (41 CFR) 101–11.206

"smoking gun" memo came into my possession. This is one of many important memos that were removed from the aspartame Docket File before I was allowed to review it in 1983. Figure 12.1 is an image of the ticket that gave me access to the FDA's "complete" collection of aspartame test data and it does confirm that memos had been removed.

Importance of the Collins Memo: Government Collusion Uncovered

Of the several million chemicals, pesticides and herbicides now in use only an exceedingly small percentage have ever tested positive for causing birth defects. Barely 800 chemicals are known teratogens, producing birth defects in laboratory animals, and "only about twenty of these are known to cause birth defects in the human."[466] Nature has numerous methods, the exact details of which are still unknown to us, for protecting the developing infant. As a last resort she will often call upon the macrophages to destroy a fetus that becomes unfit for life well before the time of birth, in a process called resorption. This is why the occurrence of a deformed fetus in the testing of any chemical is a rare phenomenon and would normally raise a "red flag" to any scientist concerned with public safety. It would be particularly significant if that chemical was being tested for use as a food additive.

It was not until 20 years after the 1978 FDA memo that methanol was first tested again and found to cause neural tube birth defects in rats[626] and eventually in many other species of laboratory animal.[104] To this day aspartame is not listed as a teratogen because the FDA and G.D. Searle covered up the tests that were performed in 1974 and 1975. Worse yet, during the time they were in possession of this proof of aspartame's teratogenicity, Searle paid to have a faux scientific paper written by one of their employees published in an international fertility journal (which is read by many gynecologists and pediatricians) stressing the safety of aspartame and falsely proclaiming that "aspartame posed no risk" from consumption during pregnancy.[100]

U. S. Environmental Protection Agency Admits Methanol Is a Probable Cause of Birth Defects

Although it was many years before the details could be determined with any certainty, it did not take a great deal of time for exposure to aspartame to adversely affect the rate of birth defects in the United States and its trading partner, the United Kingdom.[738] The reason for this is clear now that the Center for the Evaluation of Risks to Human Reproduction of the U.S. National Institutes of Health has determined methanol to be a potential developmental toxicant (teratogen) in humans. In an extensive multi-year review of the toxicity of methanol, finished in 2009, the Center reported numerous birth defects in animals exposed to methanol during pregnancy.[627] Stated continuously throughout their 500 page report is the mantra that "humans are much more sensitive to methanol toxicity than laboratory animals."

> "... The inhalation of methanol by pregnant rodents throughout the period of embryogenesis induces a wide range of concentration-dependent teratogenicity and embryolethal effects. Treatment-related malformations, primarily extra or rudimentary cervical ribs and urinary or cardiovascular defects, were found in fetuses of rats ... Increased incidences of exencephaly and cleft palate (neural tube birth defects) were found in the offspring of ... mice ... There was increased embryo/fetal death ... and an increasing incidence of resorptions. Reduced fetal weight was observed ... Fetal malformations ... included neural and ocular defects, cleft palate, hydrocephalus and limb anomalies."[685]

Tragically, the US Food and Drug Administration (FDA) kept the Collins memo secret from the Center for the Evaluation of Risks to Human Reproduction (CERHR) throughout its entire two-year investigation of methanol's potential to cause birth defects. This was done despite the fact that both the FDA and the CERHR are part of the same public agency – the Department of Health and Human Services. The final CERHR report published in September of 2009 mentions aspartame no fewer than 93 times and raises many questions about its potential for teratogenicity. These questions could have been answered by giving the committee access to the Collins memo and other studies to which the Collins memo refers that are still hidden in the vaults of the FDA.[627] It is noteworthy that two of the 11 voting members of the expert panel, both representing the US Environmental Protection Agency, refused to sign off on the summary of the CERHR methanol report and, in fact, initiated a formal dissent that warned of "a greater risk to vulnerable populations of pregnant women" than the compromised final report of the CERHR expert panel alleged.[551] The most senior of the dissenting scientists, J. Michael Davis, Ph.D. reveals in his strongly worded five page formal dissent[551] that "factual errors and omissions" prompted him not to sign the final report. He goes on:

> *"As just one example, the missing pages from the 1986 NEDO (New Energy Development Organization) report, which I identified and provided to the CERHR contractor, were evidently never provided to members of the Panel. The pages in question included a table showing reductions in brain weight in a two-generation rat study that had been replicated in a special ancillary study... If nothing else, omission of this information creates the impression that the Panel failed to consider all relevant information."* (I must point out here that autistic children often present with a reduced brain size at birth.[739])

The other courageous dissenter, Dr. Stanley Barone, a research biologist from the Neurotoxicology Division of the US EPA, explains that "the panel could not agree about the significance of the outcomes of the primate study of Burbacher et. al.[92]" He goes on:

> *"Again, I reiterate that I do not think that the process that the panel went through for the evaluation of methanol adequately addressed susceptible populations concerns. ...e.g., pregnant women with genetic polymorphisms that limit detoxification capacity of methanol."*[551]

These strong statements from the two most qualified environmental scientist members of the committee, who also happen to be civil servants, should catch your attention because it seldom happens. I listened patiently during the years that this important committee was scuffling amongst themselves to come to the conclusion which must have been so very obvious to everyone from day one: "Methanol is a potential cause of human birth defects." The fact that this statement is not considered a strong enough warning in the minds of the best scientists on the committee means, in this day and age, that the statement should have read, "Methanol causes birth defects and we need to learn more."

The tragedy is that by keeping this information secret for all these years, the FDA and the EPA have become culpable and, to my mind, complicit in allowing companies like Rumsfeld's G.D. Searle and Monsanto companies, and now the Ajinimoto company of Japan, to profit from producing and selling a product that has tested positively to damage the brains of the unborn. The extent of the human misery that has resulted will be the subject of the remainder of this chapter. Some readers may find this material very disturbing.

Ode to Joy

During the fall term of the 1984-85 school year at Arizona State University I received a call from my department chairman that a distraught woman was in his office crying uncontrollably and all he could get out of her was that she wanted to see me. By that time aspartame, despite my best efforts, had been added to carbonated beverages and the controversy of its FDA acceptance was still being debated. I had participated in interviews and debates on the subject, particularly on the local television stations, which is how this woman probably got my contact details (although I didn't ask her). When I heard the knock at my office door I wondered what to expect. I opened the door to a well-dressed, obviously intelligent young woman with tears in her eyes, an empty liter bottle of Diet Coke® in one hand and a manila envelope in the other. Two hours later we said goodbye, and were never to meet again. But that brief encounter changed my life and redirected my research like nothing else, before or since.

In short, this woman had been pregnant throughout the long, hot Arizona summer and had consumed an average of two liters of diet soda sweetened with aspartame per day. Just weeks prior to our meeting she had delivered Joy, a live full-term infant girl who appeared perfect from her little nose down to her toes, but who was born blind, deaf and unconscious. The autopsy (which was in that envelope) reported that Joy's greatly enlarged hydrocephalic skull contained very little brain tissue and diagnosed the child, who died the very day of her birth, with the neural tube birth defects anencephaly and hydrocephalus, the same birth defects that Dr. Collins found significant in infant rabbits whose mothers had been fed aspartame during their pregnancy. When I opened the manila envelope to review the details of the autopsy, a small birth photograph

Figure 12.2

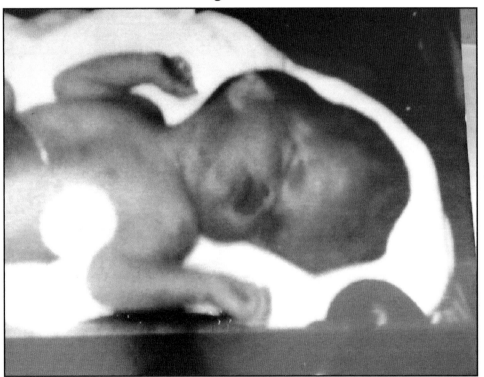

of her child fell to the floor (Figure 2). Her mother carefully retrieved the small picture (Figure 12.2), took one last loving look and insisted I take it for my research. I share this picture now because you need to be able to compare this tiny human girl with the lab animals that suffered the same fate from methanol in my laboratory.[177]

One thing that Joy's mom stressed throughout our discussion was that her intuition told her, and in "her heart she knew," the cause of her daughter's death was "in that bottle," pointing always to the empty Diet Coke® container, which never left her hand. It was as if she had caught the scoundrel and wasn't about to let it go. Thanks to the FDA's removal of the Collins memo from the docket file, I had no idea at the time that hidden from public view was considerable scientific evidence that she was probably correct. By then I was used to hearing horror stories of aspartame consumption, but this child was to inspire me and my graduate students to immediately undertake a series of feeding studies of pregnant rats to see whether methanol could cause fetal damage.

Had the FDA made the memo and the scientific studies it reviewed available to me, as is their fiduciary responsibility to the public, my meeting with Joy's mother would have allowed me to inform her immediately that animal studies of aspartame done ten years before her pregnancy had shown exactly the birth defect to which Joy had succumbed. In fact, it was very likely that the cause of Joy's disfigurement and death had indeed been "in that bottle." Had I known of the Collins memo, I would have suggested that she retain legal counsel and send a letter to the FDA with a copy of the memo. Within weeks, a class-action product liability lawsuit might have been filed against Donald Rumsfeld's G.D. Searle, the Coca-Cola Bottling Company and the Food and Drug Administration for putting this unreasonably dangerous substance into the nation's food supply and not warning women of the risk to their unborn children.

What Might Have Been

The above hypothetical chain of events might have led to the removal of a dangerous food additive before it wreaked havoc on the minds and bodies of our children. I have never been one to dwell on the past or lament on "what if" scenarios. In fact, I believe that everything happens for a purpose and usually see no reason for such exercises. In this particular case, however, imagining an alternative version of the past helps one to see the importance of having impartial government oversight of the chemical and food industry. The Collins memo was kept secret from us, and because of that deceit it would take years before the scientific community would first hear of either methanol or aspartame as teratogens and causative agents of birth defects.[124]

The Laboratory

Early in my doctoral studies I apprenticed an entire summer at the laboratory of Dr. H. Peter Chase at the University of Colorado Medical Center learning the art of working with pregnant and lactating rats in order to study the effect of diet on the details of the development of the brains of their offspring.[740] Peter was a born teacher and I learned quickly what to expect from animals stressed by such experimentation and the proper protocols to follow to study the critical times of their brain growth. This training made my study of methanol as a teratogen an easy transition that I was determined to pursue after meeting Joy's mother.

My laboratory at Arizona State University performed teratogenic testing of methanol on many litters of rat pups and we discovered its powerful teratological potential and its particular proclivity for production of neural tube defects which were identical to Joy's.[177] This poisoning and malformation of the developing pups in the womb with no visible damage to the mother animal has since been confirmed in many other laboratories and on many other species.[278] In fact, during a methanol inhalation experiment performed on pregnant monkeys, the head of one of the hydrocephalic infants who died in the womb of her methanol exposed mother was so large (much like Joy) she had to be removed via C-section.[538] Of utmost importance is that all these other species that were tested, including the monkey, are up to 100 times less sensitive to methanol than human infants like Joy.

See Appendix 2, page 231, for selected images from the slide show for this chapter, which you can find in its entirety on my website www.whilesciencesleeps.com. It gives examples of the various types of neural tube and other birth defects that we could expect from the average litter of pups whose mother was exposed to methanol in the early stages of pregnancy. Our argument against the use of aspartame in carbonated beverages would have probably succeeded if we had obtained the Collins memo and had Joy's autopsy in hand. At the very least, the revelation of the memo, along with the ongoing lawsuit, would have alerted other concerned scientists to the real reason that the incidence of three major human birth defects would suddenly rise dramatically after the introduction of what would then have been a suspected teratogen, aspartame.

A Fire of Mysterious Origin

All that remains with me of the night my home exploded in flames is the aftermath. I have a recurring memory of lying on a gurney in a hospital emergency room in Tempe, Arizona, with a physician repeatedly jabbing me in my left hand with a large gauge hypodermic needle. He was looking for an artery from which to extract a blood sample in order to prove that I had actually been in a fire, despite the fact that an ambulance had taken me directly from the fire to the hospital. The pain was excruciating, far worse than my burns. The rude awakening brought clarity to the fact that I had barely escaped a possible attempt on my life that had to be taken seriously. I vowed then that I would stay alive long enough to reveal the truth about aspartame and resolve the question of whether Joy had been killed by this deadly component of diet sodas.

The fire was officially determined to be of mysterious origin. One of the investigators discovered cigarette butts extinguished in a pile under a tree near the house, which indicated to him that some surveillance of the property was going on prior to the fire. This was before DNA techniques were available for forensic work, so that clue could not be pursued. Prior to the fire, the ASU campus police had caught a prowler snooping around my campus laboratory intimidating one of my technicians. It turned out he was a private investigator who refused to divulge who had employed him. Besides, "the university was public property, after all."

The conflagration came at a time when we were just completing our teratogen studies. We had made some fascinating, yet extremely troubling discoveries. In a display case alongside my main laboratory door, I posted pictures of the birth defects that were being produced by methanol exposure of the pregnant rats. I often posted research results to keep colleagues and students informed of our progress. The local branch of an international soft drink beverage company had some time earlier placed one of its vending machines, stocked primarily with aspartame-sweetened diet products, right next to the laboratory's primary entrance. Controversy arose over the juxtapositioning of the two displays, and ultimately the vending machine was relocated to a more aspartame-friendly neighborhood.

The vast majority of the birth defects we found during our feeding study were of the neural tube type.[177] In several cases stillborn rat pups took on an uncanny resemblance to little Joy. This was highly unusual. At that time I had worked for over twelve years with this variety of laboratory rat, feeding them various experimental chemicals, yet this was the first time I had ever encountered any birth defects in the thousands of rat pups I had examined.

By viewing now the birth defect slide show in Appendix 2, page 231, which may also be found and downloaded from the book's website (www.whilesciencesleeps.com), you will get a feel for just how destructive methanol was to the developing fetus.[177] Mother rats do not tolerate defects. Even now, after more than 20 years, I still have the occasional nightmare flashback of entering our rat room very early in the morning on the day that we were expecting our methanol-fed mothers to give birth. As I scrutinized the special cages that were supplied with straw for the rats to build their birthing nests I noticed one mother sitting up on her hind legs nibbling ever so diligently on what remained of one of her spina bifida-inflicted pups. We took great care from then on to either have a researcher present at the time of every delivery, or to sacrifice the pregnant mother just prior to birthing the pups so they could be delivered via Cesarean.

The Hidden Epidemic of Neural Tube Defects

After learning of Joy I began paying attention to the Neural Tube Birth Defect (NTD) statistics coming out of the US Centers for Disease Control. The CDC statistics showed clearly that the incidence of neural tube birth defects had steadily declined since the late 1960s. Searching this data from the years following the introduction of aspartame lulled me into thinking that perhaps there was no reason for my concern that the methanol from aspartame would cause an increase in this tragic outcome. Though occasionally minor increases in the NTD incidence could be observed as the intake of aspartame increased, no strong, statistically significant increase could be found that would prove that aspartame was causing a sea change in the number of infants born with neural tube birth defects.

From prior chapters you know how these curves are drawn and the data trend that I require to be convinced of an association between a poison and a toxic response. The dance of the slope of the curves of aspartame consumption versus neural tube birth defects was not sufficiently in synchrony to be at all convincing. To this day a review of the CDC statistics for neural tube defects in the years following the introduction of aspartame into carbonated beverages will show no statistically apparent increase in the percentage of children "born" with this outcome.

A number of laboratories including ours were revealing that methanol was a cause of neurological birth defects in animals but without human correlation this work would not be heeded. I could not be convinced that the risk was a real one to humans and was unwilling to publish my speculation with insufficient human evidence, particularly when the emotional impact of such a claim might put an undue burden of guilt on pregnant women with untoward gestational outcomes. It was many years before it was finally revealed that these numbers belied the horror of what was really being done with precious evidence.

Aborted Neural Tube Fetuses – and Their Statistics – Incinerated

The bombshell didn't become public information until ten years after aspartame had been on the market. The article appeared in the summer of 1995. Within the CDC's *Weekly Morbidity and Mortality Reports* (MMWR) were two sentences that will never be lost to my memory:

> *"Each year in the United States about 2,500 infants are born with the neural tube defects (NTDs) spina bifida and anencephaly. In addition, an **unknown number** of fetuses affected by these birth defects are aborted."*[720]

Who would have imagined that the government agency charged with keeping records of birth defects does not, to this day, require physicians aborting birth defect-ravaged fetuses to report these deaths for statistical use in the nation's birth defect surveillance program? With advances in the accuracy of prenatal screening, the CDC undoubtedly knew full well that this "oversight" has given a false low estimation of the rate of serious birth defects in the US population.

The unfortunate children for which I had been searching were being aborted and destroyed with no record kept of their suffering.[721] Exactly ten years after aspartame first began releasing its deadly payload of methanol into the developing brains of an entire generation of our children came the revelation that the evidence of their poisoning was being destroyed and the incidence was on its way toward going forever unnoticed. The 1995 CDC article states:

> *"Pregnancies that are prenatally diagnosed with neural tube birth defects and subsequently terminated in an outpatient setting or before the specified gestational age are not included in U.S. birth defects surveillance data."*[721]

The article goes on to talk about Joy's condition specifically, anencephaly, claiming that in the mid-1980s at least 80% of pregnancies so affected in England, France and Scotland were electively terminated; similar published estimates indicated that this percentage may be even higher in the United States. The researchers went on to say they were only able to study, in retrospect, a handful of US states during the period 1985-94 where the aborted fetus data was available from other sources. Though these states reported relative stability of live births suffering neural tube defects, the unreported rates of termination for these very defects increased dramatically during this same time period. Thus when the aborted fetuses were added to the live births, as logic would demand it should have been done in the first place, the rate of neural tube defects in these states increased dramatically during the period when aspartame consumption was skyrocketing after its allowance in carbonated beverages.

Quoting the article:

> *"Among all pregnancies ascertained in which the infant or fetus had anencephaly or spina bifida, the percentages that were electively terminated were available for each year of surveillance for Arkansas, Hawaii, and Iowa (Table 3). In Arkansas, this percentage more than tripled from 1985 (7%) to 1989 (23%); in Iowa, the percentage doubled from 1985 (13%) to 1990 (27%); in Hawaii, the percentage varied over the years without a discernible trend (range: 30% to 67%). However, in Hawaii, the adjusted prevalence of these defects almost doubled from the earlier years of surveillance (1988-1991, range: 0.28 to 0.57 per 1,000) to the later years (1992-1994, range: 0.97 to 1.11)."*

The article only gives us enough data to apply our graphing method comparing the actual neural tube defects to average US aspartame consumption in the state of Hawaii. I present that graph to you as Figure 12.3. Here at long last was some proof that the true incidence of neural tube birth defects did rise as the consumption of methanol from aspartame increased in the population. All that was required was to count, not discard, the bodies of the unfortunate victims. Who would have thought such valuable evidence would have been discarded?

The CDC article essentially admitted the truth about its decision not to count fetuses if the infants were aborted due to having a birth defect. They had to admit that this method was just not a good way to keep track of neural tube defect incidence in the United States.

To recap, the evidence of increased incidence of neural tube birth defects in the US population after the introduction of aspartame has been destroyed. The 1995 CDC article admits that the statistics to this day that are distributed by the Centers for Disease Control for that critical time period between 1980 and 1995 underestimate the prevalence of anencephaly (Joy's disease) by "approximately 60% to 70%." The article concludes that the comprehensive surveillance for neural tube birth defects can no longer be conducted without ascertaining pregnancies that are prenatally diagnosed and then electively terminated – advice never taken by those who administer the US Centers for Disease Control, even to the date of publication of this book. As strange and tragic as this appears to be, it gets worse – much worse.

The Rush to Mandate Vitamin B9 (Folic Acid) Consumption to "Reduce Neural Tube Birth Defects"

My first indication that something might be amiss with the neural tube birth defect numbers coming out of Washington, DC was a wakeup call in 1992 in the form of an urgent plea from

Figure 12.3

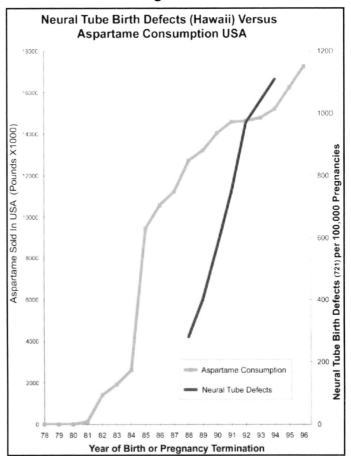

Neural Tube Birth Defects (Hawaii) Versus Aspartame Consumption USA

the Centers for Disease Control directed at **"All women of childbearing age in the United States who are capable of becoming pregnant"** that they immediately start supplementing their diet with the maximum allowed dosage of the vitamin folacin (folic acid).[720] The sole reason given for this <u>first ever</u> "vitamin alert" in the history of the federal government was that this would reduce the incidence of neural tube birth defects.

This approach was unusual for two reasons. First and foremost, we were being told that the incidence of neural tube defects had been steadily declining since 1960. Second, folic acid is a dangerous form of B9 and is not considered a safe and easy supplement. Even moderately high doses are capable of hiding pernicious anemia until it does fatal damage. Folic acid itself is considered a carcinogen[722] because of its direct involvement with methylation. Folic acid, in fact, was the only vitamin that had a legal maximum dosage level in all vitamin supplements, including prenatal vitamins. Nevertheless, the Centers for Disease Control recommended that all women of child bearing age in the United States increase their folic acid intake to 400 micrograms a day in order to prevent "neural tube defects."[720]

It is important to note that the <u>only</u> physiological use for folic acid is its service as a cofactor in the metabolism of formaldehyde and other single-carbon molecules, such as methanol, and as a requirement for controlled methylation within the living cell.[722] In other words, folic acid is primarily used by the body to give some protection from methanol and perhaps formaldehyde poisoning – *and little else*. If the CDC was trying to prevent young women from methanol or formaldehyde poisoning, it would arguably be much easier and safer to merely ban their consumption of aspartame. By 1995, aspartame was indeed the major source of methanol in the food supply.

Folic Acid, the Dangerous Form of a Little-Known Vitamin

The second alarm came directly from the US Food and Drug Administration. Remember them, the same government agency that chose to keep secret the fact that aspartame had caused neural tube defects when tested on laboratory animals? The FDA decided to do the CDC one better when it came to protecting the US from neural tube birth defects – they made it illegal for flour companies to produce enriched flour without adding folic acid. The last time the FDA had substantially added a new required nutrient to the enrichment program was in 1946.

To put things into perspective here, I was being told for fifteen years that the incidence of neural tube birth defects was steadily declining, yet suddenly, two powerful government agencies were acting impetuously to prevent a disease after having hidden the evidence of the sea change in its incidence that I had been expecting from my research and study.

Since mandatory folic acid fortification has been in effect, it has been reported that as much as 50% of the incidence of neural tube birth defects have been prevented.[719] The truth, however, is that we will never really know because we have no good records of how many of these defects to have expected in a world contaminated with methanol from aspartame. Not all cases of neural-tube defect can be prevented by increasing the intake of folic acid.[729] It is still controversial and not at all clear that the taking of the vitamin around the time of conception can reduce a woman's risk of having a child with a neural tube defect.[728]

The Chemistry of Folic Acid (Folate) Is Inseparable from Methanol and Formaldehyde

The "sole biochemical function" of folic acid appears to be the metabolism of the formic acid produced from formaldehyde.[722] Don't confuse folic acid (a man-made form of vitamin B9 sometimes called folacin) with our old friend formic acid. This is one of the main reasons I have not mentioned this connection earlier. Please study Figure 12.4 and you will see exactly how this vitamin fits into the way methanol is metabolized by the body.

Page 203

I have waited a long time to bring up the issue of the vitamin folic acid. This was purposeful on my part. The reason I have kept this vitamin from the discussion thus far, even though it is involved in the metabolism of methanol, is that neural tube birth defects are the only methanol poisoning outcome that appears to be affected by folic acid status. I have found no evidence that an insufficiency of folic acid can have a major effect even on the status of the other two birth defects associated with methanol – Autism or Fetal Alcohol Syndrome. This is a mystery for which I have no explanation.

Figure 12.4 shows that the important conversion of methanol to formaldehyde can proceed without the folate vitamin. Folate does not become necessary until after the formaldehyde has been converted to formic acid and it is necessary for the formic acid to be further burned to carbon dioxide. This is long past the time when the formaldehyde has begun its damage to tissue in all of the methanol diseases that we have discussed. Because folate comes so long after the production of formaldehyde it can only give us limited protection from diseases caused by formaldehyde itself. Nevertheless, it is generally believed that folic acid plays a role in the protection of the fetus from neural tube defects; still, since folic acid fortification has been in effect, only 27% of the incidence of neural tube birth defects have been prevented in the US.[719]

Birth Defects Caused by Methanol from Cigarette Smoke

Every laboratory species to which methanol has been fed in order to determine its teratogenic potential has revealed methanol's persistent ability to cause birth defects – including rats,[177] mice,[105] rabbits,[677] and primates.[538] The possibility that humans would be somehow immune to this one aspect of methanol poisoning experienced by animals who are in all ways and by every mechanism more resistant to all other of methanol's chronic effects is highly unlikely. This pattern, in fact, should constitute sufficient evidence to caution against exposure of pregnant women to any form of methanol, including cigarette smoke. We have, in previous chapters, seen how cigarette smoke has been just such a toxic harbinger of most of the other methanol-induced diseases of civilization. Recently, smoking has been linked to a statistically significant 260% increased occurrence of neural tube defects in the children of women exposed during the first trimester of their pregnancy. This was confirmed in a study that showed that neither street drug use or alcohol intake increased the risk. The same study also showed that folic acid intake had no relation to neural tube defect risk when adjusted for cigarette smoking.[724]

It has long been known that perinatal smoking has been linked to children with attention problems, rule-breaking and aggressive behavior.[572] A comprehensive study of all children diagnosed with infantile autism in Sweden during an eight year period has concluded that a 140% increased risk of autism was associated with daily smoking in early pregnancy.[573] The study confirmed conclusively the "smoking mother's link to autism."

An important complication of

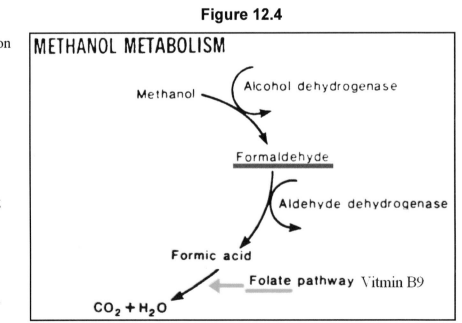

Figure 12.4

METHANOL METABOLISM

Methanol — Alcohol dehydrogenase

Formaldehyde

Aldehyde dehydrogenase

Formic acid

Folate pathway Vitmin B9

$CO_2 + H_2O$

pregnancy and the leading cause of perinatal morbidity and mortality is preterm delivery. On July 16th, 2006 a panel of experts convened by the Institute of Medicine of the National Academies of Science in the US announced that the incidence of babies born prematurely had "been creeping up for no apparent reason since 1981." Dr. Jennifer Howse, president of the March of Dimes and cofounder of a 600-page analysis, warned that the rate had been going up year by year to rise over 30% over the "past 25 years." The cause of preterm pregnancy has been linked to a number of possible causes including stress and induced fertility; however, only two factors have been successfully tested in large populations. Smoking during pregnancy increased the risk for preterm birth in a study of well over 1.2 million pregnancies presented at the Annual meeting of the American College of Preventive Medicine in Crystal City, Virginia on February 26, 2010. Mothers who smoked during pregnancy has a 24%, 23%, and 28% greater risk for very preterm, spontaneous and medically indicated preterm birth, respectively, than nonsmokers. In addition, the risk for medically indicated preterm birth increased according to the number of cigarettes smoked a day. The only other cause of preterm delivery shown to be statistically valid in as experimental population of almost 60,000 pregnant women in Denmark is the intake of artificially sweetened soft drinks.[617]

Birth defects are not natural occurrences; they are all caused by a mere handful of chemicals that attack the fetus during a critical time in its development. Methanol is one of those rare chemicals.

Autism

All the one carbon chemistry you have learned comes together in understanding autism. Autism is not a brand new disease of civilization, but it is a recent birth defect. Most likely blossoming during the Second World War, it was first described in the scientific literature in 1943 and for four decades its prevalence in the US population had maintained a narrow range of 40 to 50 per 100,000 births – until aspartame's introduction in the early1980s.[738]

It is interesting that autism's discovery coincides with the last years of the Second World War. More than any other war, World War II brought independence for women. Many of them went to work out of the home and started smoking for the first time while their husbands were overseas in the armed services being plied with free daily cigarettes provided with their rations by the American tobacco companies. Women who didn't smoke cigarettes in those years had the concentration and dosage of their methanol limited to the considerably diluted variety found in canned fruits and vegetables often diluted further with the contents of their meals. Office workers or teachers were beginning to inhale the occasional methanol whiff from the copy paper coming off their recently-introduced Ditto machines at work (see Chapter 9, slide show 2 found on the website www.whilesciencesleeps.com). This juxtaposition of several unusual events that would coincide to cause a considerable increase in methanol exposure of a large percentage of the US population, particularly women, was amazingly to be repeated again only 40 years later with the quick orchestrated acceptance of yet another popular consumer product – aspartame.

Methanol is now universally accepted as a birth defect-causing substance (teratogen).[124] More specifically, methanol has been determined to be one of the rare chemicals capable of causing "neural tube" birth defects. The question still to be asked is what other more subtle birth defects would a known neurotoxin such as methanol be capable of causing in a human, particularly since humans are, at the very least, ten (and more likely 100) times more sensitive to it as a poison than any animal (Chapter 5)?

Silly Rat Pups

It was clear after the birth of our first experimental litter of rat pups whose mothers were fed methanol that the molecule was wreaking havoc on the brains of their poisoned offspring.[177] A small, but statistically important percentage of rat infants was being born with severely damaged, or in some circumstances, nonexistent brains.[278] Something else was happening that took some time for us to notice and that has not, until this writing, been resolved to my satisfaction. Some of the pups were born looking and testing healthy in the usual ways, but their behavior gave pause. Subtle behavioral anomalies made them stand out from their littermates. I had never observed these behaviors exhibited in rats, even though at that time I had worked with this rat strain for years.

These subtle differences would probably never have been noticed in most large commercial testing laboratories where such work is done under strict protocol for pharmaceutical companies in modern sterile laboratory settings. My laboratory at Arizona State University had its own small rat room that we ran ourselves under supervision of the university veterinarian. I had technical support available day or night from the central animal care services of the university, but for the most part graduate students from our program, along with technicians and undergraduate volunteers, would help us care for the mother rats and their pups and occasionally some would take a real interest and actually get to know the little animals as pets. Modern procedures would usually not condone such intimacy between experimenters and their animal subjects.

This all became very important one day when I heard one of the student volunteers calling some of the experimental animals by her pet names. She seemed to favor the Seven Dwarfs with Sleepy and Dopey and such. When I asked her why she picked such names she said that some of the methanol pups acted so "silly" she thought it was cute. We soon started paying closer attention to the methanol litters. The occasional pups that stood out from the others did not appear to respond in a natural way to their immediate environment; they seemed disinterested even to life and death issues such as suckling on their mother's teat or finding their nests when their litter mates would jostle them out. They often had to be coaxed by us to drink from their mother's teat.

Since that time, I have noted in the scientific literature over the years that others have reported that prenatal methanol exposure may occasionally cause similar behavioral abnormalities. Newborn rat pups of mothers fed methanol required longer than controls to begin sucking and more time to locate nesting material from their home cage.[103] Another feeding study done on a different species showed that maternal aspartame exposure of mice caused aspartame-fed offspring to fail to perform a "visual placing test" in which they were simply required to raise both their forearms in attempt to grab at a taut string that lay directly in their path as they were being lowered by their tail. The researchers admitted that this might indicate "the possibility of brain dysfunction as a viable result of excessive aspartame exposure."[96] To me, what we were all observing in some animals exposed early to methanol was a disconnect between the animal and its environment. The methanol and aspartame poisoned pups were not paying attention to important environmental clues and the cause was not apparent.

Autism and Methanol – the Same Target

I scheduled an autopsy for one of the odd methanol treated pups from our laboratory when it reached weaning at 21 days of age. After gentle euthanasia we removed the brain from the skull. This was something I had done thousands of times before, but I wasn't prepared for what I saw. The little brain appears in Figure 4 below. You may never have seen a rat pup's brain, but I would think that intuitively the one pictured here would appear damaged to you. The red blotches are blood vessels whose linings have been damaged sufficiently that they are no longer able to keep blood from leaking into the tissue, thus producing small (petechial) hemorrhages. The hardest hit portion of this methanol-damaged brain is the segment which shows the most red blotches and internal bleeding – its cerebellum.

This is very significant inasmuch as the cerebellum is a region of the brain that plays a vital role in motor control. It is also involved in some cognitive functions, such as attention and language, and probably in some emotional functions, such as regulating fear and pleasure responses. Its movement-related functions are the most clearly understood. The cerebellum does not initiate movement, but it contributes to coordination, precision, and accurate timing. It receives input from the sensory systems and other parts of the brain and spinal cord and integrates these inputs to finely tuned motor activity – all activities known to be altered during autism. Damage to the cerebellum produces disorders in fine movement, equilibrium, posture, and motor learning. The methanol pup's cerebellum in Figure 12.5 looks for all intents and purposes as if someone has melted its vermis[571] with a blowtorch.

Figure 12.5

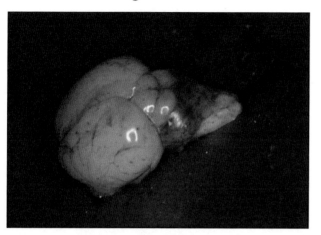

When this pup's brain was examined under a microscope, cells of the cerebellum and hippocampus were found preferentially damaged and missing. The particular type of cells showing the most damage were the specialized cells called purkinje cells. These cells from the cerebellum are some of the only cells of the brain known to contain concentrations of ADH enzyme,[637] thus making them unique in being able to convert methanol directly into formaldehyde. This may explain why purkinje cell[526] death and damage is commonly found during the autopsies of brain tissue from people who have died of methanol poisoning,[119,143] as well as during pathological examination of individuals dying for unrelated reasons while suffering with autism.[526] Perhaps even more important was our discovery that our methanol poisoned rat pups lost purkinje cells preferentially from a very specific area of the cerebellum called the vermis. This meant little to me at the time but it has now been discovered the cerebellum is known to be preferentially damaged in human autism,[622] and the vermis[570] and hippocampus are the particular areas of the cerebellum most damaged and reduced in volume by the disease.[571] A recent study of suckling rats fed aspartame showed "severe" major enzyme changes specifically in their hippocampus.[623]

Another finding in the damaged area of our rat brain was an overabundance of macrophages. We have spent a great deal of time showing how methanol's formaldehyde can lead to autoimmune diseases. Perhaps our strongest evidence for this can be found in Chapter 9 where the path from methanol consumption to multiple sclerosis is difficult to deny. There is good evidence to suggest that immune dysfunction is an important factor contributing to autism.[711] A number of reports have identified antibodies in children with autism directed against brain proteins, including the myelin basic protein[711] which plays such a prominent part in development of multiple sclerosis. The path leading from methanol's formaldehyde to macrophage activation and eventual autoantibody proliferation is now well within your scope of understanding.

The Chemistry of Autism? One Word: Methylation

The only generally accepted chemical change found consistently in excess in most autistic brain tissue thus far studied is methylation.[559] Methylation requires formaldehyde. (See Chapter 4.) The notion that autism is an epigenetic disease is now well-established. DNA methylation patterns are formed by the presence of formaldehyde attached along the entire length of the DNA double helix. Scientists have been studying DNA methylation much longer than they have any other type of epigenetic control mechanism. In fact, it was the connection between cancer and aberrant DNA methylation – a discovery made in the early 1980s – that served as one of the initial major drivers of the field, stirring both academic and pharmaceutical interest.

Initially, the notion of any possible epigenetic etiology to cancer was met with considerable skepticism, but a still-mounting body of evidence has washed away disbelief. Many cancers have been associated with hypermethylation of tumor suppressor genes; generally, the presence of too many methyl molecules (hypermethylation) results in gene silencing. Not only do scientists today recognize the epigenetic etiology of cancer, they are increasingly discovering epigenetic etiologies underlying a wide range of human health disorders, from Alzheimer's disease to infertility.

You might by now have heard of the excitement in the scientific community surrounding the discovery that our genetic makeup is more than just the composition of the genes coded on our DNA. The science of epigenetics is evolving from the observation of the differences that can occur in the health outlook of identical twins. Individuals who are identical in the coding of their DNA makeup can each develop very different diseases patterns and outcomes. One twin may remain healthy while the other develops cancer, Alzheimer's disease or, perhaps most astonishing of all, autism. I would like to recommend that you view the National Public Television

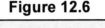

Figure 12.6

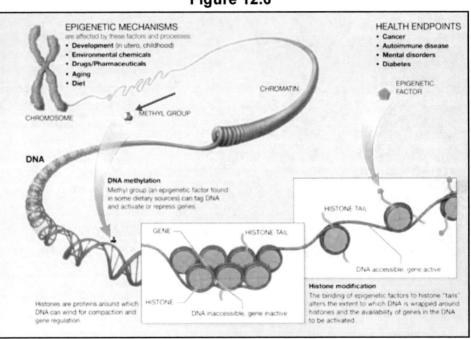

program *Ghost in Your Genes* that first appeared on NOVA in 2006. The cornerstone to this presentation is a pair of identical twin girls, one of whom was quite normal, had friends and played well with others, and the other who spent most of her waking hours rubbing her own spittle over the screen of a TV monitor. The program tells us that the difference between these two young girls is that the one with autism has "ghosts in her genes."

I had paid little attention to epigenetics until I viewed the ghost program for the first time. While viewing it my curiosity was piqued when the first series of animated graphics showed just how the so-called ghosts turned off the genes in the autistic girl's brain. Luckily I was watching the show alone in the privacy of my own home, for when the chemical nature of the ghost was revealed I yelled, at the top of my lungs in a full resonant tenor developed over 30 years of lecturing, an expletive that I had never used in public. The molecules to which they repeatedly referred, with the chemically meaningless term "methyl molecule," was, in fact, an old friend of ours. You guessed it – the ghost that turns off genes and is most likely the major cause of cancer, Alzheimer's and autism is formaldehyde. See Figure 12.6.

Formaldehyde, or More Correctly, the Methylation It Causes, Is the "Ghost in Your Genes"

Like most scientists devoted to a particular and specific field of interest, I keep up with what goes on in my narrow field by doing periodic searches for the key words most associated with methanol and formaldehyde. Why were epitgenomists using this scientifically meaningless and misleading term for formaldehyde? No one seems to know who made the decision to rename formaldehyde the "methyl molecule." We do know that the science of epigenetics is heavily funded and apparently controlled by Big Pharma. Could the name change have been done at the behest of the Formaldehyde Council? NOVA is, after all funded by Dow Chemical, a founding member of the Formaldehyde Council. Ultimately, what is really important is that whenever you hear the term "methyl molecule" or "methyl tag," you should correct it to "formaldehyde" (our "Crazy Hawk").

You now know that the only way to get formaldehyde into the nucleus of a cell is by using methyl alcohol. When a pregnant woman takes a sip of diet soda and the aspartame reaches her stomach, it releases methanol into her bloodstream. Methanol can quickly pass through her placenta and into the blood and brain of her developing fetus. From there, all that is required is that the methanol make contact with an ADH enzyme somewhere deep in the cytoplasm near the nucleus of a purkinje cell in the child's cerebellum. At that point, it can be converted into formaldehyde. Once one of the "Crazy Hawks" is out and flying, it can land on the wrong strand of DNA and attach to it. If a repair enzyme is close by, the bond will be turned into a proper methylation and a gene that was never meant to be turned off will have been turned off. That gene can never ever again be turned on; it is lost to the developing child forever. This simplistic rendition will have to hold for now until science reveals the exact details of the chemistry of Autism's methylation.

Figure 12.7

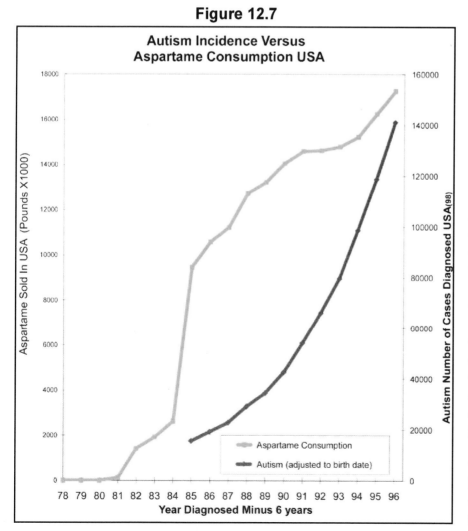

Does Aspartame Cause Autism?

Autism today, 30 years after aspartame's introduction, is "considered an epidemic" with a prevalence measured in the year 2009 of 1,100 per 100,000.[735] The exact timing of the beginning of this epidemic would be a very important date if it could be elucidated. The dramatic increase in incidence appears to have began in the early 1980s, but the nature of the disease makes it time-consuming to diagnose and the magnitude of the increase of the incidence has drawn considerable controversy to its study.

The incidence of autism began to rise with the first wave of births that followed the addition of aspartame to the US food supply. Its incidence grew precipitously after aspartame's addition to carbonated beverages. Unfortunately, researchers had no means by which to recognize this at the time, due to the unexpected nature of the teratological interaction and the years required for the diagnosis of the disease. We will soon see that mitigating circumstances are often associated with birth defects, making it more difficult than one would first expect to obtain the data necessary to interpret a dangerous trend in their incidence.

When I charted the crude data of autism diagnoses in the United States in the years after aspartame I made the decision to adjust the dates I was given by the Center of Disease Control to treat the disease as if it was a birth defect caused by aspartame consumption. To do this I took the raw data that represented numbers of diagnoses of the disease which represented children who were diagnosed at an average age of 6 years and moved the entire diagnosis curve to the left 6 years.[98] This displacement reflects that exposure to methanol occurred in the womb. Of course this is not the perfect way to do this association but it certainly does appear that there is definitely a connection between aspartame and autism. See Figure 12.7.

We had to wait until late in 2011 for the publication of two wonderful autism review articles by Helen Ratajczak.[735] Dr Ratajczak's data comes from the US Department of Education, which has only one autism classification for use by its Department of Special Education Programs to categorize students for the purpose of disability program establishment. This data was extrapolated for each child back to his or her birth date, thereby eliminating the confusion between cohorts who might have early or late diagnoses.[738] More importantly, it is the only way to discover the exact timing of the insult that might have caused the disease. In Figure 12.8, the Department of Education data indicates with some clarity that the birth date of the autism epidemic appears to tragically coincide with the allowance of aspartame into carbonated beverages.

Figure 12.8

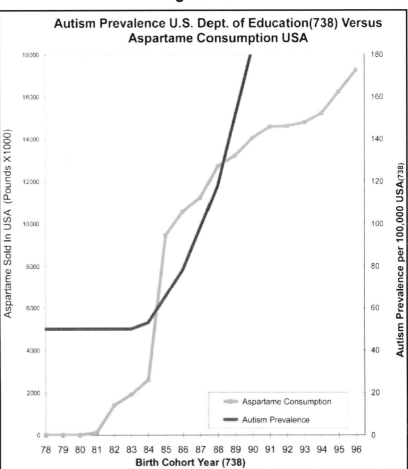

Fetal Alcohol Syndrome: "The American Paradox"

Women are constantly being cautioned against consuming any alcoholic beverage during their pregnancies – even just one drink – lest they risk bearing children with fetal alcohol syndrome. The American College of Obstetricians and Gynecologists, the American Academy of Pediatrics, and all public health officials in the United States recommend that pregnant women, as well as women who are trying to conceive, avoid all alcohol and cigarette smoking entirely. Yet the exact cause of Fetal Alcohol Syndrome (FAS) is unknown, with more than a little indication that ethanol may not be the only alcohol suspect. In fact, ethanol more often proves not to be a teratogen, even at very high concentrations, in animals that have similar toxic sensitivity to it as humans.[124] When studies do show teratological effects of ethanol, the details of the malformations are not identical to those peculiar to the human expression of FAS.[731] On the other hand, it is methanol terata in laboratory animals[96] that can be more reminiscent of the human presentation of FAS.[206] The fact that higher FAS incidence does not correspond to any measure of higher average consumption of alcohol is puzzling. For instance, the very high incidence rate for FAS in the USA and the relatively low rate in other countries does not correspond to the average alcohol consumption rate of the general population of these respective countries since the US has a "relatively low level of alcohol consumption." This has been referred to as the "American Paradox."[492]

The fact is that it was not until the introduction of aspartame into the US diet, particularly into carbonated beverages, that, as the chart below indicates, the incidence of FAS more than trebled to make the "American Paradox" a reality. It is now thought that it might be binge drinking and not occasional drinking that may be the real cause of FAS.[733] This, if proved true, greatly reinforces the evidence pointing to methanol as the causative agent. Remember, it was the human experimentation done by Dr. Edward Majchrowicz of the U.S. National Institute for Alcohol Abuse and Alcoholism that elegantly proved that methanol accumulation in the blood during binging was responsible for the most serious of the alcohol withdrawal symptomology[134] (See The Diversion of Dr. Majchrowicz: Chapter 5). The study of FAS is complex and it is not my intention to review it here, but I would be remiss if I didn't bring to your attention the abrupt change in the incidence of FAS since the introduction of aspartame.

Figure 12.9

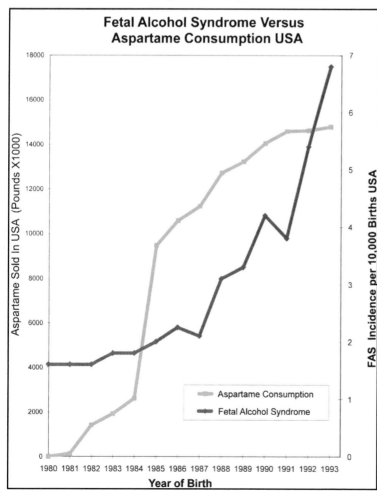

Another long-term neurological malfunction has recently been linked to methanol exposure during pregnancy. Attention deficit hyperactivity disorder (ADHD) is a common childhood psychiatric disorder that affects between 3% and 5% of school aged children. The majority of scientific studies identify maternal smoking during pregnancy as a risk factor for ADHD behaviors. In fact, the risk for a diagnosis of ADHD in those individuals whose mothers smoked during pregnancy is a highly statistically significant two-fold increase.[572] A liter of diet soda sweetened with aspartame provides to the maternal bloodstream an equal amount of methanol as does smoking a pack of cigarettes.

What you see represented in Figure 12.9 is the tripling of a disorder that is alleged to be linked directly to alcohol consumption. One that has been well-known and the subject of strong warnings for the last thirty years, subject to a plethora of media attention with what appears to be considerable compliance among the population of pregnant women; yet the effect is inverse to what would be predicted. Why?

Frank, the Friendly Face of Big Pharma

You need to know just a little of how Big Pharma gets things done. During the course of my many public debates with the G.D. Searle Company, which invented aspartame, I became acquainted with a tall, silver-grey haired, affable individual who worked for them and who we will call Frank. I was taken by surprise one day when he invited me to have a drink with him and some friends. Frank had recognized me while I attended a welcoming session of the national convention of a public health organization. We were both on the docket to be debating the topic of aspartame. His two friends were young ladies, a blond and a brunette with some considerable style and surprising intelligence. We spoke for an hour or two over drinks in a bar of the same hotel in which we were to be debating the next evening. I was invited to dinner with the three of them but declined as I laid on the table sufficient funds to cover my drinks and something for a tip. That didn't go over well, and from then on Frank was the man who would counter me at any debate and would represent aspartame during any television or radio interview, no matter where in the world that might be. Frank would always show up for the debate in the biggest stretch limo available at the destination where we would be lecturing. His chauffeur would also always accompany him in an apparent bodyguard capacity.

Frank was not very good at countering my arguments and did not have much respect for the truth, but he carried himself with practiced style and made a great deal of his statesmanlike qualities. I tried to be respectful of his age and bad memory, which at every opportunity I jokingly blamed on aspartame. One time I just could not take it any longer and called him a "liar" during a Los Angeles television interview. That was the first and last time he ever lost his cool and confronted me in an angry tone. Following that interview he dismissed his bodyguard and took me aside and said sternly, "Well, it looks as if we will be looking at a libel suit. I will need to contact our corporate attorneys the minute I get back." My answer was as matter of fact, "Frank, you lied, you always lie!" He turned white but his expression was not anger – it was more introspective. From that day on, no bodyguards accompanied Frank and we grew chummy, exchanging pleasantries and chatting about the time we spent on various vacations in unusual places as we killed time in waiting rooms before appearing on our debates.

At one point I thought that Frank might be redeemable and really only needed some education to be won over. I began doing just that and would come to our debates with literature that I thought would show Frank my side of the issue. I had uncovered an article that I thought would finally show that methanol turned into formaldehyde in the living brain. A scientist had been able to show a reaction in the brain of a laboratory animal that caused some brain chemicals to change under certain circumstances when they consumed methanol. The only cause of this would have been formaldehyde. What made the experiment fascinating was that the researcher was not intending to show this and it was merely an aside in an abstract at the time of the work's presentation.[397] I naively but proudly handed Frank the abstract at our very next chat.

It was to be six months before I met Frank for the last time at yet another interview about the safety of aspartame. I was anxious to ask him what he thought of the science I presented him previously. I will never forget his response – it shook me to my very core. Frank said that it was indeed interesting, but that he wasn't particularly concerned now that they knew where the investigator "had gone wrong." My reply was "how do you know that?" To which Frank answered with a sinister smirk, "Well, Woodrow, he works for us now." A ringing started in my ears that drowned out the rest of our dialogue, probably an indication of extremely low blood pressure. I remember nothing more of the debate that night and I never saw Frank again. I found out later that Frank was one of the people who worked on Dr. Edward Majchrowicz to get him to give up his quest for methanol as the cause of alcohol withdrawal. Edward even allowed Frank to write a chapter in Edward's book.[383] Frank was the author of the article published in the fertility journal that encouraged pregnant woman to consume aspartame.[100]

Tidy Up

We are asked to accept that in a period of about thirty years in the health history of the richest nation in the world – during a time when cigarette smoking in general, and alcoholic beverage consumption during pregnancy specifically, had been reduced significantly and healthy eating, organic lifestyle, and proper nutrition during pregnancy had developed as the mantra of the age – that during this period the incidence of at least three of the most egregious known birth defects has skyrocketed. The one purportedly caused exclusively by the drinking of alcoholic beverages during pregnancy, Fetal Alcohol Syndrome, has increased 300%. Autism is up 2000%. All of this has occurred with no lead up time, no early plateau or warning period, and only what appears to be a conspicuous start in or shortly after the year 1981, the very year aspartame was first used in foods and recommended for use during pregnancy. Indeed, the incidence charts of these diseases show, wherever the frequency data has not been tragically destroyed, that the timing and magnitude of these birth defect increases generally mirrors the dosage of aspartame consumed by the affected populations.

Further, US government health agency evaluations of privately performed experimentation presenting evidence that aspartame could cause birth defects was purposefully kept secret by a pact between the corporation that invented aspartame and the governmental agency that should have been acting as the infant's only protection from just such threats. The egregious nature of this pact is compounded by the fact that the government agency scientists knew at the time that no published scientific literature-reported tests had ever been done to show aspartame was safe for pregnant animals. As of 2005, the Department of Health and Human Services Center For the Evaluation of Risks to Human Reproduction has officially recognized the poisonous component of aspartame, concluding, "methanol is a probable human developmental teratogen capable of causing human birth defects."[551]

Woodrow C. Monte, PhD
Emeritus Professor of Nutrition
Arizona State University
woodymonte@gmail.com

Chapter 12

Epilogue

Reading this book may have various outcomes, depending on your determination and perseverance. Some of you may suffer or love someone who suffers from one of the diseases discussed here who can, on a superficial level, glide through the text, lighting easily on all the important facts and find the evidence needed to justify and commence the simple change of diet that will begin the ending of the damage done to the body and mind by methanol. I wrote this book with such individuals in mind and sincerely hope this information comes in time to help.

Those who choose to read more deeply will come away with sufficient scientific knowledge to peruse professional publications that will help them answer their many additional questions and perhaps afford a greater respect for the breadth of the natural world.

The third level is a darker encounter requiring several readings with considerable concentration on the meaning of every word, illustration and graph, the sounding of the full depth of every sentence. The reader must test the references for their appropriateness and veracity and become satisfied of the entire truth set out here. The result of all of this effort will have a different effect on each of you but it will be disconcerting for you, to say the least. The warriors of you will want blood, the scholars will want change, the parents will want revenge, and the politicians will want sanctuary. At that point of clarity, you will know what I know.

Kindest Regards,

Woodrow C. Monte PhD.

Index

headache, 3, 39, 57, 60, 75, 80, 112, 133, 159, 163

Health Consultation, 152, 153

hemodialysis, 57, 77, 82

hemorrhaging, 75, 77, 190

Henzi, 142, 151, 153

histology, 132

hydrocephalus, 196, 198

I

Iceland, 149, 150

incidence, 1, 8, 9, 12, 13, 34, 36, 52, 54, 83, 97, 98, 99, 110, 114, 116, 117, 121, 125, 139, 140, 142, 144-148, 151, 152, 153, 155, 159, 161, 162, 171, 173, 177-181, 184-191, 193, 196, 199-205, 209-211, 213

infant, 28, 72, 165, 172, 193, 194, 196, 198, 202, 213

influenza, 168

injected, 37, 45, 54, 85, 86, 167

innate, 34, 74, 75, 78, 79, 85-91, 110, 118, 144

intima, 41, 83, 87-90, 92-94, 96, 97, 110, 118, 119, 121, 129

intracranial catastrophe, 193

Inuit, 80, 112, 149, 176

Invercargill, 27

Iowa, 20-22, 52, 56, 58, 72, 202

Italian, 11, 12, 56, 155

J

Japan, 120, 144, 145, 149, 184, 197

Joy, 197-202

juice, 4, 10-12, 14, 53, 115, 139, 146, 184

K

Kurtzke, 145, 149, 150, 183

L

Langerhans, 172

latitude, 144, 149

Lauer, 151

LDL, 31, 46, 83, 84, 86, 88-94, 96, 108, 110, 118, 119

leather, 131, 140, 141, 146, 154-156

leathery, 36, 43, 101, 131

lethal dose, 22-24, 27, 28, 37, 56, 58, 59, 65, 68, 71, 98, 102, 133, 137

lipoprotein, 46, 84, 86, 92

liver, 6, 7, 10, 16, 18, 32, 41, 52, 55-67, 69, 71, 73, 76, 77, 80, 85, 86, 101, 107-109, 119, 129, 176, 186, 190

lungs, 7, 9, 25, 34, 37, 57, 68, 71, 77, 85, 98, 101, 117, 138, 146, 158, 169, 186, 190, 191, 208

lupus, 1, 8, 10, 31, 35, 46, 54, 108, 153, 160, 165, 168-171

M

macrophage, 31, 34, 35, 39, 40, 46, 47, 74, 75, 79, 83-94, 96, 97, 101, 103, 108-110, 118, 119, 121, 127-130, 134, 135, 137, 141, 144, 165-168, 171, 172, 187, 188, 196, 207

Majchrowicz, 56-60, 66, 75, 102, 211, 212

mammary, 180, 182, 185

Manhattan, 39-41, 91, 97, 166

MBP, 35, 44, 49, 128, 130, 134-137, 161

McAlpine, 125

media, 41, 83, 87, 92-94, 99, 116, 119-121, 129, 132, 178, 211

Melanoma, 187

memory, 25, 26, 36, 41, 75, 79, 111, 112, 117, 121, 133, 162, 166, 193, 199, 201, 212

Methanol Institute, 25, 65

methyl molecule, 5, 37, 54, 97, 134, 177, 208, 209

methylation, 18, 37, 47, 53, 96, 97, 135, 137, 161, 177, 203, 207, 209

Metzenbaum, 22

Mexico, 145, 147, 149, 157

microsomal, 108

migraines, 188

mitochondria, 5, 18, 26, 34, 40, 72-74, 120, 137, 187

MLD, 22,-24, 28

monkey, 21, 23, 52, 199

Monsanto, 197

Monte, 56, 178, 213

mother's love, 22

MRI, 75, 81, 141

murder, 77

mutation, 16-18, 25, 53, 123

myelin, 31, 35, 44, 46, 49, 75, 120, 121, 125, 127-130, 133-135, 138, 161, 207

Soffritti, 180, 190, 192

solvent, 9, 15, 24, 25, 27, 65-67, 69, 137-139, 141, 146, 153-155, 157, 158, 185

sparrow hawk, 41, 43, 44, 48, 49, 96, 120

species, 16, 22, 23, 33, 56, 123, 192, 196, 199, 204, 206

spiking, 37, 178

Stegink, 22

stroke, 83-86, 97, 99, 110, 182

suicide, 23, 70, 164, 165, 178

Sweden, 156, 204

symptoms, 2, 3, 15, 18, 19, 21, 24, 28, 39, 46, 52, 57-60, 65, 69, 70, 72-76, 78-81, 84, 102, 109, 111, 115, 123, 126-128, 133, 137-139, 141, 142, 148, 154, 158, 159, 161, 168, 169, 193

T

teachers, 9, 157-160, 162, 165, 180, 181, 191, 205

terata, 211

thiamine, 3

thyroid, 159, 191

tobacco, 10, 117, 118, 138, 140, 145, 205

tomato, 11, 12, 14, 147

toxic syndrome, 15, 21, 24, 25

toxicity, 15, 16, 18, 19, 21, 59, 65, 67, 72, 76, 80, 98, 99, 116, 121, 127, 135, 141, 147, 161, 163, 172, 175, 180, 191, 192, 195, 196

toxin, 67, 111, 132, 137, 146, 150

toxins, 22, 56, 85

toxoid, 167

transfusions, 160

Trojan horse, 39, 69, 177

tumor, 175, 179, 191, 208

U

United States, 1, 14, 91, 97, 99, 111, 112, 115, 116, 138, 140, 142-146, 155, 157, 159, 172, 175-178, 181, 184, 187, 189, 191, 193, 196, 201-203, 210

urine, 7, 36, 56, 77, 120

urticaria, 103

U-Shaped Curve, 103, 104, 108

V

vaccine, 28, 35, 46, 165, 167, 168

vapor, 38, 68, 153, 158, 181, 191

vegetables, 4, 10, 11-14, 27, 53, 67, 96, 139-141, 143, 144, 146-149, 151, 161, 205

venom, 167

Venus, 39-41, 44, 49, 91, 93, 166

vermis, 207

vessels, 40, 41, 44, 86, 87, 93, 98, 99, 118-120, 127, 129-134, 161, 206

vinegar, 5, 18, 20, 50, 55, 67, 86, 181

virus, 32, 35, 72, 79, 87, 150, 166, 167

visual, 18, 57, 60, 65, 70, 72, 75, 100, 133, 206

vitamin D, 80, 81, 149

vodka, 27, 65, 66, 68

W

Walton, 163

war, 35, 53, 54, 130, 140, 150, 151, 168, 205

Weisberg, 58, 157

Wellington, 131, 152-154, 162, 171

withdrawal, 56, 57, 59, 72, 76, 102

Wolfgram, 111, 137, 138

wood, 4, 9, 13, 15, 19, 27, 36, 126, 138-141, 151, 155, 156

Y

yeast, 12, 13

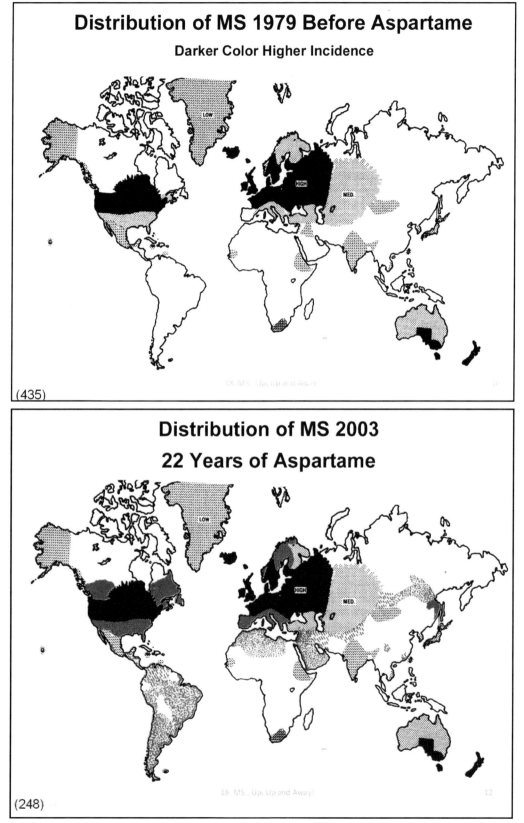

Distribution of MS 1979 Before Aspartame

Darker Color Higher Incidence

(435)

Distribution of MS 2003

22 Years of Aspartame

(248)

Editorial

Neuroepidemiology 2006;26:1–3
DOI: 10.1159/000089230

Published online: October 25, 2005

Multiple Sclerosis in Latin America

Teresa Corona[a] Gustavo C. Román[b]

[a]National Institute of Neurology and Neurosurgery, Mexico City, Mexico; [b]University of Texas Health Science Center at San Antonio, San Antonio, Tex., USA

Key Words

Multiple sclerosis, geographic distribution · Latin America

Introduction

The epidemiology of multiple sclerosis (MS) has been thoroughly studied in developed countries, particularly in areas traditionally known for their high prevalence. However, there is a dearth of epidemiological information on MS from large areas of the world. It is generally accepted that MS incidence and prevalence are higher in latitudes north and south of the Equator with prevalences ranging from 80 to 300/100,000. In contrast, its prevalence in Africa, Asia and South America has been estimated around 5/100,000 [1, 2]. However, lack of adjustment of crude incidence and prevalence rates to a common standard population creates problems in the comparison and interpretation of geographic data [3]. Nonetheless, recent studies indicate an increasing risk of developing MS over time in areas such as Sardinia [4], Norway [5], and Sweden [6], as well as in countries previously considered to have low MS prevalence such as Mexico [7].

MS in Latin America

published epidemiological studies begin to provide a reasonable estimate of the frequency and characteristics of MS in Latin America.

In Mexico, hospital-based and population-based studies indicate an increase in the incidence and prevalence of MS. In 1970, Alter and Olivares [8] reported a relatively low prevalence of 1.6/100,000. This study was not confirmed by community-based data. More recent studies based on referrals to a tertiary neurological center demonstrate an important increase in MS incidence [9–11]. A study in northern Mexico (25° north) found a prevalence of 13/100,000 inhabitants [9]. However, this study included only patients with social security benefits, representing 51% of the population. Other studies performed in central areas of the country have registered lower prevalences of about 5/100,000 at latitudes 16–20° north [10]. Clearly, MS has become one of the main causes of neurological consultation in Mexico. For instance, optic neuritis represents 12% of the patients referred to a specialized neuro-ophthalmology clinic [12]; about 40% of them are eventually diagnosed as having MS [12, 13]. Potential risk factors responsible for the increase in MS in Mexico include a decrease in breastfeeding for large segments of the society and an increased incidence of varicella and childhood eczema [14]. Research conducted at the National Institute of Neurology and Neurosurgery of Mexico has demonstrated activation of varicella-zoster virus during MS relapses [15], suggesting that this herpes virus could be an etiological agent of MS

Journal of Rehabilitation Research and Development
Vol. 39 No. 2, March/April 2002
Pages 175–186

Epidemiology and current treatment of multiple sclerosis in Europe today

Carlo Pozzilli, MD, PhD; Silvia Romano, MD; Stefania Cannoni, MD

Department of Neurological Science, University of Rome, "La Sapienza," Italy

Abstract—Multiple sclerosis (MS) is a chronic disease affecting the central nervous system, usually leading to early disablement in young adults. At least 350,000 persons in Europe have the disease. Wide variations exist both between and within European countries in the incidence and prevalence of the disease as well as in the general standard of care for MS patients. The needs, well-being, and social participation of people with MS are systematically influenced by their physical and cultural environment and the nature of the community services. Moreover, the rate of introduction of the new disease-modifying therapy also widely differs from country to country. This article helps clinical researchers to understand better the differences in epidemiology and in the current treatment of MS in Europe.

Most recent descriptive studies based on more appropriate methods contradicted the accepted belief that the distribution of MS in Europe is related to latitude (1). Until 1980, European countries from 36° to 46° north latitude were regarded as having a much lower prevalence rate of MS, about 5 to 25 cases per 100,000, compared to countries of central and northern Europe. This view was mainly based on old surveys done in Italy between 1959 and 1975. More recent studies performed in Italy and in other countries of southern Europe showed that MS prevalence is, in fact, much higher than had been previously believed (2). Therefore, the MS distribution in Europe appears to be more complex than supposed in the past,

1: Mult Scler. 2003 Aug;9(4):387-92.

Increasing frequency of multiple sclerosis in Padova, Italy: a 3 year epidemiological survey.

Ranzato F, Perini P, Tzintzeva E, Tiberio M, Calabrese M, Ermani M, Davetag F, De Zanche L, Garbin E, Verdelli F, Villacara A, Volpe G, Moretto G, Gallo P.

Department of Neurological and Psychiatric Sciences, First Neurology Clinic, University of Padova, Via Giustiniani, Padova, Italy.

OBJECTIVE: To determine the incidence and prevalence rates of multiple sclerosis (MS) and their temporal profiles over the last 30 years in the province of Padova (northeast Italy) BACKGROUND: In the early 1970s an epidemiological survey in the province of Padova showed a MS prevalence and incidence of 16/100 000 and 0.9/100 000 population, respectively; these figures are much lower than current estimates in other regions of Italy and Central Europe. METHODS: The population of the study area was approximately 820 000 (422 028 women, 398 290 men) in the 1991 census. All possible sources of case collection were used, but only clinically definite/probable and laboratory-supported definite/probable MS were considered in the analysis of incidence and prevalence trends from 1971 to 1999 RESULTS: On 31 December 1999, the crude prevalence rate was 80.5/100 000 (95% CI 70.3-90.7); prevalence was higher in women (111.1/100 000; 95% CI 99.0-123.1) than in men (49.7/100 000; 95% CI 41.3-58.1). This difference was significant (F/M = 2.43; z = 10.1, P < 0.00001); a rate adjusted for the European population was 81.4/100 000. On 31 December 1980 and on 31 December 1990 the estimated prevalence rates were 18/100 000 and 45.7/100 000, respectively. Thus, a fivefold increase in prevalence was observed from the 1970s The mean annual incidence was 2.2/100 000 in the period 1980-89, 3.9 in the period 1990-94 and 4.2 in the period 1995-99. Thus, incidence increased more than fourfold from the 1970s through 1994 and remained quite stable in the last several years. Mean age at onset was 31.3 +/- 9.88 years. Mean diagnostic

Original Paper

Increasing Incidence of Multiple Sclerosis in the Province of Sassari, Northern Sardinia

Maura Pugliatti[a, b], Trond Riise[b], M. Alessandra Sotgiu[a], Stefano Sotgiu[a], Wanda M. Satta[a], Luisella Mannu[a], Giovanna Sanna[a], Giulio Rosati[a]

[a]Institute of Clinical Neurology, University of Sassari, Sassari, Italy;
[b]Department of Public Health, Section for Occupational Medicine, University of Bergen, Bergen, Norway

Address of Corresponding Author

Neuroepidemiology 2005;25:129-134 (DOI: 10.1159/000086677)

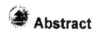 **Key Words**

- Multiple sclerosis
- Epidemiology
- Sardinia

Abstract

Sardinia is a high-risk area for multiple sclerosis (MS), with prevalence rates of 150 per 100,000 population. The study included 689 MS patients (female-male ratio 2.6) with disease onset between 1965 and 1999 in the province of Sassari. The mean annual incidence rate increased significantly from 1.1 per 100,000 population in 1965-1969 to 5.8 in 1995-1999, with no significant difference for gender and province sub-areas. The mean age at onset increased significantly during the same period from 25.7 to 30.6 years, while the proportion of patients with progressive initial course declined over time. The marked increase of MS incidence and the change of MS clinical phenotype over time cannot be explained by ascertainment bias only, thus pointing to a corresponding change in the distribution of exogenous risk factors in this highly genetically stable population.

Neuro -epidemiology

Vol. 28, No. 1, 2007

Free Abstract   Article (References)   Article (PDF 117 KB)

Original Paper

High Prevalence and Fast Rising Incidence of Multiple Sclerosis in Caltanissetta, Sicily, Southern Italy

Luigi M.E. Grimaldi[a], Barbara Palmeri[b], Giuseppe Salemi[b], Giuseppe Giglia[b], Marco D'Amelio[b], Roberto Grimaldi[a], Gaetano Vitello[a], Paolo Ragonese[b], Giovanni Savettieri[b]

[a]Unità Operativa di Neurologia, Fondazione Istituto San Raffaele G. Giglio, Cefalù, e [b]Dipartimento di Neuroscienze Cliniche, Palermo, Italia

idence of Multiple Sclerosis in Caltanissetta, Sicily, Southern Italy

♠ Abstract

Background: Epidemiological studies conducted in Sicily and Sardinia, the two major Mediterranean islands, showed elevated incidence and prevalence of multiple sclerosis (MS) and a recent increase in disease frequency. *Objective:* To confirm the central highlands of Sicily as areas of increasing MS prevalence and elevated incidence, we performed a follow-up study based on the town of Caltanissetta (Sicily), southern Italy. *Methods:* We made a formal diagnostic reappraisal of all living patients found in the previous study performed in 1981. All possible information sources were used to search for patients affected by MS diagnosed according to the Poser criteria. We calculated prevalence ratios, for patients affected by MS who were living and resident in the study area on December 31, 2002. Crude and age- and sex-specific incidence ratios were computed for the period from January 1, 1993, to December 31, 2002. *Results:* The prevalence of definite MS rose in 20 years from 69.2 (retrospective prevalence rate) to 165.8/100,000 population. We calculated the incidence of definite MS for the period 1970-2000. These rates calculated for 5-year periods increased from 2.3 to 9.2/100,000/year. *Conclusion:* This survey shows the highest prevalence and incidence figures of MS in the Mediterranean area and confirms central Sicily as a very-high-risk area for MS.

NEUROLOGY

Temporal trends in the incidence of multiple sclerosis: A systematic review
Alvaro Alonso and Miguel A. Hernán
Neurology 2008;71;129-135

Temporal trends in the incidence of multiple sclerosis

A systematic review

ABSTRACT

Background: Multiple sclerosis (MS) has been traditionally considered to be more frequent in women and in regions more distant from the equator. However, recent reports suggest that the latitude gradient could be disappearing and that the female-to-male ratio among patients with MS has increased in the last decades. We have conducted a systematic review of incidence studies of MS to assess the overall incidence of MS and explore possible changes in the latitude gradient and the female-to-male ratio over time.

DISCUSSION Our findings suggest an attenuation of the latitude gradient in MS incidence over the last 25 years, apparently as a result of increased incidence of MS in regions closer to the equator, and an increase of the female-to-male ratio of MS over time.

Finally, our review does not provide direct evidence regarding the causes of the attenuation in the latitude gradient or the increase in the female-to-male ratio.

1: Rinsho Shinkeigaku. 2006 Nov;46(11):859-62.

[Epidemiology of multiple sclerosis in Japanese: with special reference to opticopsinal multiple sclerosis]

[Article in Japanese]

Kira J.

Department of Neurology, Neurological Institute, Graduate School of Medical Sciences, Kyushu University.

The fourth nationwide survey of multiple sclerosis (MS) disclosed that the estimated number of MS patients in Japan was 9,900, and the estimated prevalence rate of MS is 7.7 per 100,000, indicating that the number of MS patients has been rapidly increasing for the past 30 years. The demographic features of the present series were compared with those of the three past nationwide surveys. The ratio of female to male patients has increased from 1.3 to 2.9. As to distribution of age at onset, in 2004, the peak of the age at onset curve shifted from the 30s to 20s and the second

Appendix 2

The FDA Knew of Birth Defects

MEMORANDUM

DEPARTMENT OF HEALTH, EDUCATION, AND WELFARE
PUBLIC HEALTH SERVICE
FOOD AND DRUG ADMINISTRATION

TO : Charles J. Kokoski, Ph.D.   DATE: September 11, 1978
Chief, Food Additives Evaluation Branch, HFF-185

FROM : Thomas F.X. Collins, Ph.D. *Thomas F.X. Collins*
Whole Animal Toxicology Branch, HFF-155

SUBJECT: Aspartame (SC-18862). Review of four studies submitted by G.D. Searle as entries to Food Additive Master File 134, in response to your memo of September 1, 1978.

1. E-79. SC-18862: Segment II, an evaluation of the teratogenic potential in the rabbit. Final report. Hazleton Laboratories, Inc., Vienna, Virginia. October 8, 1974.

At the high dose level, there was an increase in the number of fetuses with abnormalities and an increase in the number of litters affected. No abnormalities were observed in the control animals (19 litters). At the low dose level, 1 of 198 fetuses (24 litters) showed gastroschisis with associated rotation of hindlimbs, rotation of the eye, and other anomalies. At the high dose level, 7 of 343 fetuses (6 litters out of 45) showed major and minor anomalies consisting in part of: bi-clefted lip, cleft palate, fused mandible, short maxillary bones, fusion and misalignment of caudal vertebrae, reduced ossification of thoracic and caudal vertebrae and phalanges, hydrocephalus, missing ribs, and ectrodactyly.

FDA Warned on September 11, 1978

A decrease in the number of litters having completely viable fetuses was noted at the high level aspartame and with L-phen. The number of litters completely resorbed and the number of resorption sites per litter were increased at the high dose level of aspartame. Mean litter size was not affected by aspartame dosage. Fetal body weight and crown-rump lengths were significantly decreased in both sexes at 2.0 g/kg aspartame and L-phen.

The number of litters containing pups with grossly visible abnormalities was increased in the 2.0 g/kg aspartame and L-phen groups. Cleft palate appeared to be significantly increased at the high dose level of aspartame. There was a significant increase in the number of rabbits with an extra pair of ribs, as well as a significant decrease in ossification of the second sternebral center, increased absence of the 6th sternebral center, increase in unossified metacarpals, and an increase in unossified tarsals.

Conclusion. There were deleterious affects at the high dose level of aspartame, 2.0 g/kg, in rabbits. Dosage up to 1.0 g/kg/day did not appear to affect pregnant rabbits.

General conclusions. 1. Aspartame appeared to be non-teratogenic in the mouse feeding study at dose levels of 1.4, 2.7, and 5.7 g/kg.

2. In both rabbit studies, aspartame appeared to cause birth defects at the high level (2 g/kg).

Birth Defects Caused by Methanol In My ASU Laboratory Rats

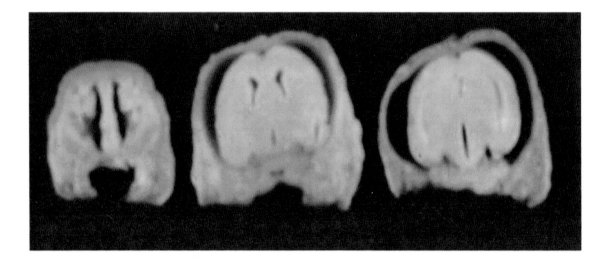

Classic Methanol Neural Tube Defect

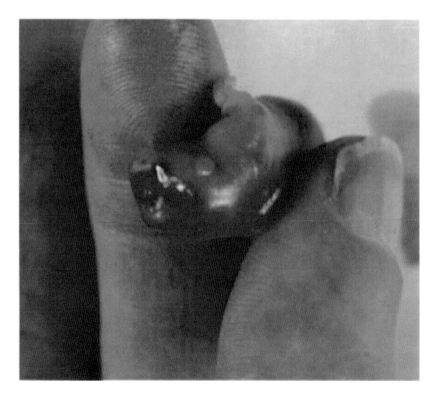

Methanol Litter Mates Normal Pup
Left Neural Tube Defect on Right

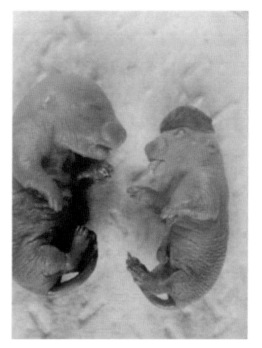

Exencephaly and Anencephaly (Neural
Tube Defects) Caused by Methanol

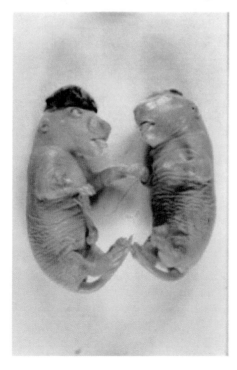

Methanol Induced Exencephaly on left
Hydrocephalus on right

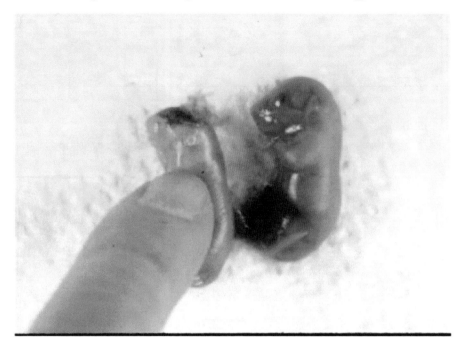

Methanol Spina Bifida Terata

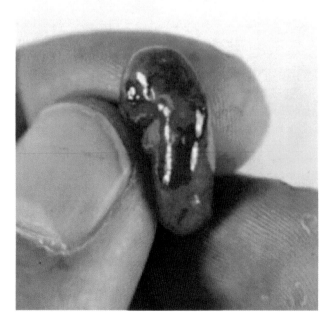

Methanol Induced Fetal Resorption

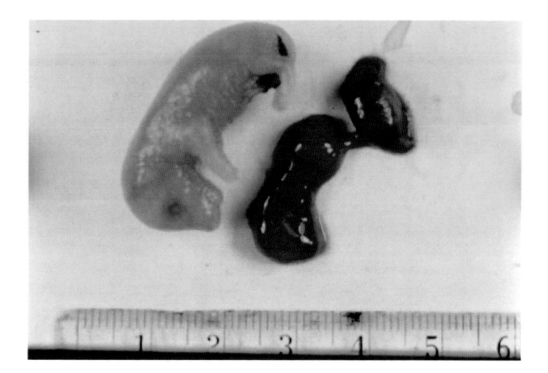

Methanol Pups Born With No Eyes

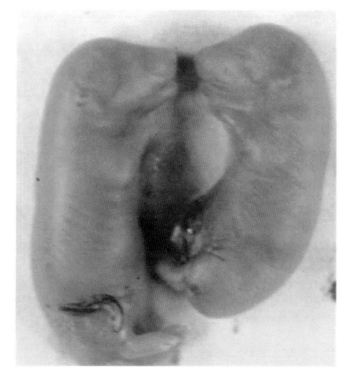

Normal Rat Verses Methanol Placenta

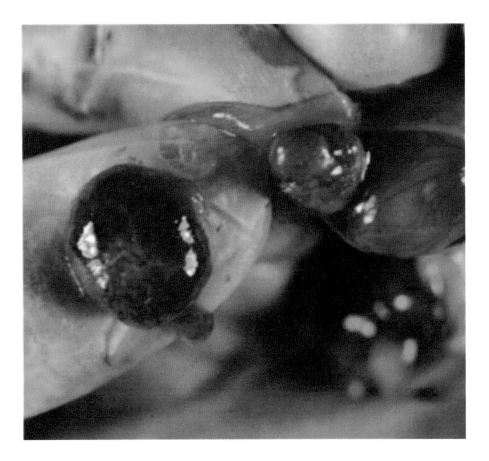

Made in the USA
Lexington, KY
30 June 2012